DIMENSIONAL ANALYSIS
for MEDS

Third Edition

DIMENSIONAL ANALYSIS for MEDS

Third Edition

Anna M. Curren

**Former Associate Professor
of Nursing,
Long Beach City College,
Long Beach, California**

THOMSON
DELMAR LEARNING

Australia Canada Mexico Singapore Spain United Kingdom United States

THOMSON

™

DELMAR LEARNING

Dimensional Analysis for Meds, Third Edition
by Anna M. Curren

Vice President, Health Care Business Unit:
William Brottmiller

Editorial Director:
Cathy L. Esperti

Executive Editor:
Matthew Kane

Developmental Editor:
Maria D'Angelico

Editorial Assistant:
Michelle Leavitt

Marketing Director:
Jennifer McAvey

Marketing Coordinator:
Michele Gleason

Technology Director:
Laurie Davis

Technology Production Coordinator:
Carolyn Fox

Assistant to Production/Technology Directors:
Kate Kaufman

Production Director:
Carolyn Miller

Art and Design Specialist:
Robert Plante

Production Coordinator:
Mary Ellen Cox

Senior Project Editor:
David Buddle

Library of Congress Cataloging-in-Publication Data

Curren, Anna M.
 Dimensional analysis for meds / Anna M. Curren.—3rd ed.
  p. cm.
 Includes index.
 ISBN 1-4018-7801-6
 1. Pharmaceutical arithmetic. 2. Dimensional analysis. I. Title.
 RS57.C868 2006
 615'.14'01513—dc22

2005013643

Contents

Preface

Dimensional Analysis for Meds, Third Edition, instructs learners in the increasingly lauded, unforgettably simple dimensional analysis dosage calculation method. This method totally eliminates the multiple steps and outdated formulas of alternative calculation instruction. The text is completely self-instructional and is successfully used in all levels of nursing programs from LPN/LVN to baccalaureate, in medical and dental assistant programs, in emergency medical technology programs, and in additional health-related programs as diverse as veterinary medicine. As educators become familiar with the simplicity of dimensional analysis, this method is increasingly being adopted.

I approached this revision of my text with the same philosophical tenets I have adhered to throughout my years of authorship. I have kept the content realistic and uncluttered and concentrated on those sequential instructional steps that consistently dispel the learner's natural apprehension to this subject. I included multiple learning exercises to cement the basic math and related skills. I have structured the content from simple to complex, in a seamless progression that has been my lifelong trademark.

Since the last edition, considerable progress has been made in addressing the ongoing problem areas leading to dosage errors. Recommendations for acceptable drug measure abbreviations have, for the first time, made it possible to all but delete content on the outdated and error-ridden apothecaries' measures that were the source of many errors. All of these important changes are integrated into this new edition.

A revised and updated CD-ROM, the *Dimensional Analysis for Meds Learning Program*, has been prepared to accompany the text. The format of this important instructional aid, at the request of numerous educators, follows its inaugural format, which was found to be so invaluable to learners. To enhance the tried-and-true format and instructional method, improvements have been made to the software design and navigation of the *Learning Program*.

With this edition I have passed the thirtieth year in my writing career in clinical dosage calculations texts. I look back with wonder on two persistent facts: how much the content needs to be updated to remain current, and the sad difficulty in reaching educators who have not yet been exposed to the tremendous advantage that dimensional analysis offers in the ease, accuracy, and safety of clinical calculations. Dimensional analysis is the future in clinical calculations. In my opinion not to use it is to deprive learners of an invaluable instructional tool.

Educator evaluation remains an ongoing factor in fueling content change, and I receive many suggestions every year. To those educators who kindly shared their expertise I once again extend my sincere thanks. If this is your introduction to the DA method, I invite you to join me in gifting your learners by using this approach. To my returning users I ask a favor: spread the word. Our learners deserve only the best. Let's give it to them.

Anna M. Curren

Acknowledgments

These reviewers gave valuable comments during the development of the manuscript:

Susan Bruce, PhD (c), RN, ANP
Clinical Assistant Professor
University at Buffalo
Buffalo, New York

Paul Clements, PhD, APRN, BC, DF-IAFN
Assistant Professor
University of New Mexico
Albuquerque, New Mexico

M. Joyce Dienger, DNSc, RN
Assistant Professor
University of Cincinnati
Cincinnati, Ohio

Marilyn C. Handley, RN, PhD
Assistant Professor
University of Alabama
Tuscaloosa, Alabama

Mary Hibbert, RN, MS
Assistant Professor
Southern Nazarene University
Bethany, Oklahoma

Bernadette Madara, EdD, APRN, CS
Associate Professor
Southern Connecticut State University
New Haven, Connecticut

Cathy Renz, BSN, MEd
Instructor of Nursing
Iowa Western Community College
Council Bluffs, Iowa

Phyllis Rowe, RN, MSN, ANP
Associate Professor, Nursing
Assistant Chair, Vocational Nursing Program
Riverside Community College
Riverside, California

Anna Sanford, MSN, ARNP, BC, AOCN
Associate Professor
Northern Michigan University
Marquette, Michigan

Lori Stutte, MSN, RN
Assistant Professor
Cardinal Stritch University
Milwaukee, Wisconsin

Directions to the Learner

Welcome to what we anticipate will be one of the most enjoyable texts you have ever used. *Dimensional Analysis for Meds*, Third Edition is about to reassure you that math is nothing to be afraid of; that even the most difficult clinical calculations you encounter will present no problem for you; and that, on completion of your instruction, you will not only have the calculation skills you need, but ones that you can share with more experienced nurses and allied health personnel who have not had the benefit of learning the simplified dimensional analysis method.

Your instruction will be in two parts: your text, a portable self-instructional tutorial that can be used anywhere, anytime; and an exciting and unique *Learning Program* CD-ROM, a full-color audiovisual presentation that takes a slightly different instructional approach to dimensional analysis (DA) from your text. The CD-ROM is a mandatory part of your instruction, as it demonstrates DA with animations that are impossible to present on a printed page. Besides, you will love it.

The instructions for the Learning Program are included in the program and in the following section, "How to Use the Learning Program."

The directions for using your text are quite simple:

1. You will need to gather a pencil or pen, plenty of scratch paper, and a calculator. Take these to a quiet spot where you will not be disturbed, and be prepared to be surprised and pleased as you travel with your author on a mutually enjoyable teaching and learning experience.

2. Record the answers to calculations on scratch paper as well as in your text. This will make checking answers against those provided much easier.

3. As you work your way through the text, do exactly as you are instructed to do, and no more. Programmed learning proceeds in small steps, and skipping steps may cause confusion. The programs are designed to let you move at your own speed. If you already know some of the basics, you will move through them more quickly than you can imagine.

4. You will discover that most medication calculations are fairly simple and can be done, or at least simplified, without using a calculator. Your text stresses manual solution because, quite frankly, it's much quicker. But it also points out when a calculator should be used and reminds you that all answers must be routinely double-checked. Answers must also be evaluated to see if they make sense, and your text provides guidelines throughout on making common-sense appraisals of the answers obtained.

5. Some medication calculations require rounding in decimal fraction answers, and instruction on rounding is provided on a chapter-by-chapter basis. Be aware, however, that calculator settings vary, and you may occasionally experience fractional answers that differ by a hundredth. Your instructor will advise you of specific hospital or clinical policies regarding rounding that you need to be aware of.

Once you have completed your program, keep *Dimensional Analysis for Meds* in your personal library. As you move to different clinical areas during your career, you will encounter different types of calculations. A quick refresher with *Dimensional Analysis for Meds* will be invaluable when that occurs.

Instructional Elements of the Text

The step-by-step, building-block approach of this text is designed to accommodate the needs of learners at all levels and with every range of basic skills and knowledge. It begins with a math pretest and progresses through the math instruction basic to clinical dosage calculations, for example working with fractions and decimals. This is followed by instruction in reading actual drug labels, hypodermic syringe calibrations, and commonly used drug measurement units, such as the metric system units and their symbols. Dosage calculation instruction begins after the basics have been completed and follows a simple-to-complex approach to cover the full range of clinical calculations used in all pertinent clinical arenas. Each calculation is illustrated with multiple examples and is followed by problem sets, with correct answers provided. Successful mastery of calculation skills has been a predictable outcome of this leading instructional method for over 30 years.

> **The symbols μ, for micro, and cc and ml for mL, are officially obsolete, and must not be used in transcribing dosages.**

Key Points

A key icon identifies the important facts to be memorized for safe clinical performance in the calculation and measurement of drug dosages.

EXAMPLE 2

A dosage of **50,000 units** is ordered to be added to an IV solution. The strength available is **10,000 units/1.5 mL**. Calculate how many **mL** will contain this dosage.

Write the mL being calculated to the left of the equation followed by an equal sign.

$$\text{mL} =$$

The mL being calculated must be matched in the numerator of the first ratio entered. Look back at your problem and locate the complete ratio containing mL, the 10,000 units in 1.5 mL dosage strength available. Enter this ratio now with 1.5 mL as the numerator to match the mL numerator being calculated; 10,000 units becomes the denominator.

$$\text{mL} = \frac{1.5\ \text{mL}}{10,000\ \text{units}}$$

The units denominator of the first ratio must now be matched in the next numerator. This is provided by the 50,000 units ordered. Enter this now as the next numerator to complete this one-step equation.

$$\text{mL} = \frac{1.5\ \text{mL}}{10,000\ \text{units}} \times \frac{50,000\ \text{units}}{}$$

Cancel the alternate denominator/numerator units entries to double-check for correct ratio entry. Only the mL unit being calculated remains in the equation. Do the math.

$$\text{mL} = \frac{1.5\ \text{mL}}{10,000\ \text{units}} \times \frac{50,000\ \text{units}}{}$$

Examples

Each calculation is introduced using multiple examples that include a corresponding step-by-step narrative explanation.

PROBLEM

Refer to the label in Figure 6-6 and answer the questions about this drug.

1. What is the generic name? _____
2. What is the trade name? _____
3. What is the dosage strength? _____
4. What company manufactured this drug? _____
5. How many tablets are in this container? _____

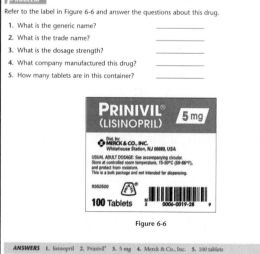

Figure 6-6

ANSWERS 1. lisinopril 2. Prinivil® 3. 5 mg 4. Merck & Co., Inc. 5. 100 tablets

Problem Sets

Each calculation presented includes sets of problems to allow for immediate practice. Answers follow each problem set to provide immediate feedback of accuracy in all problems.

Dosage Labels

Real, full-color drug labels are an integral part of all examples and problems, challenging the user to read and interpret all information common to actual dosage calculation.

Syringe Photographs

Photos showing hypodermic syringes in their actual sizes are included to allow for realistic practice in reading calibrations and accurate measurement of dosages calculated.

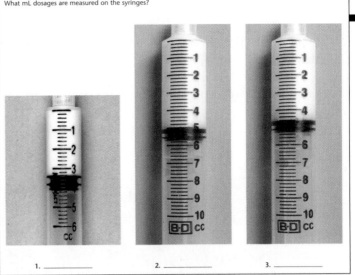

PROBLEM

What mL dosages are measured on the syringes?

1. _____ 2. _____ 3. _____

Combined Syringe and Drug Label Questions

Over a thousand problems use actual drug labels and appropriately sized hypodermic syringes to measure the dosages calculated. These ensure total integration of both math concepts and clinical reality in dosage calculation and measurement.

Dosage Ordered	mL Needed
28. Terramycin® 0.1 g	_____

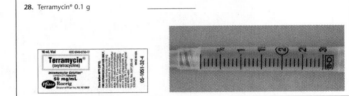

Summary Self-Tests

Each chapter ends with a comprehensive summary self-test, which provides both review and integration of entire chapter instruction.

Summary Self-Test

You are to assist with some IV procedures. Answer the situational questions concerning IV procedures.

1. An adult is admitted and an IV of 1000 mL D5RL is started. These initials identify what type of solution?

    This is referred to as what type of line?

2. All roller clamps on the IV tubing are closed before connection to the solution bag. Why?

3. The IV is started in the back of the left hand. This makes it what type of line?

4. You are asked to check the fluid level in the drip chamber, and you observe that it is correct, which is

5. You are then asked to adjust the flow rate. You will use what type of clamp to do this?

6. A decision was made to use an electronic infusion control device to administer this IV. The device used is a

7. An IV antibiotic is ordered. This is sent from the pharmacy already prepared in a small-volume IV solution bag. The setup used to infuse this medication is referred to as an IV

8. This is abbreviated how?

9. In order for the antibiotic to infuse first, how must it be hung in relation to the original solution bag?

10. Some days later the IV is to be discontinued, but IV antibiotics are to be continued. What is the site used for this intermittent administration called?

11. A PCA was used for one day. What do these initials mean?

    What symptoms is this device designed to control?

Answer the questions as briefly as possible.

12. A small-volume IV medication is to be diluted in 20 mL and infused. This can be most accurately measured using a _____.

13. These devices are calibrated in _____ increments.

How to Use the Learning Program CD-ROM

We are pleased to present the third edition of the *Dimensional Analysis for Meds Learning Program* CD-ROM. The CD-ROM is a proven tool for reinforcing important instructional content in your text in a unique and interactive way. This edition maintains the audio and visual presentation of content while improving the navigation, animations, and visual appeal. You will enjoy the following features:

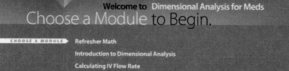

Main Menu

The *Learning Program* presents five modules of content, each of which contains three to six lessons. The modules are:
• Refresher Math
• Introduction to Dimensional Analysis
• Calculating IV Flow Rate
• Calculating IV Infusion Time
• Calculating Dosage Infusing During Titration

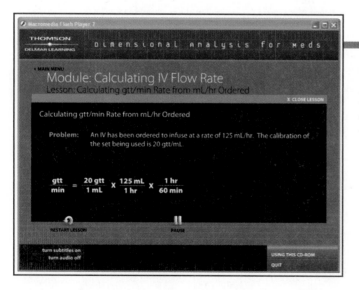

Problems

Each didactic presentation is followed by a series of problems. Audio and visuals are used together to explain each step of solving the problem.

Subtitles

The audio presentation clearly describes each step in solving DA problems. You can listen to the narration or read it in subtitles at the bottom of the screen. Simply click a button to turn subtitles on or off.

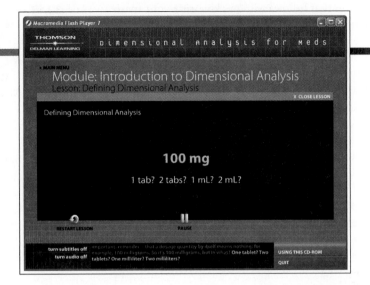

Summary Self-Tests

Each module includes a brief test of all of the concepts presented. You have the option to print the test and complete it on the hard copy or take the test on the screen. You can also view the answers on a separate screen to check your work.

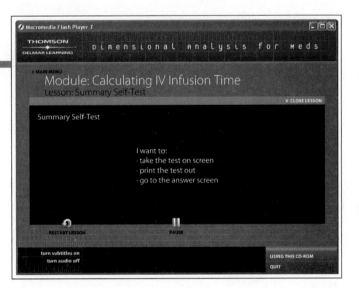

Refresher Math Pretest

If you can complete the following pretest with 100% accuracy, you are off to an excellent start. However, don't be alarmed if you make some errors, because the Refresher Math section that follows will quickly bring your math skills up to date. Regardless of your proficiency, **it's important to complete the entire Refresher Math section**. It includes many memory cues and shortcuts for simplifying and solving clinical calculations that are used throughout the text, and you will need to be familiar with these.

Identify the decimal fraction with the highest value.

1.	a) 4.4	b) 2.85	c) 5.3
2.	a) 6.3	b) 5.73	c) 4.4
3.	a) 0.18	b) 0.62	c) 0.35
4.	a) 0.2	b) 0.125	c) 0.3
5.	a) 0.15	b) 0.11	c) 0.14
6.	a) 4.27	b) 4.31	c) 4.09

Add the decimals.

7. $0.2 + 2.23$ =

8. $1.5 + 0.07$ =

9. $6.45 + 12.1 + 9.54$ =

10. $0.35 + 8.37 + 5.15$ =

Subtract the decimals.

11. $3.1 - 0.67$ =

12. $12.41 - 2.11$ =

13. $2.235 - 0.094$ =

14. $4.65 - 0.7$ =

15. If tablets with a strength of 0.2 mg are available and 0.6 mg is ordered, how many tablets must you give?

16. If tablets are labeled 0.8 mg and 0.4 mg is ordered, how many tablets must you give?

17. If the available tablets have a strength of 1.25 mg and 2.5 mg is ordered, how many tablets must you give?

18. If 0.125 mg is ordered and the tablets available are labeled 0.25 mg, how many tablets must you give?

Express the numbers to the nearest tenth.

19. 2.17 =

20. 0.15 =

21. 3.77 =

22. 4.62 =

23. 11.74 =

24. 5.26 =

Express the numbers to the nearest hundredth.

25. 1.357 =

26. 7.413 =

27. 10.105 =

28. 3.775 =

29. 0.176 =

30. Define "product."

_____

_____

Multiply the decimals. Express your answers to the nearest tenth.

31. 0.7×1.2 = _____

32. 1.8×2.6 = _____

33. $5.1 \times 0.25 \times 1.1$ = _____

34. 3.3×3.75 = _____

Divide the fractions. Express your answers to the nearest hundredth.

35. $16.3 \div 3.2$ = _____

36. $15.1 \div 1.1$ = _____

37. $2 \div 0.75$ = _____

38. $4.17 \div 2.7$ = _____

39. Define "numerator."

_____

_____

40. Define "denominator."

_____

_____

41. Define "highest common denominator."

_____

_____

Solve the equations. Express your answers to the nearest tenth.

42. $\dfrac{1}{4} \times \dfrac{2}{3}$ = _____

43. $\dfrac{240}{170} \times \dfrac{135}{300}$ = _____

44. $\dfrac{0.2}{1.75} \times \dfrac{1.5}{0.2}$ = _____

45. $\dfrac{2.1}{3.6} \times \dfrac{1.7}{1.3}$ = _____

46. $\dfrac{0.26}{0.2} \times \dfrac{3.3}{1.2}$ = _____

47. $\dfrac{750}{1} \times \dfrac{300}{50} \times \dfrac{7}{2}$ = _____

48. $\dfrac{50}{1} \times \dfrac{60}{240} \times \dfrac{1}{900} \times \dfrac{400}{1}$ = _____

49. $\dfrac{35,000}{750} \times \dfrac{35}{1}$ = _____

50. $\dfrac{50}{2} \times \dfrac{450}{40} \times \dfrac{1}{900} \times \dfrac{114}{1}$ = _____

ANSWERS

1. c	15. 3 tab	29. 0.18	39. The top number in a common fraction
2. a	16. ½ tab	30. The answer obtained from the multiplication of two or more numbers	40. The bottom number in a common fraction
3. b	17. 2 tab		41. The highest number that can be divided into two numbers to reduce them to their lowest terms (values)
4. c	18. ½ tab		42. 0.2
5. a	19. 2.2		43. 0.6
6. b	20. 0.2	31. 0.8	44. 0.9
7. 2.43	21. 3.8	32. 4.7	45. 0.8
8. 1.57	22. 4.6	33. 1.4	46. 3.6
9. 28.09	23. 11.7	34. 12.4	47. 15,750
10. 13.87	24. 5.3	35. 5.09	48. 5.6
11. 2.43	25. 1.36	36. 13.73	49. 1633.3
12. 10.3	26. 7.41	37. 2.67	50. 35.6
13. 2.141	27. 10.11	38. 1.54	
14. 3.95	28. 3.78		

SECTION ONE
Refresher Math

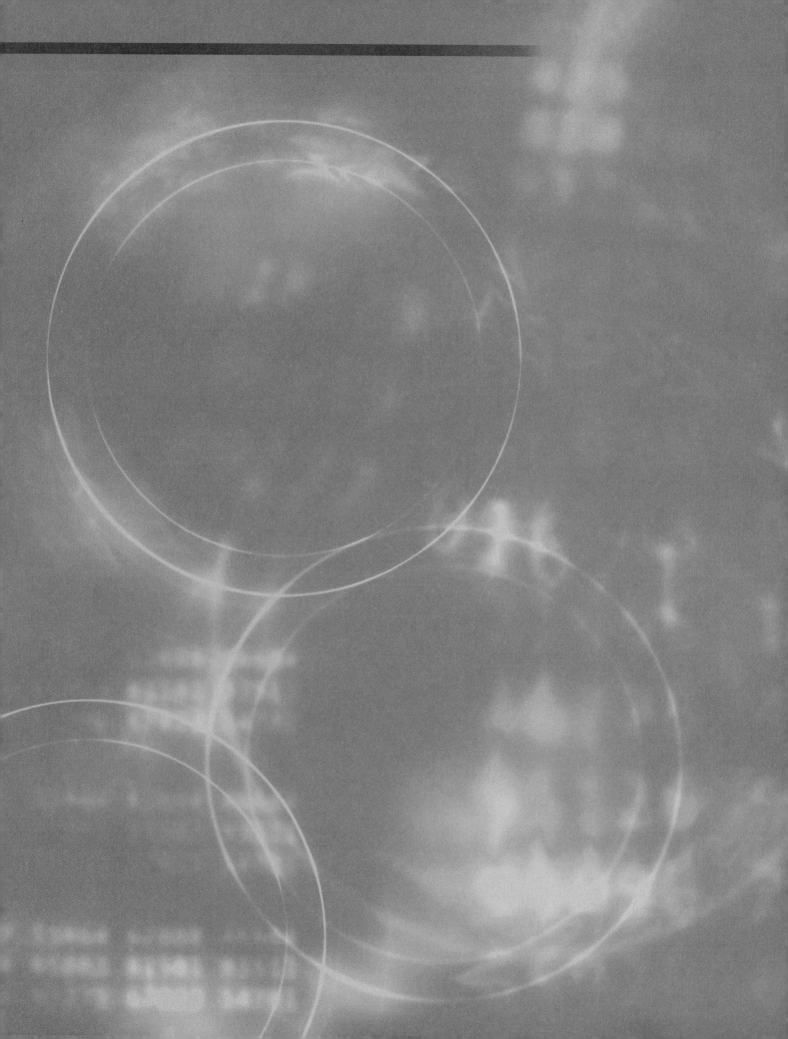

Relative Value, Addition, and Subtraction of Decimals

In the course of administering medications, you will be dealing with decimal fraction dosages on a daily basis. The first two chapters of this text provide a complete and easy refresher of everything you need to know about decimals, including safety measures when you do calculations both manually and with a calculator. We'll start with a review of the range of decimal values you will see in dosages. This will enable you to immediately recognize which of two or more numbers has the highest (and lowest) value—knowledge you will use constantly in your professional career.

Relative Value of Decimals

The most helpful fact to remember about decimals is that our **monetary system of dollars and cents is a decimal system.** The whole numbers in dosages have the same relative value as dollars, and decimal fractions have the same value as cents: **the higher the number, the higher the value.** If you keep this constantly in mind, you will already have learned the most important safety measure in dealing with decimals.

The range of drug dosages stretches from millions on the whole number side to thousandths on the decimal side. Refer to the decimal scale in Figure 1-1, and locate the decimal point, which is slightly to the right on this scale. Notice first the whole numbers on the left of the scale, which rise increasingly in value from ones (units) to millions, which is the largest whole number drug dosage in use.

OBJECTIVES

The learner will:
1. identify the relative value of decimals
2. add decimals
3. subtract decimals
4. list precautions in calculator use
5. list the steps in dosage calculation

Prerequisite

Recognize the abbreviations mg, for milligram, and g, for gram, as drug measures.

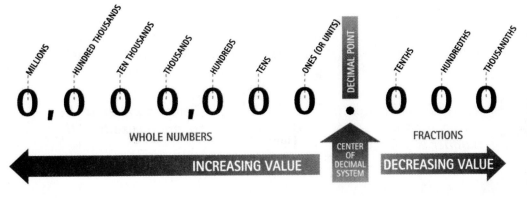

Figure 1-1

3

The first key point in determining relative value of decimals is the presence of whole numbers. The higher the whole number, the higher the value.

EXAMPLE 1   10.1 is higher than 9.15

EXAMPLE 2   3.2 is higher than 2.99

EXAMPLE 3   7.01 is higher than 6.99

PROBLEM

Identify the number with the highest value.

1.	a)	3.5	b)	2.7	c)	4.2	_____
2.	a)	6.15	b)	5.95	c)	4.54	_____
3.	a)	12.02	b)	10.19	c)	11.04	_____
4.	a)	2.5	b)	1.75	c)	0.75	_____
5.	a)	4.3	b)	2.75	c)	5.1	_____
6.	a)	6.15	b)	7.4	c)	5.95	_____

ANSWERS 1. c 2. a 3. a 4. a 5. c 6. b

If, however, the whole numbers are the same, for example, **10**.2 and **10**.7, or there are no whole numbers, for example, **0**.25 and **0**.35, **then the fraction will determine the relative value.** Let's take a closer look at the fractional side of the scale (refer to Figure 1-2).

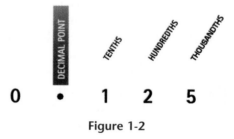

Figure 1-2

It is necessary to consider only three figures after the decimal point on the fractional side because drug dosages measured as decimal fractions do not contain more than three digits, for example, 0.125 mg. First notice that a **zero is used to replace the whole number** in this decimal fraction and in all other dosages that do not contain a whole number.

 If a decimal fraction is not preceded by a whole number, a zero is used in front of the decimal point to emphasize that the number is a fraction.

EXAMPLE   **0.125   0.1   0.45**

Look once again at Figure 1-2. The numbers on the right of the decimal point represent **tenths, hundredths,** and **thousandths** in that order. When you see a dosage quantity in which the **whole numbers are the same,** or there are **no whole numbers,** stop and look first at the fractional number representing **tenths.**

 When the whole numbers are identical, the fraction with the higher number representing tenths has the higher value.

EXAMPLE 1   0.3 is higher than 0.27 (0.3 is the same as 0.30)

EXAMPLE 2   0.4 is higher than 0.29 (0.4 is the same as 0.40)

EXAMPLE 3   1.2 is higher than 1.19 (1.2 is the same as 1.20)

PROBLEM

Which decimal has the highest value?

1.	a)	0.4	b)	0.2	c)	0.5
2.	a)	2.73	b)	2.61	c)	2.87
3.	a)	0.19	b)	0.61	c)	0.34
4.	a)	3.5	b)	3.75	c)	3.25
5.	a)	0.3	b)	0.25	c)	0.4
6.	a)	1.35	b)	1.29	c)	1.4

ANSWERS 1. c. 2. c 3. b 4. b 5. c 6. c

If in decimal fractions the numbers representing **the tenths are identical,** for example, 0.25 and 0.27, then **the number representing the hundredths will determine the relative value.**

 When the tenths are identical, the decimal fraction with the higher number representing hundredths will have the higher value.

EXAMPLE 1   0.27 is higher than 0.2**5**

EXAMPLE 2   0.15 is higher than 0.1 (0.1 is the same as 0.1**0**)

 Extra zeros on the end of decimal fractions are omitted in drug dosages because they can easily be misread.

EXAMPLE 1   2.25 is higher than 2.2 (same as 2.2**0**)

EXAMPLE 2   9.77 is higher than 9.7 (same as 9.7**0**)

Which decimal has the highest value?

1.	a)	0.12	b)	0.15	c)	0.17	_____
2.	a)	1.21	b)	1.24	c)	1.23	_____
3.	a)	0.37	b)	0.32	c)	0.36	_____
4.	a)	3.27	b)	3.25	c)	3.21	_____
5.	a)	0.16	b)	0.11	c)	0.19	_____
6.	a)	4.23	b)	4.2	c)	4.09	_____

ANSWERS   1. c   2. b   3. a   4. a   5. c   6. a

The number of figures on the right of the decimal point is not an indication of relative value. Always look at the figure representing the tenths first, and if these are identical, look at the figure representing the hundredths to determine which has the higher value.

PROBLEM

Which fraction has the higher value?

    a) 0.125   b) 0.25

ANSWER   The correct answer is b) 0.25. The decimal fraction that has the higher number representing the **tenths** has the higher value. **2** is higher than **1**; therefore 0.25 has a higher value than 0.125. Medication errors have been made in this **identical** decimal fraction, so remember it well.

This completes your introduction to the relative value of decimals. The key points just reviewed will cover all situations in dosage calculations in which you will have to recognize high and low values. Therefore, you are now ready to test yourself more extensively on this information.

PROBLEM

Identify the decimal with the highest value.

1.	a)	0.24	b)	0.5	c)	0.125	_____
2.	a)	0.4	b)	0.45	c)	0.5	_____
3.	a)	7.5	b)	6.25	c)	4.75	_____
4.	a)	0.3	b)	0.25	c)	0.35	_____
5.	a)	1.125	b)	1.75	c)	1.5	_____
6.	a)	4.5	b)	4.75	c)	4.25	_____
7.	a)	0.1	b)	0.01	c)	0.04	_____
8.	a)	5.75	b)	6.25	c)	6.5	_____
9.	a)	0.6	b)	0.16	c)	0.06	_____
10.	a)	3.55	b)	2.95	c)	3.7	_____

ANSWERS   1. b   2. c   3. a   4. c   5. b   6. b   7. a   8. c   9. a   10. c

Addition and Subtraction of Decimals

Most addition and subtraction dosage problems can be done more quickly, and quite safely, without a calculator. So, let's start by reviewing a few rules for basic addition and subtraction.

 When you write the numbers down, line up the decimal points.

EXAMPLE To add 0.25 and 0.27

$$0.25$$
$$+0.27 \text{ is safe}$$

$$0.25$$
$$+0.27 \text{ may be unsafe; it could lead to errors}$$

 Always add or subtract from right to left.

If you decide to write the numbers down, **don't confuse yourself by trying to "eyeball" the answer.** Also, write any numbers that you carried, or rewrite those reduced by borrowing, if you find this helpful.

EXAMPLE 1 When adding 0.25 and 0.27

$$\begin{array}{r} 1 \\ 0.25 \\ +0.27 \\ \hline 0.52 \end{array}$$ Add the 5 and 7 first, then the 2, 2, and the 1 you carried. Work from right to left.

EXAMPLE 2 When subtracting 0.63 from 0.71

$$\begin{array}{r} 6\,1 \\ 0.\!\not{7}1 \\ -0.63 \\ \hline 0.08 \end{array}$$ Borrow 1 from 7 and rewrite as 6.
Write the borrowed 1. Subtract 3 from 11.
Subtract 6 from 6. Work from right to left.

Add zeros as necessary to make the fractions equal in length.

This does not alter the value of the fractions, and it helps prevent confusion and mistakes.

EXAMPLE When subtracting 0.125 from 0.25

$$\begin{array}{r} 0.25 \\ -0.125 \end{array} \text{ becomes } \begin{array}{r} 0.250 \\ -0.125 \end{array} \qquad \text{Answer} = 0.125$$

If you follow these simple rules and make them a habit, you will automatically reduce calculation errors. The following problems will give you an excellent opportunity to practice these rules.

Add the decimals.

1.	0.25 + 0.55	= _____	**6.**	3.75 + 1.05	= _____
2.	0.1 + 2.25	= _____	**7.**	6.35 + 2.05	= _____
3.	1.74 + 0.76	= _____	**8.**	5.57 + 4.03	= _____
4.	1.4 + 0.02	= _____	**9.**	0.33 + 2.42	= _____
5.	2.3 + 1.45	= _____	**10.**	1.44 + 3.06	= _____

Subtract the decimals.

11.	1.25 − 1.125	= _____	**16.**	7.33 − 4.03	= _____
12.	3.25 − 0.65	= _____	**17.**	4.25 − 1.75	= _____
13.	2.3 − 1.45	= _____	**18.**	0.07 − 0.035	= _____
14.	0.02 − 0.01	= _____	**19.**	0.235 − 0.12	= _____
15.	5.5 − 2.5	= _____	**20.**	5.75 − 0.95	= _____

ANSWERS **1.** 0.8 **2.** 2.35 **3.** 2.5 **4.** 1.42 **5.** 3.75 **6.** 4.8 **7.** 8.4 **8.** 9.6 **9.** 2.75 **10.** 4.5 **11.** 0.125 **12.** 2.6 **13.** 0.85 **14.** 0.01 **15.** 3 **16.** 3.3 **17.** 2.5 **18.** 0.035 **19.** 0.115 **20.** 4.8 **Note:** If you did not add a zero in front of the decimal point in answers that do not contain a whole number, or you failed to eliminate unnecessary zeros from the end of decimal fractions, your answers are incorrect.

Summary

This concludes the refresher on relative value, addition, and subtraction of numbers containing decimals. The important points to remember from this chapter are:

If the decimal fraction contains a whole number, the value of the whole number is the first determiner of relative value.

If the fraction does not include a whole number, a zero is placed in front of the decimal point to emphasize that the number is a fraction.

If there is no whole number, or if the whole numbers are the same, the number representing the tenths in the decimal fraction will be the next determiner of relative value.

If the tenths values in decimal fractions are identical, the number representing hundredths will determine relative value.

When adding or subtracting decimal fractions, first line up the decimal points, then add or subtract from right to left.

Extra zeros on the end of decimal fractions can be a source of error and are routinely eliminated.

Summary Self-Test

Choose the decimal with the highest value.

1.	**a)**	2.45	**b)**	2.57	**c)**	2.19		_____
2.	**a)**	3.07	**b)**	3.17	**c)**	3.71		_____
3.	**a)**	0.12	**b)**	0.02	**c)**	0.01		_____
4.	**a)**	5.31	**b)**	5.35	**c)**	6.01		_____

5.	**a)**	4.5	**b)**	4.51	**c)**	4.15	_____
6.	**a)**	0.015	**b)**	0.15	**c)**	0.1	_____
7.	**a)**	1.3	**b)**	1.25	**c)**	1.35	_____
8.	**a)**	0.1	**b)**	0.2	**c)**	0.25	_____
9.	**a)**	0.125	**b)**	0.1	**c)**	0.05	_____
10.	**a)**	13.7	**b)**	13.5	**c)**	13.25	_____

11. If you have medication tablets whose strength is 0.1 mg and you must give 0.3 mg, you will need

    a) 1 tablet   **b)** less than 1 tablet   **c)** more than 1 tablet   _____

12. If you have tablets with a strength of 0.25 mg and you must give 0.125 mg, you will need

    a) 1 tablet   **b)** less than 1 tablet   **c)** more than 1 tablet   _____

13. If you have an order to give a dosage of 7.5 mg and the tablets have a strength of 3.75 mg, you will need

    a) 1 tablet   **b)** less than 1 tablet   **c)** more than 1 tablet   _____

14. If the order is to give 0.5 mg and the tablet strength is 0.5 mg, you will give

    a) 1 tablet   **b)** less than 1 tablet   **c)** more than 1 tablet   _____

15. The order is to give 0.5 mg and the tablets have a strength of 0.25 mg. You must give

    a) 1 tablet   **b)** less than 1 tablet   **c)** more than 1 tablet   _____

Add the decimals.

16. $1.31 + 0.4 =$ _____		**20.** $1.3 + 1.04 =$ _____
17. $0.15 + 0.25 =$ _____		**21.** $4.7 + 3.03 =$ _____
18. $2.5 + 0.75 =$ _____		**22.** $0.5 + 0.5 =$ _____
19. $3.2 + 2.17 =$ _____		**23.** $5.4 + 2.6 =$ _____

24. You have just given two tablets with a dosage strength of 3.5 mg each. What was the total dosage administered?   _____

25. You are to give one tablet labeled 0.5 mg and one labeled 0.25 mg. What is the total dosage of these two tablets?   _____

26. If you give two tablets labeled 0.02 mg, what total dosage will you administer?   _____

27. You are to give one tablet labeled 0.8 mg and two tablets labeled 0.4 mg. What is the total dosage?   _____

28. You have two tablets: one is labeled 0.15 mg and the other is labeled 0.3 mg. What is the total dosage of these two tablets?   _____

Subtract the decimals.

29. $4.32 - 3.1 =$ _____		**33.** $1.3 - 0.02 =$ _____
30. $2.1 - 1.91 =$ _____		**34.** $0.2 - 0.07 =$ _____
31. $3.73 - 1.93 =$ _____		**35.** $3.95 - 0.35 =$ _____
32. $5.75 - 4.05 =$ _____		**36.** $1.9 - 0.08 =$ _____

37. You are to prepare a dosage of 7.5 mg and you have only one tablet labeled 3.75 mg. How many more milligrams do you need? _____

38. You have a tablet labeled 0.02 mg and you are to give 0.06 mg. How many more milligrams do you need for this dosage? _____

39. The tablet available is labeled 0.5 mg, but you must give a dosage of 1.5 mg. How many more milligrams will you need to obtain the correct dosage? _____

40. Your client is to receive a dosage of 1.2 mg and you have one tablet labeled 0.6 mg. What additional dosage in milligrams will you need? _____

41. You must give your patient a dosage of 2.2 mg, but you have only two tablets labeled 0.55 mg. What additional dosage in milligrams will you need? _____

Determine how many tablets are needed to give the correct dosages.

42. Tablets are labeled 0.01 mg. You must give 0.02 mg. _____

43. Tablets are labeled 2.5 mg. You must give 5 mg. _____

44. Tablets are labeled 0.25 mg. Give 0.125 mg. _____

45. Tablets are 0.5 mg. Give 1.5 mg. _____

46. A dosage of 1.8 mg is ordered. Tablets are 0.6 mg. _____

47. Tablets available are 0.04 mg. You are to give 0.02 mg. _____

48. The dosage ordered is 3.5 mg. The tablets available are 1.75 mg. _____

49. Prepare a dosage of 3.2 mg using tablets with a strength of 1.6 mg. _____

50. You have tablets labeled 0.25 mg, and a dosage of 0.375 mg is ordered. _____

ANSWERS				
1. b	**11.** c	**21.** 7.73	**31.** 1.8	**41.** 1.1 mg
2. c	**12.** b	**22.** 1	**32.** 1.7	**42.** 2 tab
3. a	**13.** c	**23.** 8	**33.** 1.28	**43.** 2 tab
4. c	**14.** a	**24.** 7 mg	**34.** 0.13	**44.** ½ tab
5. b	**15.** c	**25.** 0.75 mg	**35.** 3.6	**45.** 3 tab
6. b	**16.** 1.71	**26.** 0.04 mg	**36.** 1.82	**46.** 3 tab
7. c	**17.** 0.4	**27.** 1.6 mg	**37.** 3.75 mg	**47.** ½ tab
8. c	**18.** 3.25	**28.** 0.45 mg	**38.** 0.04 mg	**48.** 2 tab
9. a	**19.** 5.37	**29.** 1.22	**39.** 1 mg	**49.** 2 tab
10. a	**20.** 2.34	**30.** 0.19	**40.** 0.6 mg	**50.** 1½ tab

Note: If you did not add a zero in front of the decimal point in answers that did not contain a whole number, or you failed to eliminate unnecessary zeros from the end of decimal fractions, your answers are incorrect.

Multiplication
and Division
of Decimals

Multiplication and division are integral parts of dosage calculations. As is the case with addition and subtraction, many multiplication and division problems involving dosages can be done more quickly manually than by using a calculator. The basic steps in multiplication and division are reviewed in this chapter. In addition, a number of preliminary shortcuts will be introduced that will make numbers, especially those containing decimal fractions, quite simple to work with. And for those limited number of calculations that are more safely handled with a calculator, safety in calculator use will be introduced.

Multiplication of Decimals

The main precaution in multiplication of decimals is the **placement of the decimal point in the answer**, which is called the **product**.

The decimal point in the product of decimal fractions is placed the same number of places to the left in the product as the total of numbers after the decimal points in the fractions multiplied.

EXAMPLE 1   Multiply 0.35 by 0.5

Begin by lining up the numbers to be multiplied on the right side, because this is safer. Then disregard the decimals during multiplication.

$$
\begin{array}{r}
0.35 \\
\times\ \underline{0.5} \\
175
\end{array}
$$

0.35 has two numbers after the decimal and 0.5 has one. Place the decimal point three places to the left in the product to make it .175, then add a zero (0) in front of the fraction to emphasize the decimal point.

Answer = **0.175**

EXAMPLE 2   Multiply 1.61 by 0.2

$$
\begin{array}{r}
1.61 \\
\times\ \ 0.2 \\
\hline
322
\end{array}
$$

1.61 has two numbers after the decimal point and 0.2 has one. Place the decimal point three places to the left in the product, so that 322 becomes .322, then add a zero in front of the fraction to emphasize it.

Answer = **0.322**

If the product contains insufficient numbers for correct placement of the decimal point, add as many zeros as necessary to the left of the product to correct this.

EXAMPLE 3   Multiply 1.5 by 0.06

$$
\begin{array}{r}
1.5 \\
\times\ 0.06 \\
\hline
90
\end{array}
$$

1.5 has one number after the decimal point and 0.06 has two. To place the decimal three places to the left in the product, a zero must be added, making it 0.090. The excess zero is then eliminated from the end of the fraction; thus 0.090 becomes 0.09

Answer = **0.09**

EXAMPLE 4   Multiply 0.21 by 0.32

$$
\begin{array}{r}
0.21 \\
\times\ 0.32 \\
\hline
42 \\
\times\ 63\ \ \\
\hline
672
\end{array}
$$

In this example 0.21 has two numbers after the decimal point and 0.32 also has two. Add a zero in front of the product to allow correct placement of the decimal point, making it .0672, then add a zero in front of the fraction to emphasize it.

Answer = **0.0672**

EXAMPLE 5   Multiply 0.12 by 0.2

$$
\begin{array}{r}
0.12 \\
\times\ \ 0.2 \\
\hline
24
\end{array}
$$

In this example there are a total of three numbers after the decimal points in 0.12 and 0.2. Add a zero in front of the product for correct decimal placement in the answer, making it .024, then add a zero in front of .024 to emphasize the fraction.

Answer = **0.024**

Multiply the decimal fractions.

1. 0.45×0.2 = _____

2. 0.35×0.12 = _____

3. 1.3×0.05 = _____

4. 0.7×0.04 = _____

5. 0.4×0.17 = _____

6. 2.14×0.03 = _____

ANSWERS 1. 0.09 2. 0.042 3. 0.065 4. 0.028 5. 0.068 6. 0.0642

Division of Decimal Fractions

Decimal fractions occur frequently in calculations as common fractions, which require division. Our first example includes a commonly seen dosage calculation that illustrates this point.

EXAMPLE $\dfrac{0.25}{0.125} = \dfrac{\text{numerator}}{\text{denominator}}$

Before actual decimal fraction (or any) division is done, the numbers in common fractions are routinely simplified by using **three preliminary reduction steps:**

1. **elimination of decimal points**
2. **reduction of the numbers using common denominators**
3. **reduction of numbers ending in zero**

We will begin by practicing these three important steps, which you will discover quite frequently complete a calculation and actually make final division unnecessary. You'll recall the pertinent common fraction terminology of **numerator**, the **top number** in a fraction, and **denominator**, which is the **bottom number**.

Elimination of Decimal Points

Decimal points can be eliminated from the numbers in a decimal fraction without changing its value.

To eliminate the decimal points from decimal fractions, move them the same number of places to the right in the numerator and in the denominator until they are eliminated from both. Zeros may have to be added to accomplish this.

EXAMPLE 1 $\dfrac{0.25}{0.125}$ becomes $\dfrac{250}{125}$

The decimal point must be moved three places to the right in the denominator 0.125 to make it 125. Therefore, it must be moved three places to the right in the numerator 0.25, which requires the addition of one zero to make it 250.

EXAMPLE 2 $\dfrac{0.3}{0.15}$ becomes $\dfrac{30}{15}$

The decimal point must be moved two places in the denominator 0.15 to make it 15, so it must be moved two places to the right in the numerator 0.3, which requires the addition of one zero to become 30.

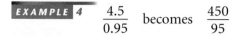

EXAMPLE 3　$\dfrac{1.5}{2}$　becomes　$\dfrac{15}{20}$

Move the decimal point one place in 1.5 to make it 15; add one zero to 2 to make it 20.

EXAMPLE 4　$\dfrac{4.5}{0.95}$　becomes　$\dfrac{450}{95}$

> *Eliminating the decimal points from a decimal fraction before final division does not alter the value of the fraction or the answer obtained in the final division.*

PROBLEM

Eliminate the decimal points from the decimal fractions.

1. $\dfrac{17.5}{2}$ = _____		6. $\dfrac{0.1}{0.05}$ = _____	
2. $\dfrac{0.5}{25}$ = _____		7. $\dfrac{0.9}{0.03}$ = _____	
3. $\dfrac{6.3}{0.6}$ = _____		8. $\dfrac{10.75}{2.5}$ = _____	
4. $\dfrac{3.76}{0.4}$ = _____		9. $\dfrac{0.4}{0.04}$ = _____	
5. $\dfrac{8.4}{0.7}$ = _____		10. $\dfrac{1.2}{0.4}$ = _____	

ANSWERS　1. $\dfrac{175}{20}$　2. $\dfrac{5}{250}$　3. $\dfrac{63}{6}$　4. $\dfrac{376}{40}$　5. $\dfrac{84}{7}$　6. $\dfrac{10}{5}$　7. $\dfrac{90}{3}$　8. $\dfrac{1075}{250}$　9. $\dfrac{40}{4}$　10. $\dfrac{12}{4}$

Reduction of Fractions

Once the decimal points are eliminated, a second simplification step is to reduce the numbers as far as possible using common denominators.

> *To reduce fractions, divide the numerator and the denominator by their highest common denominator (the highest number that will divide into both).*

The **highest common denominator** is usually **2, 3, 4, 5, or multiples of these numbers,** such as 6, 8, 25, and so on.

EXAMPLE 1　$\dfrac{175}{20}$　The highest common denominator is 5

$$\dfrac{\cancel{175}}{\cancel{20}} = \dfrac{35}{4}$$

EXAMPLE 2 $\dfrac{63}{6}$ The highest common denominator is 3

$$\dfrac{\cancel{63}}{\cancel{6}} = \dfrac{21}{2}$$

EXAMPLE 3 $\dfrac{1075}{250}$ The highest common denominator is 25

$$\dfrac{\cancel{1075}}{\cancel{250}} = \dfrac{43}{10}$$

There is a second way you can reduce fractions in examples with large numbers such as this one, and it is equally correct. Divide by 5, then 5 again.

$$\dfrac{\cancel{1075}}{\cancel{250}} = \dfrac{\cancel{215}}{\cancel{50}} = \dfrac{43}{10}$$

If the highest common denominator is difficult to determine, reduce several times using smaller common denominators.

EXAMPLE 4 $\dfrac{376}{40} = \dfrac{47}{5}$ Reduce by 8

or divide by 4, then 2 $\dfrac{\cancel{376}}{\cancel{40}} = \dfrac{\cancel{94}}{\cancel{10}} = \dfrac{47}{5}$

or divide by 2, 2, then 2 $\dfrac{\cancel{376}}{\cancel{40}} = \dfrac{\cancel{188}}{\cancel{20}} = \dfrac{\cancel{94}}{\cancel{10}} = \dfrac{47}{5}$

Remember that **simple numbers are easier to work with**, and the time spent doing extra reductions may be well worth the payoff in safety.

PROBLEM

Reduce the fractions as much as possible in preparation for final division.

1. $\dfrac{84}{8}$ = _____   6. $\dfrac{40}{14}$ = _____

2. $\dfrac{20}{16}$ = _____   7. $\dfrac{82}{28}$ = _____

3. $\dfrac{250}{325}$ = _____   8. $\dfrac{100}{75}$ = _____

4. $\dfrac{96}{34}$ = _____   9. $\dfrac{50}{75}$ = _____

5. $\dfrac{175}{20}$ = _____   10. $\dfrac{60}{88}$ = _____

ANSWERS 1. $\dfrac{21}{2}$ 2. $\dfrac{5}{4}$ 3. $\dfrac{10}{13}$ 4. $\dfrac{48}{17}$ 5. $\dfrac{35}{4}$ 6. $\dfrac{20}{7}$ 7. $\dfrac{41}{14}$ 8. $\dfrac{4}{3}$ 9. $\dfrac{2}{3}$ 10. $\dfrac{15}{22}$

Reduction of Numbers Ending in Zero

The third type of simplification is not related solely to decimal fractions, but it is best covered at this time. This type of simplification concerns reductions when both numbers in the fraction end in zeros.

EXAMPLE $\dfrac{800}{250}$

 Numbers that end in a zero or zeros may initially be reduced by crossing off the same number of zeros in both the numerator and the denominator.

EXAMPLE 1 $\dfrac{800}{250}$

In this fraction, the numerator, 800, has two zeros and the denominator, 250, has one zero. The number of zeros crossed off must be the same in both the numerator and the denominator, so only one zero can be eliminated from each.

$$\frac{800}{250} = \frac{80}{25} \quad \text{Reduce by } 5 = \frac{16}{5}$$

EXAMPLE 2 $\dfrac{2400}{2000} = \dfrac{24}{20}$ Reduce by $4 = \dfrac{6}{5}$

Two zeros can be eliminated from the denominator and the numerator in this fraction.

EXAMPLE 3 $\dfrac{15,000}{30,000} = \dfrac{15}{30}$ Reduce by $5 = \dfrac{3}{6}$

In this fraction three zeros can be eliminated.

PROBLEM

Reduce the fractions to their lowest terms in preparation for final division.

1. $\dfrac{50}{250}$ = _____

2. $\dfrac{120}{50}$ = _____

3. $\dfrac{2500}{1500}$ = _____

4. $\dfrac{1,000,000}{750,000}$ = _____

5. $\dfrac{800}{150}$ = _____

6. $\dfrac{110}{100}$ = _____

7. $\dfrac{200,000}{150,000}$ = _____

8. $\dfrac{1000}{800}$ = _____

9. $\dfrac{60}{40}$ = _____

10. $\dfrac{150}{200}$ = _____

ANSWERS 1. $\frac{1}{5}$ 2. $\frac{12}{5}$ 3. $\frac{5}{3}$ 4. $\frac{4}{3}$ 5. $\frac{16}{3}$ 6. $\frac{11}{10}$ 7. $\frac{4}{3}$ 8. $\frac{5}{4}$ 9. $\frac{3}{2}$ 10. $\frac{3}{4}$

Calculator Use for Final Division

Final division of a fraction or equation is one area where using a calculator may be preferable to manual division. So it's appropriate that calculator use be introduced at this juncture. **Calculator use does not guarantee accuracy.** Mistakes have been made in all types of calculations when calculators were used, so their use should be regarded as an adjunct to, not a replacement for, manual solution.

> *Manual solution is the essential first step of clinical calculations. Calculator use, when necessary, is a second, adjunct step.*

That said, let's review calculator use in clinical calculations. Calculators vary in how they function, so the necessary first step is to **be sure you know how to use the calculator available to you.** If you find yourself in a situation where you must do frequent calculations, it would be wise to buy and use your own calculator.

The next precaution, and this is critical, is to **enter the functions (add, subtract, multiply, divide) and all numbers correctly**, especially those numbers containing decimal points. The next most important caution is to **visually check each entry, but not the running totals**, which can cause confusion. And finally, be aware that **calculator errors tend to be repetitive.** If you find yourself making a mistake be extremely careful to be sure you don't repeat it.

> *Use of a calculator does not guarantee correct answers in dosage calculations. All entries, and all answers obtained, must be double-checked.*

Expressing to the Nearest Tenth

When a fraction has been reduced as much as possible, it is ready for final division. This is done by **dividing the numerators by the denominators.** Answers are most often rounded off and expressed as decimal numbers to the nearest tenth. If the division is simple this can be done manually, or you can use a calculator.

> *To express an answer to the nearest tenth, the division is carried to hundredths (two places after the decimal). When the number representing hundredths is 5 or larger, the number representing tenths is increased by one.*

EXAMPLE 1 $\dfrac{0.35}{0.4}$ = 0.35 ÷ 0.4 = 0.87

Answer = **0.9**

The number representing hundredths is 7, so the number representing tenths is increased by one: 0.87 becomes 0.9

EXAMPLE 2 $\dfrac{0.5}{0.3}$ = 0.5 ÷ 0.3 = 1.66 = **1.7**

The number representing hundredths, 6, is larger than 5, so 1.66 becomes 1.7

EXAMPLE 3 $\dfrac{0.16}{0.3}$ = 0.53 = **0.5**

The number representing hundredths, 3, is less than 5, so the number representing tenths, 5, remains unchanged, and the 3 is dropped.

EXAMPLE 4 $\dfrac{0.2}{0.3}$ = 0.66 = **0.7**

EXAMPLE 5 An answer of 1.42 remains **1.4**

EXAMPLE 6 An answer of 1.86 becomes **1.9**

PROBLEM

Divide the decimal numbers. Express your answers to the nearest tenth. A calculator can be used for final division, if necessary.

1. $\dfrac{5.1}{2.3}$ = _____

2. $\dfrac{0.9}{0.7}$ = _____

3. $\dfrac{3.7}{2}$ = _____

4. $\dfrac{6}{1.3}$ = _____

5. $\dfrac{1.5}{2.1}$ = _____

6. $\dfrac{2.7}{1.1}$ = _____

7. $\dfrac{4.2}{5}$ = _____

8. $\dfrac{0.5}{2.5}$ = _____

9. $\dfrac{5.2}{0.91}$ = _____

10. $\dfrac{2.4}{2.7}$ = _____

ANSWERS **1.** 2.2 **2.** 1.3 **3.** 1.9 **4.** 4.6 **5.** 0.7 **6.** 2.5 **7.** 0.8 **8.** 0.2 **9.** 5.7 **10.** 0.9

Expressing to the Nearest Hundredth

Some drugs are administered in dosages carried to the nearest hundredth. This is common in pediatric dosages and in drugs that alter the body's vital functions, for example, the heart rate.

 To express an answer to the nearest hundredth, the division is carried to thousandths (three places after the decimal point). When the number representing thousandths is 5 or larger, the number representing hundredths is increased by one.

EXAMPLE 1 0.736 becomes **0.74**

The number representing thousandths, 6, is larger than 5, so the number representing hundredths, 3, is increased by one to become 4.

EXAMPLE 2 0.777 becomes **0.78**

EXAMPLE 3 0.373 remains **0.37**

The number representing thousandths, 3, is less than 5, so the number representing hundredths, 7, remains unchanged.

EXAMPLE 4 0.934 remains **0.93**

PROBLEM

Express the numbers to the nearest hundredth.

1.	0.175	= _____	7.	1.081	= _____
2.	0.344	= _____	8.	1.327	= _____
3.	1.853	= _____	9.	0.739	= _____
4.	0.306	= _____	10.	0.733	= _____
5.	3.015	= _____	11.	2.072	= _____
6.	2.154	= _____	12.	0.089	= _____

ANSWERS 1. 0.18 2. 0.34 3. 1.85 4. 0.31 5. 3.02 6. 2.15 7. 1.08 8. 1.33 9. 0.74 10. 0.73 11. 2.07 12. 0.09

Summary

This concludes the chapter on multiplication and division of decimals. The important points to remember from this chapter are:

When decimal fractions are multiplied manually, the decimal point is placed the same number of places to the left in the product as the total of numbers after the decimal points in the fractions multiplied.

Zeros must be placed in front of a product if it contains insufficient numbers for the correct placement of the decimal point.

To simplify fractions for final division, the preliminary steps of eliminating decimal points, reducing the numbers by common denominators, and reducing numbers ending in zeros can be used.

The use of a calculator does not eliminate the need for preliminary manual simplification steps.

Practice using a calculator until proficiency is achieved.

All calculator entries must be double-checked.

Calculator running totals should be disregarded, because they can cause confusion.

A personal calculator is a must if frequent calculations are necessary.

To express to tenths, increase the answer by one if the number representing the hundredths is 5 or larger.

To express to hundredths, increase the answer by one if the number representing the thousandths is 5 or larger.

Summary Self-Test

Multiply the following decimals manually.

1. $1.49 \times 0.05 = $ _____

2. $0.15 \times 3.04 = $ _____

3. $0.025 \times 3.5 = $ _____

4. $0.55 \times 2.5 = $ _____

5. $1.31 \times 2.07 = $ _____

6. $5.3 \times 1.02 = $ _____

7. $0.35 \times 1.25 = $ _____

8. $4.32 \times 0.05 = $ _____

9. $0.2 \times 0.02 = $ _____

10. $0.4 \times 1.75 = $ _____

11. You are to administer 4 tablets with a dosage strength of 0.04 mg each. What total dosage are you giving? _____

12. You have given 2½ (2.5) tablets with a strength of 1.25 mg per tablet. What total dosage is this? _____

13. Tablets are labeled 0.1 mg and you are to give 3½ (3.5) tablets. What total dosage is this? _____

14. You gave 3 tablets labeled 0.75 mg each, and the dosage ordered was 2.25 mg. Was this the correct dosage? _____

15. The tablets available are labeled 12.5 mg, and you are to give 4½ (4.5) tablets. What total dosage will this be? _____

16. A dosage of 4.5 mg is ordered. The tablets available are labeled 3.5 mg, and there are 2½ tablets in the medication drawer. Is this a correct dosage? _____

Reduce and divide the fractions. Express answers to the nearest tenth. A calculator can be used for final division.

17. $\dfrac{1.3}{0.7} = $ _____

18. $\dfrac{1.9}{3.2} = $ _____

19. $\dfrac{32.5}{9} = $ _____

20. $\dfrac{0.04}{0.1} = $ _____

21. $\dfrac{1.45}{1.2} = $ _____

22. $\dfrac{250}{1000} = $ _____

23. $\dfrac{0.8}{0.09} = $ _____

24. $\dfrac{2,000,000}{1,500,000} = $ _____

25. $\dfrac{4.1}{2.05} = $ _____

26. $\dfrac{7.3}{12} = $ _____

27. $\dfrac{150,000}{120,000} = $ _____

28. $\dfrac{0.15}{0.08} = $ _____

29. $\dfrac{2700}{900} = $ _____

30. $\dfrac{0.25}{0.15} = $ _____

Reduce and divide the fractions. Express answers to the nearest hundredth. A calculator can be used for final division.

31. $\dfrac{900}{1700} = $ _____

32. $\dfrac{0.125}{0.3} = $ _____

33. $\dfrac{1450}{1500} = $ _____

34. $\dfrac{65}{175} = $ _____

35. $\dfrac{0.6}{1.35}$ = _____

36. $\dfrac{0.04}{0.12}$ = _____

37. $\dfrac{750}{10,000}$ = _____

38. $\dfrac{0.65}{0.8}$ = _____

39. $\dfrac{3.01}{4.2}$ = _____

40. $\dfrac{4.5}{6.1}$ = _____

41. $\dfrac{0.13}{0.25}$ = _____

42. $\dfrac{0.25}{0.7}$ = _____

43. $\dfrac{3.3}{5.1}$ = _____

44. $\dfrac{0.19}{0.7}$ = _____

45. $\dfrac{1.1}{1.3}$ = _____

46. $\dfrac{3}{4.1}$ = _____

47. $\dfrac{62}{240}$ = _____

48. $\dfrac{280,000}{300,000}$ = _____

49. $\dfrac{115}{255}$ = _____

50. $\dfrac{10}{14.3}$ = _____

2

ANSWERS

1. 0.0745	**11.** 0.16 mg	**21.** 1.2	**31.** 0.53	**41.** 0.52
2. 0.456	**12.** 3.125 mg	**22.** 0.3	**32.** 0.42	**42.** 0.36
3. 0.0875	**13.** 0.35 mg	**23.** 8.9	**33.** 0.97	**43.** 0.65
4. 1.375	**14.** Yes	**24.** 1.3	**34.** 0.37	**44.** 0.27
5. 2.7117	**15.** 56.25 mg	**25.** 2	**35.** 0.44	**45.** 0.85
6. 5.406	**16.** No	**26.** 0.6	**36.** 0.33	**46.** 0.73
7. 0.4375	**17.** 1.9	**27.** 1.3	**37.** 0.08	**47.** 0.26
8. 0.216	**18.** 0.6	**28.** 1.9	**38.** 0.81	**48.** 0.93
9. 0.004	**19.** 3.6	**29.** 3	**39.** 0.72	**49.** 0.45
10. 0.7	**20.** 0.4	**30.** 1.7	**40.** 0.74	**50.** 0.7

3

Solving Common Fraction Equations

OBJECTIVES

The learner will solve equations containing:
1. whole numbers
2. decimal numbers
3. multiple numbers

Prerequisites

Chapters 1 and 2

The majority of clinical calculations involve solving an equation containing one to five common fractions. Two examples are:

$$\frac{2}{5} \times \frac{3}{4} \quad \text{and} \quad \frac{20}{1} \times \frac{1000}{60,000} \times \frac{1200}{1} \times \frac{1}{60}$$

Two options are available to solve common fraction equations: initial fraction reduction, then calculator use as necessary for final division; or calculator use throughout. The first option was stressed in Chapter 1, and it is recommended again in this chapter.

Do the math **for all the examples** yourself, and **compare it** with the math provided. Simply reading the examples will not help you understand why initial reduction of the fractions is so important, nor will it help you develop an appreciation for why calculator entries require particular care. Do each example very carefully.

Don't forget the calculator use precautions stressed in Chapter 2. Make sure you understand how the calculator you are using actually functions; double-check each entry for accuracy; and do not become confused by the running totals that register and change throughout the calculation.

Whole Number Equations

The examples start with whole number equations because they are somewhat less complicated. Answers are expressed in tenths and in hundredths for all examples.

EXAMPLE 1   **Option 1: Initial Reduction of Fractions**

$$\frac{2}{5} \times \frac{3}{4}$$

$$\frac{\overset{1}{\cancel{2}}}{5} \times \frac{3}{\underset{2}{\cancel{4}}}$$ Divide the numerator, 2, and the denominator, 4, by 2 (to become 1 and 2)

$$1 \times 3 \div 5 \times 2$$ Multiply the remaining numerators, 1 and 3, to obtain 3; then the remaining denominators, 5 and 2, to obtain 10

$$3 \div 10$$ Divide the numerator, 3, by the denominator, 10

$$= 0.3$$

Answer = **0.3 (tenth)** or **0.3 (hundredth)**

22

Option 2: Calculator Use Throughout

$$\frac{2}{5} \times \frac{3}{4}$$

$2 \times 3 \div 5 \div 4$ Multiply the numerators, 2 and 3; divide by the denominators, 5 then 4, in continuous entries

$= 0.3$

Answer $= $ **0.3 (tenth)** or **0.3 (hundredth)**

EXAMPLE 2   **Option 1: Initial Reduction of Fractions**

$$\frac{250}{175} \times \frac{150}{325}$$

$$\frac{\overset{10}{\cancel{250}}}{\underset{7}{\cancel{175}}} \times \frac{\overset{6}{\cancel{150}}}{\underset{13}{\cancel{325}}}$$ Divide the numerator, 250, and the denominator, 175, by 25 (to become 10 and 7); divide the numerator, 150, and denominator, 325, by 25 (to become 6 and 13)

$10 \times 6 \div 7 \times 13$ Multiply the numerators, 10 and 6, then the denominators, 7 and 13

$60 \div 91$ Divide 60 by 91

$= 0.659$

Answer $= $ **0.7 (tenth)** or **0.66 (hundredth)**

Option 2: Calculator Use Throughout

$$\frac{250}{175} \times \frac{150}{325}$$

$250 \times 150 \div 175 \div 325$ Multiply the numerators, 250 and 150, then divide by the denominators, 175 and 325

$= 0.659$

Answer $= $ **0.7 (tenth)** or **0.66 (hundredth)**

EXAMPLE 3   **Option 1: Initial Reduction of Fractions**

$$\frac{7}{50} \times \frac{25}{3} \times \frac{120}{32}$$

$$\frac{7}{\underset{2}{\cancel{50}}} \times \frac{\overset{1}{\cancel{25}}}{3} \times \frac{\overset{15}{\cancel{120}}}{\underset{4}{\cancel{32}}}$$ Divide 25 and 50 by 25; divide 120 and 32 by 8

$7 \times 15 \div 2 \times 3 \times 4$ Multiply the remaining numerators, 7 and 15, then the remaining denominators, 2 by 3 by 4

$105 \div 24$ Divide the numerator, 105, by the denominator, 24

$= 4.375$

Answer $= $ **4.4 (tenth)** or **4.38 (hundredth)**

Option 2: Calculator Use Throughout

$$\frac{7}{50} \times \frac{25}{3} \times \frac{120}{32}$$

$7 \times 25 \times 120 \div 50 \div 3 \div 32$ Multiply the numerators, 7, 25, and 120, then divide by the denominators, 50, 3, and 32

$= 4.375$

Answer $= $ **4.4 (tenth)** or **4.38 (hundredth)**

EXAMPLE 4   **Option 1: Initial Reduction of Fractions**

$$\frac{20}{1} \times \frac{1000}{60,000} \times \frac{1200}{1} \times \frac{1}{60}$$

$$\frac{\overset{1}{\cancel{20}}}{1} \times \frac{1000}{\underset{3}{\cancel{60,000}}} \times \frac{\overset{20}{\cancel{1200}}}{1} \times \frac{1}{\cancel{60}_{\,1}}$$ Reduce 1000 and 60,000 by eliminating three zeros from each; divide 20 and 60 by 20; divide 1200 and 60 by 60

$20 \div 3$ Divide the remaining numerator, 20, by the remaining denominator, 3

$= 6.666$

Answer $= $ **6.7 (tenth)** or **6.67 (hundredth)**

Option 2: Calculator Use Throughout

$$\frac{20}{1} \times \frac{1000}{60,000} \times \frac{1200}{1} \times \frac{1}{60}$$

$20 \times 1000 \times 1200 \div 60,000 \div 60$

$= 6.666$

Answer $= $ **6.7 (tenth)** or **6.67 (hundredth)**

EXAMPLE 5   **Option 1: Initial Reduction of Fractions**

$$\frac{2000}{1500} \times \frac{2500}{3000}$$

$$\frac{\cancel{2000}}{\underset{3}{\cancel{1500}}} \times \frac{\overset{5}{\cancel{2500}}}{\cancel{3000}}$$ Eliminate three zeros in 2000 and 3000; divide 2500 and 1500 by 500

$2 \times 5 \div 3 \times 3$ Multiply the remaining numerators, 2 and 5, then the remaining denominators, 3 and 3

$10 \div 9$ Divide the numerator, 10, by the denominator, 9

$= 1.111$

Answer $= $ **1.1 (tenth)** or **1.11 (hundredth)**

Option 2: Calculator Use Throughout

$$\frac{2000}{1500} \times \frac{2500}{3000}$$

$$2000 \times 2500 \div 1500 \div 3000$$

$$= 1.111$$

Answer = **1.1 (tenth)** or **1.11 (hundredth)**

PROBLEM

Solve the equations. Express your answers to the nearest tenth and hundredth. Reduce fractions manually first, and use a calculator as necessary for the final division.

1. $\dfrac{3}{8} \times \dfrac{6}{3}$ = _____

2. $\dfrac{3}{4} \times \dfrac{10}{2}$ = _____

3. $\dfrac{3}{5} \times \dfrac{1050}{40}$ = _____

4. $\dfrac{10}{1} \times \dfrac{750}{40,000} \times \dfrac{1000}{1} \times \dfrac{1}{60}$ = _____

5. $\dfrac{12}{1} \times \dfrac{500}{2700} \times \dfrac{2000}{1} \times \dfrac{1}{60}$ = _____

6. $\dfrac{1500}{750} \times \dfrac{350}{600}$ = _____

7. $\dfrac{1000}{2700} \times \dfrac{1300}{500} \times \dfrac{70}{50}$ = _____

8. $\dfrac{15}{1} \times \dfrac{2500}{20,000} \times \dfrac{1000}{1} \times \dfrac{1}{60}$ = _____

ANSWERS 1. 0.8; 0.75 2. 3.8; 3.75 3. 15.8; 15.75 4. 3.1; 3.13 5. 74.1; 74.07 6. 1.2; 1.17 7. 1.3; 1.35
8. 31.3; 31.25

Decimal Fraction Equations

Decimal fraction equations raise an instant warning flag in calculations, because it is here that most dosage errors occur. As with whole number equations, simplifying by eliminating decimal points, then reducing the numbers, is the first step. However, if you use a calculator, be sure to take your time and double-check all entries and all answers.

 Extreme care must be taken with calculator entry of decimal numbers to include the decimal point, and entries and answers must always be double-checked.

EXAMPLE 1   Option 1: **Initial Elimination of Decimal Points and Reduction of Fractions**

$$\frac{0.3}{1.65} \times \frac{2.5}{1}$$

$$\frac{30}{165} \times \frac{25}{10}$$ Move the decimal point two places to the right in 0.3 and 1.65 (to become 30 and 165), and one place to the right in 2.5 and 1 (to become 25 and 10)

$$\frac{\overset{3}{\cancel{30}}}{\underset{33}{\cancel{165}}} \times \frac{\overset{5}{\cancel{25}}}{\underset{1}{\cancel{10}}}$$ Divide 30 and 10 by 10; divide 25 and 165 by 5

$$\frac{\overset{1}{\cancel{3}}}{\underset{11}{\cancel{33}}} \times \frac{5}{1}$$ Divide 3 and 33 by 3

$$5 \div 11$$ Divide the remaining numerator, 5, by the denominator, 11

$$= 0.454$$

Answer $=$ **0.5 (tenth)** or **0.45 (hundredth)**

Option 2: Calculator Use Throughout

$$\frac{0.3}{1.65} \times \frac{2.5}{1}$$

$$0.3 \times 2.5 \div 1.65$$ Multiply 0.3 by 2.5, then divide by 1.65

$$= 0.454$$

Answer $=$ **0.5 (tenth)** or **0.45 (hundredth)**

EXAMPLE 2   Option 1: **Initial Elimination of Decimal Points and Reduction of Fractions**

$$\frac{0.3}{1.2} \times \frac{2.1}{0.15}$$

$$\frac{3}{12} \times \frac{210}{15}$$ Eliminate the decimal points by moving them one place to the right in 0.3 and 1.2 (to become 3 and 12), and two places to the right in 2.1 and 0.15 (to become 210 and 15)

$$\frac{\overset{1}{\cancel{3}}}{\underset{4}{\cancel{12}}} \times \frac{\overset{42}{\cancel{210}}}{\underset{3}{\cancel{15}}}$$ Divide 3 and 12 by 3; divide 210 and 15 by 5

$$\frac{1}{\underset{2}{\cancel{4}}} \times \frac{\overset{21}{\cancel{42}}}{3}$$ Divide 42 and 4 by 2; multiply the denominators, 2 by 3

$$21 \div 6$$ Divide the numerator, 21, by the denominator, 6

$$= 3.5$$

Answer $=$ **3.5 (tenth)** or **3.5 (hundredth)**

Option 2: Calculator Use Throughout

$$\frac{0.3}{1.2} \times \frac{2.1}{0.15}$$

$0.3 \times 2.1 \div 1.2 \div 0.15$ Multiply 0.3 by 2.1, then divide by 1.2 and 0.15

$= 3.5$

Answer $=$ **3.5 (tenth)** or **3.5 (hundredth)**

EXAMPLE 3   **Option 1: Initial Elimination of Decimal Points and Reduction of Fractions**

$$\frac{0.15}{0.17} \times \frac{3.1}{2}$$

$\dfrac{15}{17} \times \dfrac{31}{20}$ Move the decimal point two places to the right in 0.15 and 0.17; move it one place to the right in 3.1 and 2 (requires adding a zero to 2)

$\dfrac{\overset{3}{\cancel{15}}}{17} \times \dfrac{31}{\underset{4}{\cancel{20}}}$ Divide 15 and 20 by 5

$3 \times 31 \div 17 \times 4$ Use a calculator to multiply the remaining numerators, 3 and 31, then the remaining denominators, 17 and 4

$93 \div 68$ Divide the numerator, 93, by the denominator, 68

$= 1.367$

Answer $=$ **1.4 (tenth)** or **1.37 (hundredth)**

Option 2: Calculator Use Throughout

$$\frac{0.15}{0.17} \times \frac{3.1}{2}$$

$0.15 \times 3.1 \div 0.17 \div 2$ Multiply 0.15 by 3.1, divide by 0.17 then by 2

$= 1.367$

Answer $=$ **1.4 (tenth)** or **1.37 (hundredth)**

EXAMPLE 4   **Option 1: Initial Elimination of Decimal Points and Reduction of Fractions**

$$\frac{2.5}{1.5} \times \frac{1.2}{1.1}$$

$\dfrac{25}{15} \times \dfrac{12}{11}$ Move the decimal point one place in 2.5 and 1.5; move it one place in 1.2 and 1.1

$\dfrac{\overset{5}{\cancel{25}}}{\underset{3}{\cancel{15}}} \times \dfrac{12}{11}$ Divide 25 and 15 by 5

$$\frac{5}{\underset{1}{\cancel{3}}} \times \frac{\overset{4}{\cancel{12}}}{11}$$ Divide 12 and 3 by 3

$5 \times 4 \div 1 \times 11$ Multiply the remaining numerators, 5 and 4, then the remaining denominators, 1 and 11

$20 \div 11$ Divide the numerator, 20, by the denominator, 11

$= 1.818$

Answer = **1.8 (tenth)** or **1.82 (hundredth)**

Option 2: Calculator Use Throughout

$$\frac{2.5}{1.5} \times \frac{1.2}{1.1}$$

$2.5 \times 1.2 \div 1.5 \div 1.1$ Multiply 2.5 by 1.2, divide by 1.5 then by 1.1

$= 1.818$

Answer = **1.8 (tenth)** or **1.82 (hundredth)**

PROBLEM

Solve the equations. Express your answers to the nearest tenth and hundredth. A calculator may be used for the final division.

1. $\dfrac{2.1}{1.15} \times \dfrac{0.9}{1.2} = $ _____

2. $\dfrac{3.1}{2.7} \times \dfrac{2.2}{1.4} = $ _____

3. $\dfrac{0.3}{1.2} \times \dfrac{3}{2.1} = $ _____

4. $\dfrac{0.17}{0.3} \times \dfrac{2.5}{1.5} = $ _____

5. $\dfrac{1.75}{0.95} \times \dfrac{1.5}{2} = $ _____

6. $\dfrac{0.75}{1.15} \times \dfrac{3}{1.25} = $ _____

7. $\dfrac{10.2}{1.5} \times \dfrac{2}{5.1} = $ _____

8. $\dfrac{0.125}{0.25} \times \dfrac{2.5}{1.5} = $ _____

9. $\dfrac{0.9}{0.3} \times \dfrac{1.2}{1.4} = $ _____

10. $\dfrac{0.35}{1.7} \times \dfrac{2.5}{0.7} = $ _____

ANSWERS **1.** 1.4; 1.37 **2.** 1.8; 1.8 **3.** 0.4; 0.36 **4.** 0.9; 0.94 **5.** 1.4; 1.38 **6.** 1.6; 1.57 **7.** 2.7; 2.67 **8.** 0.8; 0.83 **9.** 2.6; 2.57 **10.** 0.7; 0.74

Multiple Number Equations

The calculation steps you have already practiced are also used for multiple number equations. Reduction of numbers is frequently of particular benefit here, because calculations of this type sometimes have large numbers that either cancel or reduce dramatically. Answers are expressed to the nearest whole number in the examples and problems that follow to replicate actual clinical intravenous rate calculations.

EXAMPLE 1   **Option 1: Initial Reduction of Fractions**

$$\frac{60}{1} \times \frac{1000}{4} \times \frac{1}{1000} \times \frac{6}{1}$$

$$\frac{60}{1} \times \frac{\overset{1}{\cancel{1000}}}{\underset{2}{\cancel{4}}} \times \frac{1}{\cancel{1000}} \times \frac{\overset{3}{\cancel{6}}}{1}$$

Eliminate 1000 from the numerator and denominator; divide 6 and 4 by 2

$180 \div 2$

Multiply the numerators, 60 by 3; divide by the denominator, 6

$= 90$

Answer $= $ **90**

Option 2: Calculator Use Throughout

$$\frac{60}{1} \times \frac{1000}{4} \times \frac{1}{1000} \times \frac{6}{1}$$

$60 \times 1000 \times 6 \div 4 \div 1000$ Multiply 60 by 1000, then by 6; divide by 4 and 1000

$= 90$

Answer $= $ **90**

EXAMPLE 2   **Option 1: Initial Reduction of Fractions**

$$\frac{1}{60} \times \frac{1}{12} \times \frac{10}{1} \times \frac{750}{1}$$

$$\frac{1}{\underset{6}{\cancel{60}}} \times \frac{1}{\underset{6}{\cancel{12}}} \times \frac{\overset{1}{\cancel{10}}}{1} \times \frac{\overset{375}{\cancel{750}}}{1}$$

Divide 10 and 60 by 10; divide 750 and 12 by 2

$375 \div 36$

Divide the numerator, 375, by the denominator, 36

$= 9.86$ Round to whole number

Answer $= $ **10**

Option 2: Calculator Use Throughout

$$\frac{1}{60} \times \frac{1}{12} \times \frac{10}{1} \times \frac{750}{1}$$

$10 \times 750 \div 60 \div 12$ Multiply 10 by 750; divide by 60, then by 12

$= 9.86$ Round to whole number

Answer $= $ **10**

EXAMPLE 3   **Option 1: Initial Reduction of Fractions**

$$\frac{20}{1} \times \frac{75}{1} \times \frac{1}{60}$$

$$\frac{\overset{1}{\cancel{20}}}{1} \times \frac{\overset{25}{\cancel{75}}}{1} \times \frac{1}{\underset{1}{\cancel{60}}}$$

Divide 20 and 60 by 20 to become 1 and 3; divide 75 and 3 by 3 to become 25 and 1

$= 25$

Answer $= $ **25**

$$\frac{20}{1} \times \frac{75}{1} \times \frac{1}{60}$$

$20 \times 75 \div 60$ Multiply 20 by 75; divide by 60

$= 25$

Answer $= $ **25**

EXAMPLE 4   **Option 1: Initial Reduction of Fractions**

$$\frac{2}{0.5} \times \frac{1}{100} \times \frac{275}{1}$$

$$\frac{20}{5} \times \frac{1}{100} \times \frac{275}{1}$$ Eliminate the decimal point by moving it one place to the right in 0.5, and one place to the right in 2, which requires adding a zero to 2 (to become 5 and 20)

$$\frac{\overset{1}{\cancel{20}}}{\underset{1}{\cancel{5}}} \times \frac{1}{\underset{5}{\cancel{100}}} \times \frac{\overset{55}{\cancel{275}}}{1}$$ Divide 20 and 100 by 20; divide 275 and 5 by 5

$$\frac{1}{\underset{1}{\cancel{5}}} \times \frac{\overset{11}{\cancel{55}}}{1}$$ Divide 5 and 55 by 5

$= 11$

Answer $= $ **11**

Option 2: Calculator Use Throughout

$$\frac{2}{0.5} \times \frac{1}{100} \times \frac{275}{1}$$

$2 \times 275 \div 0.5 \div 100$ Multiply 2 by 275; divide by 0.5 and 100

$= 11$

Answer $= $ **11**

PROBLEM

Solve the equations. Express answers to the nearest whole number.

1. $\dfrac{15}{1} \times \dfrac{350}{5} \times \dfrac{1}{60} \quad = \quad$ _____

2. $\dfrac{1}{32} \times \dfrac{60}{1} \times \dfrac{7.5}{3.1} \quad = \quad$ _____

3. $\dfrac{10}{1} \times \dfrac{2500}{24} \times \dfrac{1}{60} \quad = \quad$ _____

4. $\dfrac{1.7}{2.3} \times \dfrac{15.3}{12.1} \times \dfrac{6.2}{0.3} \quad = \quad$ _____

5. $\dfrac{20}{1} \times \dfrac{1200}{16} \times \dfrac{1}{60} \quad = \quad$ _____

ANSWERS   1. 18   2. 5   3. 17   4. 19   5. 25

Summary

This concludes the chapter on solving common fraction equations. The important points to remember from this chapter are:

Most clinical calculations consist of an equation containing one to five common fractions.

Numbers in an equation are initially reduced to simplify final multiplication and division.

If an equation contains decimal fractions, the decimal points may be eliminated from numerators and denominators without altering their value.

Zeros may be eliminated from the same number of numerators and denominators without altering the value of the equation.

A calculator may be used for final division as necessary.

Answers may be expressed as whole numbers, or to the nearest tenth or hundredth, depending on the calculation being done.

Summary Self-Test

Solve the equations. Express your answers to the nearest tenth and hundredth. A calculator may be used for final division.

1. $\dfrac{0.8}{0.65} \times \dfrac{1.2}{1}$ = _____

2. $\dfrac{350}{1000} \times \dfrac{4.4}{1}$ = _____

3. $\dfrac{0.35}{1.3} \times \dfrac{4.5}{1}$ = _____

4. $\dfrac{0.4}{1.5} \times \dfrac{2.3}{1}$ = _____

5. $\dfrac{1}{75} \times \dfrac{500}{1}$ = _____

6. $\dfrac{0.15}{0.12} \times \dfrac{1.45}{1}$ = _____

7. $\dfrac{100,000}{80,000} \times \dfrac{1.7}{1}$ = _____

8. $\dfrac{1.45}{2.1} \times \dfrac{1.5}{1}$ = _____

9. $\dfrac{1550}{500} \times \dfrac{0.5}{1}$ = _____

10. $\dfrac{4}{0.375} \times \dfrac{0.25}{1}$ = _____

11. $\dfrac{0.08}{0.1} \times \dfrac{2.1}{1}$ = _____

12. $\dfrac{1.5}{1.25} \times \dfrac{1.45}{1}$ = _____

13. $\dfrac{0.5}{0.15} \times \dfrac{0.35}{1}$ = _____

14. $\dfrac{300,000}{200,000} \times \dfrac{1.7}{1}$ = _____

15. $\dfrac{13.5}{10} \times \dfrac{1.8}{1}$ = _____

16. $\dfrac{1,000,000}{800,000} \times \dfrac{1.4}{1}$ = _____

17. $\dfrac{1.3}{0.2} \times \dfrac{0.25}{1}$ = _____

18. $\dfrac{1.5}{0.1} \times \dfrac{0.25}{1}$ = _____

19. $\dfrac{1.9}{3.5} \times \dfrac{3.2}{1.4}$ = _____

20. $\dfrac{15,000}{7500} \times \dfrac{3.5}{1.2}$ = _____

21. $\dfrac{4.7}{1.3} \times \dfrac{50}{20} \times \dfrac{4}{25} \times \dfrac{8.2}{2.1}$ = _____

22. $\dfrac{40}{24} \times \dfrac{250}{5} \times \dfrac{0.375}{7.5}$ = _____

23. $\dfrac{6.9}{21.6} \times \dfrac{250}{5} \times \dfrac{0.75}{2.1}$ = _____

24. $\dfrac{1}{60} \times \dfrac{1}{25} \times \dfrac{10}{1} \times \dfrac{1000}{1}$ = _____

25. $\dfrac{50.5}{22.75} \times \dfrac{4.7}{6.3} \times \dfrac{31.7}{10.2}$ = _____

Solve the equations. Express your answers to the nearest whole number. A calculator may be used for final division.

26. $\dfrac{104}{95} \times \dfrac{20}{15} \times \dfrac{63}{1.6}$ = _____

27. $\dfrac{40,000}{10,000} \times \dfrac{30}{1} \times \dfrac{3.7}{12.5}$ = _____

28. $\dfrac{60}{1} \times \dfrac{500}{50} \times \dfrac{1}{1000} \times \dfrac{116}{1}$ = _____

29. $\dfrac{1.5}{0.6} \times \dfrac{10}{14} \times \dfrac{3.2}{5.3} \times \dfrac{100}{2}$ = _____

30. $\dfrac{60}{1} \times \dfrac{50}{250} \times \dfrac{1}{100} \times \dfrac{455}{1}$ = _____

31. $\dfrac{33.7}{15.9} \times \dfrac{19.2}{2.6} \times \dfrac{2.9}{3.85}$ = _____

32. $\dfrac{20}{4} \times \dfrac{100}{88} \times \dfrac{1200}{250} \times \dfrac{10}{30}$ = _____

33. $\dfrac{14}{7.9} \times \dfrac{88}{8}$ = _____

34. $\dfrac{10}{1} \times \dfrac{325}{1.5} \times \dfrac{1}{60}$ = _____

35. $\dfrac{60}{1} \times \dfrac{300}{400} \times \dfrac{1}{800} \times \dfrac{400}{1}$ = _____

36. $\dfrac{3.7}{1.3} \times \dfrac{12}{8} \times \dfrac{3.1}{7.4} \times \dfrac{5}{1}$ = _____

37. $\dfrac{20}{2} \times \dfrac{125}{25} \times \dfrac{2}{750} \times \dfrac{216}{1}$ = _____

38. $\dfrac{4}{3} \times \dfrac{45}{1} \times \dfrac{22.5}{37.8}$ = _____

39. $\dfrac{7.5}{12.3} \times \dfrac{55}{5} \times \dfrac{23.2}{1.2}$ = _____

40. $\dfrac{1000}{1} \times \dfrac{50}{250} \times \dfrac{20}{1} \times \dfrac{1}{60}$ = _____

41. $\dfrac{15}{1} \times \dfrac{1000}{4000} \times \dfrac{800}{1} \times \dfrac{1}{60}$ = _____

42. $\dfrac{15}{1} \times \dfrac{500}{3} \times \dfrac{1}{60}$ = _____

43. $\dfrac{25}{3} \times \dfrac{750}{8} \times \dfrac{0.1}{1}$ = _____

44. $\dfrac{40}{2} \times \dfrac{250}{50} \times \dfrac{1}{800} \times \dfrac{154}{1}$ = _____

45. $\dfrac{33}{4} \times \dfrac{75}{40} \times \dfrac{2}{150} \times \dfrac{432}{1}$ = _____

46. $\dfrac{22.5}{7} \times \dfrac{100}{5} \times \dfrac{1}{700} \times \dfrac{3}{80} \times \dfrac{3150}{1}$ = _____

47. $\dfrac{100}{250} \times \dfrac{50}{1} \times \dfrac{27.5}{1.375}$ = _____

48. $\dfrac{2.2}{0.25} \times \dfrac{3.6}{1} \times \dfrac{3.7}{7.1}$ = _____

49. $\dfrac{1.3}{0.21} \times \dfrac{0.3}{2} \times \dfrac{10.1}{0.75}$ = _____

50. $\dfrac{27.5}{10} \times \dfrac{40}{7} \times \dfrac{8.5}{1.9}$ = _____

3

ANSWERS

1. 1.5; 1.48	**11.** 1.7; 1.68	**21.** 5.6; 5.65	**31.** 12	**41.** 50
2. 1.5; 1.54	**12.** 1.7; 1.74	**22.** 4.2; 4.17	**32.** 9	**42.** 42
3. 1.2; 1.21	**13.** 1.2; 1.17	**23.** 5.7; 5.7	**33.** 19	**43.** 78
4. 0.6; 0.61	**14.** 2.6; 2.55	**24.** 6.7; 6.67	**34.** 36	**44.** 19
5. 6.7; 6.67	**15.** 2.4; 2.43	**25.** 5.1; 5.15	**35.** 23	**45.** 89
6. 1.8; 1.81	**16.** 1.8; 1.75	**26.** 57	**36.** 9	**46.** 11
7. 2.1; 2.13	**17.** 1.6; 1.63	**27.** 36	**37.** 29	**47.** 400
8. 1; 1.04	**18.** 3.8; 3.75	**28.** 70	**38.** 36	**48.** 17
9. 1.6; 1.55	**19.** 1.2; 1.24	**29.** 54	**39.** 130	**49.** 13
10. 2.7; 2.67	**20.** 5.8; 5.83	**30.** 55	**40.** 67	**50.** 70

SECTION TWO

Introduction to Drug Measures

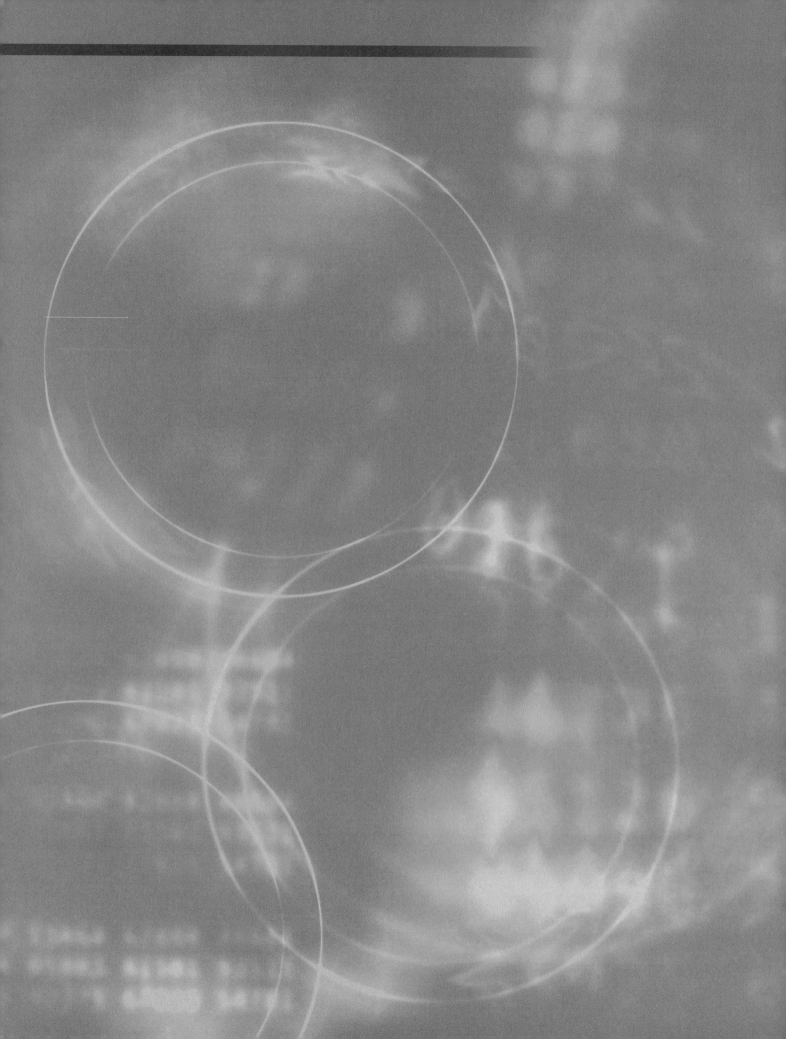

Metric, International (SI) System

The major system of weights and measures used in medicine is the metric system, which is also known as the international system or SI (from the French *Système International d'Unités*). The metric system was invented in France in 1875, and takes its name from the meter, a length roughly equivalent to a yard, from which all other units of measure in the system are derived. The strength of the metric system lies in its simplicity, because **all units of measure differ from each other in powers of ten (10). Conversions between units in the system are accomplished by simply moving a decimal point.**

Although it is not necessary for you to know the entire metric system to administer medications safely, you must understand its basic structure and become familiar with the units of measure you will be using.

Basic Units of the Metric/SI System

Three types of metric measures are in common use: those for **length**, **volume** (or capacity), and **weight**. The basic units or beginning points of these three measures are:

length — meter
volume — liter
weight — gram

You must memorize these basic units: do so now if you do not already know them. In addition to these basic units, there are both larger and smaller units of measure for length, volume, and weight. Let's compare this concept with something familiar. The pound is a unit of weight that we use every day. A smaller unit of measure is the ounce; a larger unit of measure is the ton. **However, all are units measuring weight.**

In the same way, there are smaller and larger units than the basic meter, liter, and gram. In the metric system, however, there is one very important advantage: **all other units, whether larger or smaller than the basic units, have the name of the basic unit incorporated in them.** So when you see a unit of metric measure there is no doubt what it is measuring: **meter—length, liter—volume, gram—weight.**

Indicate the appropriate category of weight, length, or volume for the metric measures.

1. milligram _____
2. centimeter _____
3. milliliter _____
4. millimeter _____
5. kilogram _____
6. microgram _____

4

ANSWERS 1. weight 2. length 3. volume 4. length 5. weight 6. weight

Metric/SI Prefixes

Prefixes are used in combination with the names of the basic units to identify larger and smaller units of measure. The same prefixes are used with all three measures. Therefore, there is a kilo**meter**, a kilo**gram**, and a kilo**liter**. Prefixes also change the value of each of the basic units by the same amount. For example, the prefix *kilo* identifies a unit of measure that is larger than (or multiplies) the basic unit by 1000. Therefore,

1 kilometer = 1000 meters
1 kilogram = 1000 grams
1 kiloliter = 1000 liters

Kilo is the only prefix you will be using that identifies a measure **larger** than the basic unit. Kilograms are frequently used as a measure for body weight, especially for infants and children.

You will see only three measures **smaller** than the basic unit in common medical use. The prefixes for these are:

centi—as in centimeter
milli—as in milligram
micro—as in microgram

Therefore, you will be working with only four prefixes: **kilo**, which identifies a larger unit of measure than the basic units; and **centi**, **milli**, and **micro**, which identify smaller units than the basic units.

Metric/SI Symbols

In medical use the basic units of metric measure are represented by symbols, which consist of their first letters. The symbol for meter and gram are a lowercase m and g. The symbol for liter is capitalized to distinguish it from the numeral 1. Therefore, liter's symbol is an uppercase L.

The first initial of their names provides the symbols for the basic units of metric measure. Lowercase letters are used for meter and gram. Liter is capitalized to distinguish it from the numeral 1.

gram is abbreviated **g**
liter is abbreviated **L**
meter is abbreviated **m**

Symbols for the prefixes used in combination with the basic units are printed using lowercase letters.

> kilo is **k** (as in kilogram—kg)
> centi is **c** (as in centimeter—cm)
> milli is **m** (as in milligram—mg)
> micro is **mc** (as in microgram—mcg)

 In combination with metric prefixes, liter remains capitalized.

> milliliter = mL
> kiloliter = kL

Two significant rule changes were recently made in the use of metric symbols. The symbol μ, for micro, was discontinued, because it resulted in a significant number of dosage errors. For example, μg was being misread as mg, resulting in dosages 1000 times larger than ordered. The second rule change was to discontinue the interchangeable use of cc and mL. A cc is actually the amount of physical space occupied by a 1 mL volume. Its use sometimes resulted in cc being misread as a number, rather than a symbol.

While it may take some time for cc and μ to disappear completely from labeling on medical supplies and drug labels, in no circumstances should these symbols continue to be used in transcribing dosages. You may also see the symbol ml used for mL, even on some labels in this text, because this symbol, with a lowercase l, is still used in Europe. However, in the United States and Canada use of the ml symbol is being phased out.

 The symbols μ, for micro, and cc and ml for mL, are officially obsolete, and must not be used in transcribing dosages.

PROBLEM

Print the abbreviations for the metric units.

1. microgram _____
2. liter _____
3. kilogram _____
4. milliliter _____
5. centimeter _____
6. milligram _____
7. meter _____
8. kiloliter _____
9. millimeter _____
10. gram _____

ANSWERS 1. mcg 2. L 3. kg 4. mL 5. cm 6. mg 7. m 8. kL 9. mm 10. g

Metric/SI Notation Rules

The easiest way to remember the rules of metric **notations**, in which **a unit of measure is expressed with a quantity**, is to memorize some prototypes (examples) that incorporate all the rules. Then, if you get confused, you can stop, think, and remember the correct way to write them. The notations for one-half, one, and one and one-half milliliters will incorporate all the rules you must know for the metric system.

Prototype notations: **0.5 mL   1 mL   1.5 mL**

RULE 1 **The quantity is written in Arabic numerals, 1, 2, 3, 4, etc.**
example: 0.5   1   1.5

RULE 2 **The numerals representing the quantity are placed in front of the symbols.**
example: 0.5 mL   1 mL   1.5 mL   (not mL 0.5, etc.)

RULE 3 **A full space is used between the quantity and the symbol.**
example: 0.5 mL   1 mL   1.5 mL   (not 0.5mL, etc.)

RULE 4 **Fractional parts of a unit are expressed as decimal fractions.**
example: 0.5 mL   1.5 mL   (not ½ mL, 1½ mL, etc.)

RULE 5 **To emphasize the decimal point, a zero is placed in front of the decimal when it is not preceded by a whole number.**
example: 0.5 mL   1 mL   1.5 mL   (not 0.50 mL)

So once again, as examples of the rules of metric notations, memorize the prototypes 0.5 mL—1 mL—1.5 mL. Just refer back to these examples if you get confused, and you will be able to write the notations correctly.

PROBLEM

Write the metric measures using official symbols and notation rules.

1. two grams   _____
2. five hundred milliliters   _____
3. five-tenths of a liter   _____
4. two-tenths of a milligram   _____
5. five-hundredths of a gram   _____
6. two and five-tenths kilograms   _____
7. one hundred micrograms   _____
8. two and three-tenths milliliters   _____
9. seven-tenths of a milliliter   _____
10. three-tenths of a milligram   _____
11. two and four-tenths liters   _____
12. seventeen and five-tenths kilograms   _____
13. nine-hundredths of a milligram   _____

14. ten and two-tenths micrograms   _____

15. four-hundredths of a gram   _____

Conversion between Metric/SI Units

When you administer medications, you will routinely be **converting units of measure within the metric system**, for example, g to mg, and mg to mcg. Learning the relative value of the units you will be working with is the first prerequisite to accurate conversions.

There are only four metric **weights** commonly used in medicine. From **highest** to **lowest** value these are:

kg	=	kilogram
g	=	gram
mg	=	milligram
mcg	=	microgram

Only two units of **volume** are frequently used. From **highest** to **lowest** value these are:

L	=	liter
mL	=	milliliter

 Each of the metric measures used in medication dosages differs from the next by 1000.

1 kg	=	1000 g
1 g	=	1000 mg
1 mg	=	1000 mcg
1 L	=	1000 mL

Once again, from highest to lowest value the units are, for weight: kg—g—mg—mcg; for volume: L—mL. Each unit differs in value from the next by 1000, and **all conversions used in dosages will be between the touching units of measure**, for example, g to mg, mg to mcg, L to mL.

Because the metric system is a decimal system, **conversions between the units are accomplished by moving the decimal point**. Also, because each unit of measure in common use differs from the next by 1000, if you know one conversion, you know them all.

How far do you move the decimal point? Here is an unforgettable memory cue that can be used with **all** metric dosage conversions. There are **three zeros in 1000**. The decimal point moves **three places**, the **same number of places as the zeros** in the conversion.

 In metric conversions between touching units of measure differing by 1000, the decimal point is moved three places, the same as the number of zeros in 1000.

This rule holds true for **all** decimal conversions in the metric system. If the difference in value is **10**, which has **one zero**, the decimal will move **one place**. If the difference is **100**, which has **two zeros**, it will move **two places**. When the difference is **1000** (as it is in dosage conversions), which has **three zeros**, the decimal point moves **three places**.

Which way do you move the decimal point? If you are converting **down** the scale to a **smaller** unit of measure, for example, g to mg or L to mL, the **quantity must get larger**, so the decimal point must move three places to the **right**.

EXAMPLE *1*   0.5 g = _____ mg

You are converting **down** the scale from **g to mg**, so the quantity must be **larger**. Move the decimal point **three places to the right**. To do this, you must **add two zeros** to the end of the quantity and **eliminate the zero in front** of it. The larger 500 mg quantity indicates that you have moved the decimal point in the correct direction.

Answer   **0.5 g = 500 mg**

EXAMPLE *2*   2.5 L = _____ mL

You are converting **down** the scale from **L to mL** so the quantity must be **larger**. Move the decimal point **three places to the right**. To do this, you must **add two zeros**. The larger 2500 mL quantity indicates that you have moved the decimal point in the correct direction.

Answer   **2.5 L = 2500 mL**

PROBLEM

Convert the metric measures.

1. 7 mg = _____ mcg		6. 1.5 mg = _____ mcg	
2. 1.7 L = _____ mL		7. 0.7 g = _____ mg	
3. 3.2 g = _____ mg		8. 0.3 L = _____ mL	
4. 0.03 kg = _____ g		9. 7 kg = _____ g	
5. 0.4 mg = _____ mcg		10. 0.01 mg = _____ mcg	

ANSWERS   1. 7000 mcg   2. 1700 mL   3. 3200 mg   4. 30 g   5. 400 mcg   6. 1500 mcg   7. 700 mg   8. 300 mL   9. 7000 g   10. 10 mcg

In metric conversions **up the scale**, from **smaller to larger units** of measurement, such as mL to L, the quantity will be **smaller**. The decimal point is moved **three places to the left**.

EXAMPLE *1*   200 mL = _____ L

You are converting **up** the scale from **mL to L** so the quantity will be **smaller**. Move the decimal point **three places to the left. Eliminate the two zeros at the end** of the 200 mL quantity, and **add a zero in front of** the decimal point to make it 0.2 L.

Answer   **200 mL = 0.2 L**

EXAMPLE *2*   500 mcg = _____ mg

You are converting **up** the scale from **mcg to mg** so the quantity will be **smaller**. Move the decimal point **three places to the left. Eliminate the two zeros at the end** of 500 and **add a zero in front of** the decimal point.

Answer   **500 mcg = 0.5 mg**

Convert the metric measures.

1. 3500 mL = _____ L

2. 520 mg = _____ g

3. 1800 mcg = _____ mg

4. 750 mL = _____ L

5. 150 mg = _____ g

6. 250 mcg = _____ mg

7. 1200 mg = _____ g

8. 600 mL = _____ L

9. 100 mg = _____ g

10. 950 mcg = _____ mg

ANSWERS 1. 3.5 L 2. 0.52 g 3. 1.8 mg 4. 0.75 L 5. 0.15 g 6. 0.25 mg 7. 1.2 g 8. 0.6 L 9. 0.1 g
10. 0.95 mg

4

Common Errors in Metric/SI Dosages

Most errors in metric dosages occur when a dosage or calculation contains a decimal. So, let's take a close look at how the basic safety rules you learned in Section 1, Refresher Math, can be used to reduce the possibility of error in metric dosages.

The first way to prevent errors is to make sure orders are interpreted and transcribed correctly. Handwritten orders can be confusing, so don't hesitate to question everything that looks suspicious. A common error is **failure to write a zero in front of the decimal point** in decimal fractions, for example, .2 mg instead of 0.2 mg. This makes the decimal easy to miss, an error that can be eliminated by strict adherence to the rule of placing a zero in front of all decimal fractions. Regardless of the presence of a zero in a written order, make sure one is added when it is transferred to a medication administration record or chart.

 Fractional dosages in the metric system must be transcribed with a zero in front of the decimal point to identify its fractional value.

The next most common error is **to include zeros where they should not be,** for example, .20 mg. An order written like this can easily be misread as 20 mg. Or, consider a dosage written 2.0 mg. The same potential for error exists. There is an unnecessary zero included in the order.

 Unnecessary zeros must be eliminated when metric dosages are transcribed.

The third error to watch for is in **calculations where decimal fractions are involved.** The presence of a decimal point in a calculation should raise a warning flag to slow down and double-check all math. Use your reasoning powers. If you misplace a decimal point, you are going to get an answer a minimum of ten times too much or too little. **Learn to question quantities that seem unreasonable.** A 1 mL dosage makes sense if you are calculating an IM injection. A 0.1 mL or 10 mL (or a 10 tab) dosage does not seem reasonable, and this is the type of error you might see. Be alert when assessing answers to determine if they seem reasonable.

 Question answers to calculations that seem unreasonably large or small.

The final error to be aware of is in **dosage conversions within the metric system**. Errors in conversions can be eliminated by thinking **three**. All conversions between the g, mg, and mcg measures used in dosages are accomplished by moving the decimal point **three** places—always and forever. There are not many instances when you can use the words *always* and *forever*, but converting between these units of measure in the metric system is one of those rare instances.

 Conversions between the units of measure g, mg, and mcg in metric dosages require moving the decimal point three places.

If you are constantly mindful of these problem areas, you can be an outstandingly safe clinical practitioner.

Summary

This concludes the refresher on the metric system. The important points to remember from this chapter are:

The meter, liter, and gram are the basic units of metric measure.

Larger and smaller units than the basic units are identified by the use of prefixes.

The largest unit you will see is the kilo; the symbol for kilo is k.

The smallest units you will see are milli–m, micro–mc, and centi–c.

Each prefix changes the value of the basic unit by the same amount.

Converting from one unit to another within the system is accomplished by moving the decimal point.

When you convert down the scale to smaller units of measurement, the quantity will get larger.

To convert down the scale from larger to smaller units, the decimal point is moved to the right.

When you convert up the scale to larger units of measurement, the quantity will get smaller.

To convert up the scale from smaller to larger units, the decimal point is moved to the left.

Conversions between g, mg, and mcg, and between mL and L, all require moving the decimal point three places.

Fractional dosages are transcribed with a zero in front of the decimal point.

Unnecessary zeros are eliminated from dosages and quantities.

The symbol μ for micro, and cc and ml to represent mL, are obsolete and being phased out.

Summary Self-Test

List the basic units of measure of the metric system and indicate what type of measure they are used for.

1. _____   _____

   _____   _____

   _____   _____

Which are official metric/SI symbols?

2. a) L   e) mg

   b) g   f) kg

   c) kL   g) ml

   d) Mgm   h) G

   _____

Express the measures using official metric symbols and notation rules.

3. six-hundredths of a milligram   _____

4. three hundred and ten milliliters   _____

5. three-tenths of a kilogram   _____

6. four-tenths of a milliliter   _____

7. one and five-tenths grams   _____

8. one-hundredths of a gram   _____

9. four thousand milliliters   _____

10. one and two-tenths milligrams   _____

List the four commonly used units of weight and the two units of volume, from highest to lowest value.

11. _____   _____   _____

    _____   _____   _____

Convert the metric measures.

12. 160 mg = _____ g	24. 2.1 L = _____ mL
13. 10 kg = _____ g	25. 475 mL = _____ L
14. 1500 mcg = _____ mg	26. 0.9 L = _____ mL
15. 750 mg = _____ g	27. 300 mg = _____ g
16. 200 mL = _____ L	28. 2.5 mg = _____ mcg
17. 0.3 g = _____ mg	29. 1 kL = _____ L
18. 0.05 g = _____ mg	30. 3 L = _____ mL
19. 0.15 g = _____ mg	31. 100 mL = _____ L
20. 1.2 L = _____ mL	32. 0.7 mg = _____ mcg
21. 150 mcg = _____ mg	33. 4 g = _____ mg
22. 2 mg = _____ mcg	34. 1000 mL = _____ L
23. 900 mcg = _____ mg	35. 2.5 L = _____ mL

36. 1000 mg = _____ g   **39.** 1.4 g = _____ mg

37. 0.2 mg = _____ mcg   **40.** 1.5 L = _____ mL

38. 2000 g = _____ kg

ANSWERS

1. gram-weight; liter-volume; meter-length	**8.** 0.01 g	**16.** 0.2 L	**25.** 0.475 L	**34.** 1 L
2. a, b, c, e, f	**9.** 4000 mL	**17.** 300 mg	**26.** 900 mL	**35.** 2500 mL
3. 0.06 mg	**10.** 1.2 mg	**18.** 50 mg	**27.** 0.3 g	**36.** 1 g
4. 310 mL	**11.** kg, g, mg, mcg, L, mL	**19.** 150 mg	**28.** 2500 mcg	**37.** 200 mcg
5. 0.3 kg	**12.** 0.16 g	**20.** 1200 mL	**29.** 1000 L	**38.** 2 kg
6. 0.4 mL	**13.** 10,000 g	**21.** 0.15 mg	**30.** 3000 mL	**39.** 1400 mg
7. 1.5 g	**14.** 1.5 mg	**22.** 2000 mcg	**31.** 0.1 L	**40.** 1500 mL
	15. 0.75 g	**23.** 0.9 mg	**32.** 700 mcg	
		24. 2100 mL	**33.** 4000 mg	

Additional Drug Measures: Unit, Percentage, Milliequivalent, Ratio, Apothecary, Household

Although metric measures predominate in medications, there are several other measures frequently used, particularly in parenteral (injectable) solutions, that are important for you to know. In addition you must be able to recognize several measures in the apothecary and household systems, because you may occasionally need to convert these to metric measures.

International Units

A number of drugs are measured in international units. Insulin, penicillin, and heparin are commonly seen examples. A unit **measures a drug in terms of its action**, not its physical weight. The quantities of dosages measured in units are unusual in that they range all the way from single digits, for example 5 units, to millions, for example 2,000,000 units. Dosage notations in units are written the same way as in the metric system, with the quantity in front of the unit measurement.

The word *unit* does not have a symbol, but is written in full in lowercase letters: units. This recent rule change eliminated the use of an uppercase U as a symbol for units because it resulted in errors when it was misread as a zero.

 The symbol U, for units, is obsolete, and its use must be discontinued.

PROBLEM

Express the dosages using correct notation rules.

1. two hundred and fifty thousand units _____

2. ten units _____

3. five thousand units _____

4. forty-four units _____

5. forty thousand units _____

6. one million units _____

7. one thousand units _____

8. twenty-five hundred units _____

OBJECTIVES

The learner will recognize dosages:
1. measured in units
2. measured as percentages
3. using ratio strengths
4. in milliequivalents
5. in apothecary measures
6. in household measures

9. thirty-four units　　　　　　　　_____

10. one hundred units　　　　　　　_____

Percentage (%) Measures

Percentage strengths are used extensively in intravenous solutions and somewhat less commonly for a variety of other medications, including eye and topical (for external use) ointments. **Percentage (%) means parts per hundred. The higher the percentage strength, the stronger the solution or ointment.** Percentage notations are made with no space between the quantity and symbol, for example, 10%.

 In solutions, percent represents the number of grams of drug per 100 mL of solution.

EXAMPLE 1　　100 mL of a 1% solution will contain 1 g of drug

EXAMPLE 2　　100 mL of a 2% solution will contain 2 g of drug

EXAMPLE 3　　50 mL of a 1% solution will contain 0.5 g of drug

EXAMPLE 4　　200 mL of a 2% solution will contain 4 g of drug

PROBLEM

Answer the true or false questions about percentage dosages.

	True	False
1. A 30% solution is stronger than a 25% solution.	_____	_____
2. A 2% ointment is not as strong as a 5% ointment.	_____	_____
3. A 1% solution is 10 parts drug.	_____	_____
4. 100 mL of a 3% solution will contain 30 grams of drug.	_____	_____
5. There is no space between a percentage strength and its symbol.	_____	_____

Milliequivalent (mEq) Measures

Milliequivalents (**mEq**) is **an expression of the number of grams of a drug contained in 1 mL of a normal solution.** This is a definition that may be quite understandable to a pharmacist or chemist, but you need not memorize it. Milliequivalent notations are also written the same way as metric measures, using Arabic numbers, with a space between the quantity and symbol, for example, 30 mEq. You will see milliequivalents used in a variety of oral and parenteral solutions; potassium chloride is a common example.

Express the milliequivalent dosages using correct symbol and notation rules.

1. sixty milliequivalents   _____

2. fifteen milliequivalents   _____

3. forty milliequivalents   _____

4. one milliequivalents   _____

5. fifty milliequivalents   _____

6. eighty milliequivalents   _____

7. fifty-five milliequivalents   _____

8. seventy milliequivalents   _____

9. thirty milliequivalents   _____

10. twenty milliequivalents   _____

ANSWERS   1. 60 mEq   2. 15 mEq   3. 40 mEq   4. 1 mEq   5. 50 mEq   6. 80 mEq   7. 55 mEq
8. 70 mEq   9. 30 mEq   10. 20 mEq

Ratio Measures

Ratio strengths are used primarily in solutions. They represent **parts of drug per parts of solution**, for example, 1 : 1000 (one part drug to 1000 parts solution).

EXAMPLE 1   A 1 : 100 strength solution has 1 part drug in 100 parts solution

EXAMPLE 2   A 1 : 5 solution contains 1 part drug in 5 parts solution

EXAMPLE 3   A solution that is 1 part drug in 2 parts solution would be written 1 : 2

The **less solution** a drug is dissolved in, the **stronger the solution**. For example, a ratio strength of 1 : 10 (1 part drug to 10 parts solution) is much stronger than a 1 : 100 (1 part drug in 100 parts solution).

Ratio strengths are always expressed in their **simplest terms**. For example, 2 : 10 would be incorrect, because it can be reduced to 1 : 5. Dosages expressed using ratio strengths are not common, but you do need to know what they represent.

PROBLEM

Express the solution strengths as ratios.

1. 1 part drug to 200 parts solution   _____

2. 1 part drug to 4 parts solution   _____

3. 1 part drug to 7 parts solution   _____

Identify the strongest solution.

4. **a)** 1 : 20   **b)** 1 : 200   **c)** 1 : 2   _____

5. **a)** 1 : 50   **b)** 1 : 20   **c)** 1 : 100   _____

6. **a)** 1 : 1000   **b)** 1 : 5000   **c)** 1 : 2000   _____

ANSWERS   1. 1 : 200   2. 1 : 4   3. 1 : 7   4. c   5. b   6. a

Apothecary and Household Measures

There is only one apothecary weight, the grain, and three apothecary volumes, the ounce, dram, and minim. There are just two household measures, the tablespoon and teaspoon. There are no longer any official symbols for these measures, although some disposable medication cups may still contain old symbols. Apothecary and household measures are officially obsolete, and in the event an order is written using one, it must immediately be converted to metric units of measure. This can be done using an apothecary/household/ metric equivalents conversion table, such as the one illustrated in Table 5-1. Notice that the line entries on this table are small and close together. If you have to use a table like this one, take any straight edge available, and position it to read safely from one column to the other.

A **drop**, whose symbol is **gtt**, is still occasionally used in some small volume pediatric dosages, and for eye or ear drops. All such medication preparations have an **integral dropper** attached to the solution bottle for accurate measurement.

 Apothecary and household measures are officially obsolete, and orders written using them must be converted and transcribed using metric equivalents.

Table 5-1

APOTHECARY / HOUSEHOLD / METRIC EQUIVALENTS							
Liquid				Weight			
ounce	mL	minim	mL	grain	mg	grain	mg
1 = 30		45 = 3		15 = 1000		1/4 = 15	
1/2 = 15		30 = 2		10 = 600		1/6 = 10	
		15 = 1		7 1/2 = 500		1/8 = 7.5	
dram	mL	12 = 0.75		5 = 300		1/10 = 6	
2 1/2 = 10		10 = 0.6		4 = 250		1/15 = 4	
2 = 8		8 = 0.5		3 = 200		1/20 = 3	
1 1/4 = 5		5 = 0.3		2 1/2 = 150		1/30 = 2	
1 = 4		4 = 0.25		2 = 120		1/40 = 1.5	
		3 = 0.2		1 1/2 = 100		1/60 = 1	
1 tablespoon = 15 mL		1 1/2 = 0.1		1 = 60		1/100 = 0.6	
1 teaspoon = 5 mL		3/4 = 0.05		1/2 = 30		1/150 = 0.4	
		1/2 = 0.03		1/3 = 20		1/200 = 0.3	
						1/250 = 0.25	

Summary

This concludes your introduction to the additional measures you will see used in dosages and in solutions. The important points to remember from this chapter are:

- *International units measure a drug by its action rather than its weight.*
- *There is no official symbol for the units measure.*
- *Percentage (%) strengths are frequently used in solutions and ointments.*
- *Percent represents grams of drug per 100 mL of solvent.*
- *The higher the percentage strength, the stronger the solution.*
- *The symbol for milliequivalent is mEq, and it is a frequently used measure in solutions.*

Ratio strengths represent parts of drug per parts of solution.

Apothecary and household measures are officially obsolete and must be immediately converted to metric symbols.

Summary Self-Test

Express the dosages using official notations and symbols.

1. three hundred thousand units   _____

2. forty-five units   _____

3. ten percent   _____

4. two and a half percent   _____

5. forty milliequivalents   _____

6. a one in two thousand ratio   _____

7. two units   _____

8. three milliequivalents   _____

9. one percent   _____

10. two thousand units   _____

11. five percent   _____

12. nine-tenths percent   _____

13. ten units   _____

14. a one in two ratio   _____

15. five percent   _____

16. twenty milliequivalents   _____

17. fourteen units   _____

18. twenty percent   _____

19. two million units   _____

20. one hundred thousand units   _____

5

ANSWERS

1. 300,000 units	6. 1 : 2000	11. 5%	16. 20 mEq
2. 45 units	7. 2 units	12. 0.9%	17. 14 units
3. 10%	8. 3 mEq	13. 10 units	18. 20%
4. 2.5%	9. 1%	14. 1 : 2	19. 2,000,000 units
5. 40 mEq	10. 2000 units	15. 5%	20. 100,000 units

SECTION THREE

Reading Medication Labels and Syringe Calibrations

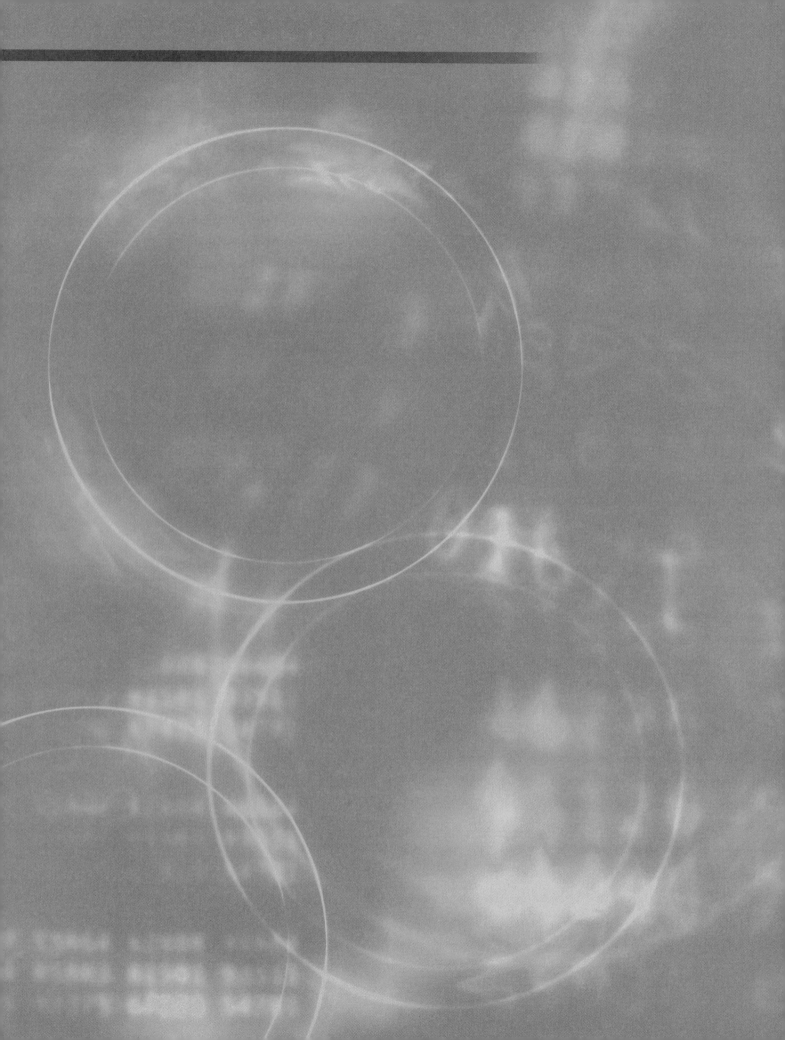

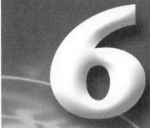

Reading Oral Medication Labels

Medication labels contain a variety of information that ranges from simple to complex. In this chapter, you will be introduced to labels of oral medications, which are generally the least complicated. With this instruction, you will be able to locate drugs and calculate simple dosages without confusion, as well as understand the more complicated labels presented in later chapters.

Let's begin with labels for solid drug preparations. These include tablets; scored tablets (which contain an indented marking to make breakage for partial dosages possible); enteric coated tablets (which delay absorption until the drug reaches the small intestine); capsules (powdered or oily drugs in a gelatin cover); and sustained or controlled release capsules (action spread over a prolonged period of time, for example, 12 hours). See illustrations in Figure 6-1.

OBJECTIVES

The learner will:
1. identify scored tablets, unscored tablets, and capsules
2. read drug labels to identify trade and generic names
3. locate dosage strengths and calculate simple dosages
4. measure oral solutions using a medicine cup

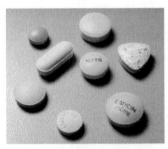

Tablets

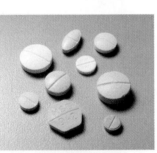

Scored Tablets

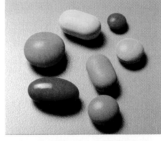

Enteric Coated Tablets

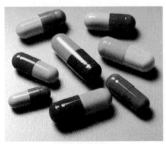

Capsules

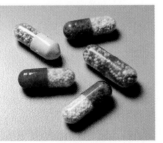

Controlled Release Capsules

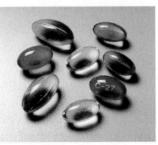

Gelatin Capsules

Figure 6-1

Tablet and Capsule Labels

The most common type of label you will see in the hospital setting is the **unit dosage label**, in which each tablet or capsule is packaged separately. However, the dosage on both unit and multiple dose labels is identical.

EXAMPLE 1

Look at the Lanoxin® label in Figure 6-2. The first thing to notice is that this drug has two names. The first, Lanoxin, is its **trade name**, which is identified by the ® registration symbol. Trade names are usually capitalized and printed first on the label. The name in smaller print, digoxin, is the **generic** or **official name** of the drug. Each drug has only one official name, but may have several trade names, each for the exclusive use of the company that manufactures it. It is important to remember, however, that most labels do contain **both** names, because drugs may be ordered by either name, depending on hospital policy or physician preference. You will frequently need to cross-check trade and generic names for accurate drug identification.

Next on the label is the **dosage strength**, 250 mcg or 0.25 mg. The dosage is often representative of the **average dosage strength, the dosage given to the average patient at one time**. This label also identifies the manufacturer of this drug, GlaxoSmithKline.

Notice that "1000 Tablets" is printed at the top of this label. This is the total number of tablets in the bottle. Be careful not to confuse the quantity of tablets or capsules in a container with the dosage strength. **The dosage strength always has a unit of measure associated with it**, in this case mcg and mg. Because label designs vary widely, this is an important point to remember.

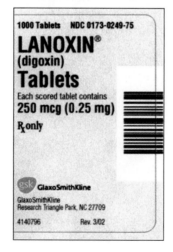

Figure 6-2

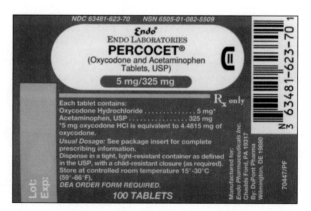

Figure 6-3

EXAMPLE 2

The Percocet® label in Figure 6-3 is for a medication that contains two different drugs, oxycodone amd acetaminophen, both of which are generic drug names. Medications that contain more than one drug would be ordered by trade name, in this case Percocet, and by the number of capsules or tablets to be given, rather than by dosage. The total number of Percocet tablets in this package, 100, is listed at the bottom of the label. The name of the drug manufacturer, Endo Laboratories, is near the top.

Tablets and capsules that contain more than one drug are ordered by trade name and by number of tablets or capsules to be given, rather than by dosage.

EXAMPLE 3

The small unit dosage (single dose) label in Figure 6-4 bears only one name, phenobarbital, which is actually the generic name of the drug. This labeling is common with drugs that have been in use for many years. The official (generic) name was so well established that drug manufacturers did not try to promote their own trade names. Also notice that immediately after the drug name are the initials **U.S.P.** This is the abbreviation for **U**nited **S**tates **P**harmacopeia, one of the two official national listings of drugs. The other is the **N**ational **F**ormulary, **N.F.** You will see U.S.P. and N.F. on drug labels and must not confuse them with other initials that identify additional drugs or specific action of drugs in a preparation.

Next, notice that this label gives the dosage strength of phenobarbital in metric, 15 mg, and an apothecary measure, ¼ grain. A few very old drugs, such as phenobarbital, may still occasionally include an apothecary measure. Because they are now officially obsolete, these dosages are scheduled to be phased out. Finally, on the right of the label, printed sideways, are the letters "Exp" This represents "expiration," the last date when the drug should be used. **Make a habit of checking the expiration date on labels.**

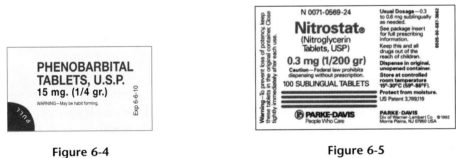

Figure 6-4   Figure 6-5

PROBLEM

Refer to the label in Figure 6-5 and answer the questions about this drug.

1. What is the generic name?   _____

2. What is the trade name?   _____

3. What is the dosage strength in metric units? _____

4. Locate the outdated apothecary dosage on this label _____

5. What does the USP on this label identify?   _____

ANSWERS 1. nitroglycerin   2. Nitrostat®   3. 0.3 mg   4. 1/200 gr   5. United States Pharmacopeia

Refer to the label in Figure 6-6 and answer the questions about this drug.

1. What is the generic name? _____

2. What is the trade name? _____

3. What is the dosage strength? _____

4. What company manufactured this drug? _____

5. How many tablets are in this container? _____

PRINIVIL® **5 mg**
(LISINOPRIL)

Dist. by:
MERCK & CO., INC.
Whitehouse Station, NJ 08889, USA

USUAL ADULT DOSAGE: See accompanying circular.
Store at controlled room temperature, 15-30°C (59-86°F),
and protect from moisture.
This is a bulk package and not intended for dispensing.

9352500

100 Tablets   N3   0006-0019-28   9

Figure 6-6

ANSWERS   1. lisinopril   2. Prinivil®   3. 5 mg   4. Merck & Co., Inc.   5. 100 tablets

Refer to the Sinemet® label in Figure 6-7. Sinemet is another example of a combined drug tablet. The generic names of the drugs it contains are carbidopa and levodopa. These are listed on the label in several places: directly under the trade name, then with the **amount** of each drug in the fine print on the right side of the label. Also notice the numbers 25-100. This again is the amount of carbidopa, 25 mg, and levodopa, 100 mg. Contrast this with the Sinemet labels in Figures 6-8 and 6-9.

SINEMET®   **25-100**   NDC 0056-0650-68
(CARBIDOPA-LEVODOPA)   **100 TABLETS**   7783/SJ

USUAL ADULT DOSAGE: See accompanying circular.

Dispense in a well-closed container.
This is a bulk package and not intended for dispensing.

Rx only
SINEMET is a registered trademark of MERCK & CO., INC.

Lot

Each tablet contains:
Carbidopa .... 25 mg*
*(Anhydrous equivalent)
Levodopa .... 100 mg

Manufactured by:
MERCK & CO., INC.
Whitehouse Station, NJ 08889, USA

Marketed by:
Bristol-Myers Squibb Company
Princeton, NJ 08543 USA

9544307   100|No. 3365

Figure 6-7

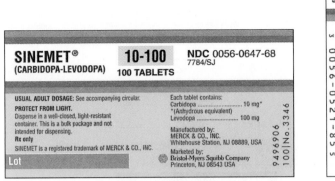

Figure 6-8

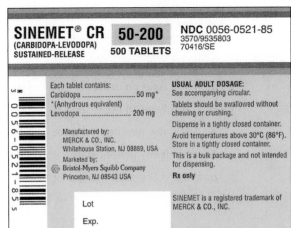

Figure 6-9

In Figure 6-8 the dosage strengths are different. To the right of the trade name are numbers that identify the strengths of carbidopa and levodopa as 10 mg and 100 mg, respectively, actually a lower dosage. And finally, Figure 6-9 is a label for Sinemet **CR**, a controlled **r**elease or sustained release tablet, with yet another dosage strength of 50-200, carbidopa 50 mg, levodopa 200 mg. Unlike the previous combined drug tablet discussed, an order for Sinemet **must** include the dosage because it is available in several strengths.

 Extra numbers after a drug name may be used to identify the dosage strengths of more than one drug in a preparation, and extra initials may be used to identify a special drug action.

Tablet/Capsule Dosage Calculation

When the time comes for you to administer medications, you will have to read a medication record or Kardex to prepare the dosage. This will tell you the name and amount of drug to be given, but **it will not tell you how many tablets or capsules contain this dosage.** You must calculate this yourself. However, this is not difficult. Most tablets and capsules are prepared in average dosage strengths, and most orders will involve giving one half to three tablets (or one to three capsules, since capsules cannot be broken in half). **Learn to question orders for more than three tablets or capsules.** Although some drugs require multiple tablets, most do not, and **an unusual number of tablets or capsules could be a warning of an error in prescribing, transcribing, or your calculations.**

 Regardless of the source of an error, if you give a wrong drug or dosage you are legally responsible for it.

Let's look at some sample orders and do some actual dosage calculations. **Assume that both tablets in our problems are scored and can be broken in half.**

PROBLEM

Refer to the Thorazine® label in Figure 6-10 and answer the questions.

1. What is the dosage strength? _____

2. If you have an order for 100 mg give _____

3. If you have an order for 150 mg give _____

4. If 300 mg are ordered give _____

5. What is the generic name of this drug? _____

6. What is the total number of tablets in this package? _____

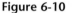

Store between 15° and 30°C (59° and 86°F).
Dispense in a tight, light-resistant container.
Each tablet contains chlorpromazine hydrochloride, 100 mg.
Dosage: This strength tablet is for use only in severe neuropsychiatric conditions. See accompanying prescribing information.
Important: Use safety closures when dispensing this product unless otherwise directed by physician or requested by purchaser.

GlaxoSmithKline
Research Triangle Park, NC 27709

100mg
NDC 0007-5077-20
THORAZINE®
CHLORPROMAZINE HCl TABLETS

100 Tablets   R̲only

gsk GlaxoSmithKline

Figure 6-10

ANSWERS **1.** 100 mg **2.** 1 tab **3.** 1½ tab **4.** 3 tab **5.** chlorpromazine HCl **6.** 100 tablets

PROBLEM

Refer to the Aricept® label in Figure 6-11 and answer the questions.

1. What is the dosage strength? _____

2. If 10 mg is ordered give _____

3. If 2.5 mg is ordered give _____

4. If 5 mg is ordered give _____

5. What is the generic name of this drug? _____

6. What is the total number of tablets in this package? _____

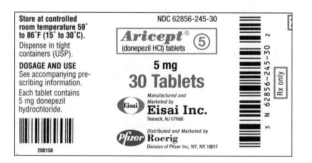

Store at controlled room temperature 59° to 86°F (15° to 30°C).
Dispense in tight containers (USP).

DOSAGE AND USE
See accompanying prescribing information.

Each tablet contains 5 mg donepezil hydrochloride.

NDC 62856-245-30

Aricept® ⑤
(donepezil HCl) tablets

5 mg
30 Tablets

Manufactured and Marketed by
Eisai **Eisai Inc.**
Teaneck, NJ 07666

Distributed and Marketed by
Pfizer **Roerig**
Division of Pfizer Inc, NY, NY 10017

N 3 62856-245-30 2   Rx only

200156

Figure 6-11

ANSWERS **1.** 5 mg **2.** 2 tab **3.** ½ tab **4.** 1 tab **5.** donepezil HCl **6.** 30 tablets

It is not uncommon to have a drug **ordered** in one unit of metric measure, for example, mg, and discover that it is **labeled** in another measure, for example, g. It will then be necessary to **convert the units to calculate the dosage**. This is not difficult because conversions will always be between touching units of measure: g and mg, or mg and mcg. Conversion is a matter of moving the decimal point three places.

EXAMPLE 1

Refer to the Halcion® label in Figure 6-12. A dosage of 250 mcg has been ordered. The label reads 0.25 mg. Convert the mg to mcg and you can mentally verify that these dosages are identical. Give 1 tablet.

EXAMPLE 2

Refer to the Carafate® label in Figure 6-13. Carafate 2000 mg is ordered. The label reads 1 gram, so you must give 2 tablets (1 tab = 1000 mg, so 2000 mg requires 2 tab).

Figure 6-12

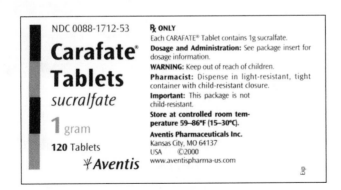

Figure 6-13

PROBLEM

Locate the appropriate labels for the dosages, and indicate how many tablets or capsules are needed to give them. Assume all tablets are scored.

1. verapamil HCl 0.12 g   _____ cap

2. Percocet 5 mg/325 1 tab   _____ tab

3. Dilatrate®-SR 0.04 g   _____ cap

4. terbutaline sulfate 5000 mcg   _____ tab

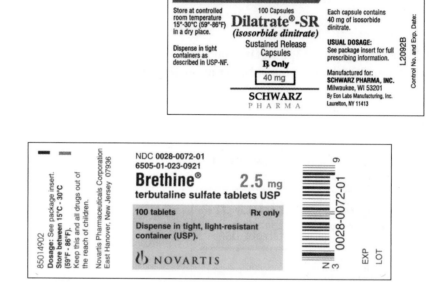

NDC 0091-0920-01

Store at controlled room temperature 15°-30°C (59°-86°F) in a dry place.

Dispense in tight containers as described in USP-NF.

100 Capsules

Dilatrate®-SR
(isosorbide dinitrate)
Sustained Release Capsules
℞ Only

40 mg

SCHWARZ
PHARMA

Each capsule contains 40 mg of isosorbide dinitrate.

USUAL DOSAGE: See package insert for full prescribing information.

Manufactured for:
SCHWARZ PHARMA, INC.
Milwaukee, WI 53201
By Eon Labs Manufacturing, Inc.
Laurelton, NY 11413

L2092B

Control No. and Exp. Date:

NDC 0028-0072-01
6505-01-023-0921

Brethine®   **2.5 mg**
terbutaline sulfate tablets USP

100 tablets   Rx only

Dispense in tight, light-resistant container (USP).

↻ NOVARTIS

Dosage: See package insert. Store between 15°C - 30°C (59°F - 86°F). Keep this and all drugs out of the reach of children.

Novartis Pharmaceuticals Corporation East Hanover, New Jersey 07936

85014902

0028-0072-01
N 3   9
EXP   LOT

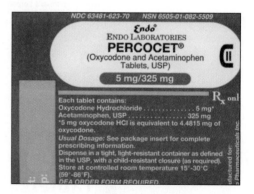

NDC 63481-623-70   NSN 6505-01-082-5509

Endo®
ENDO LABORATORIES
PERCOCET®
(Oxycodone and Acetaminophen Tablets, USP)

5 mg/325 mg

℞ onl

CII

Each tablet contains:
Oxycodone Hydrochloride . . . . 5 mg*
Acetaminophen, USP . . . . 325 mg
*5 mg oxycodone HCl is equivalent to 4.4815 mg of oxycodone.
Usual Dosage: See package insert for complete prescribing information.
Dispense in a tight, light-resistant container as defined in the USP, with a child-resistant closure (as required).
Store at controlled room temperature 15°-30°C (59°-86°F).
DEA ORDER FORM REQUIRED.

Pharmaceuticals Inc.

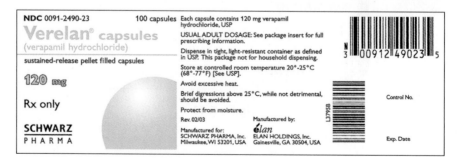

NDC 0091-2490-23   100 capsules

Verelan® capsules
(verapamil hydrochloride)

sustained-release pellet filled capsules

120 mg

Rx only

SCHWARZ
PHARMA

Each capsule contains 120 mg verapamil hydrochloride, USP

USUAL ADULT DOSAGE: See package insert for full prescribing information.

Dispense in tight, light-resistant container as defined in USP. This package not for household dispensing.

Store at controlled room temperature 20°-25°C (68°-77°F) [See USP].

Avoid excessive heat.

Brief digressions above 25°C, while not detrimental, should be avoided.

Protect from moisture.

Rev. 02/03

Manufactured for:
SCHWARZ PHARMA, Inc.
Milwaukee, WI 53201, USA

Manufactured by:
élan
ELAN HOLDINGS, Inc.
Gainesville, GA 30504, USA

N 3 00912 49023 5

L3795B

Control No.

Exp. Date

ANSWERS   **1.** 1 cap   **2.** 1 tab   **3.** 1 cap   **4.** 2 tab

Locate the appropriate labels for the drug orders and indicate the number of tablets or capsules that will be required to administer the dosages ordered. Assume that all tablets are scored. Notice that both generic and trade names are used for the orders, and a label may be used in more than one problem.

1. isosorbide dinitrate 80 mg _____ cap

2. sulfasalazine 0.5 g _____ tab

3. sulfasalazine 1 g _____ tab

4. hydrochlorothiazide 25 mg _____ tab

5. chlordiazepoxide HCl 50 mg _____ cap

6. Stelazine® 7.5 mg _____ tab

7. Minipress® 2 mg _____ cap

8. methyldopa 500 mg _____ tab

9. levothyroxine Na 0.3 mg _____ tab

10. DiaBeta® 3.75 mg _____ tab

6

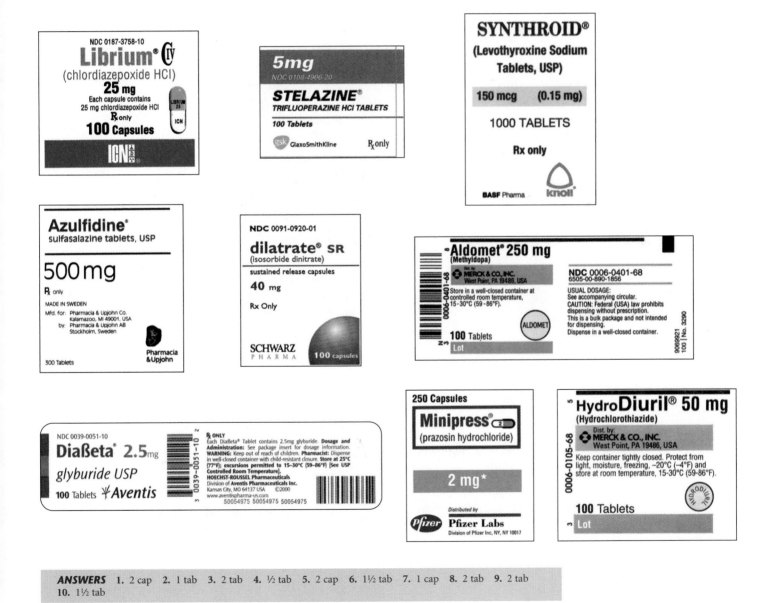

Oral Solution Labels

In liquid drug preparations the weight of the drug is contained in a certain **volume of solution**. Let's review dosages in some solid and liquid drug preparations to illustrate the difference.

EXAMPLE 1   **Solid:** 250 mg in **1 tablet**   **Liquid:** 250 mg in **5 mL**

EXAMPLE 2   **Solid:** 100 mg in **1 capsule**   **Liquid:** 100 mg in **10 mL**

EXAMPLE 3

Refer to the Lomotil® label in Figure 6-14. The information it contains will be familiar. Lomotil is the trade name, diphenoxylate is the generic or official name. The dosage strength is **2.5 mg per 5 mL**. As with solid drugs, the medication record will tell you the **dosage of the drug** to be administered, but rarely will it specify **the volume that contains this dosage**.

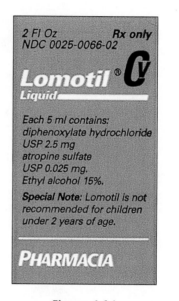

Figure 6-14

PROBLEM

Refer to the Lomotil label in Figure 6-14 again, and calculate the dosages.

1. The order is for diphenoxylate 2.5 mg.   Give _____

2. The order is for Lomotil 5 mg.   Give _____

ANSWERS   1. 5 mL   **2.** 10 mL   If you did not express your answers as mL, they are incorrect. **Numbers have no meaning unless they are expressed with a unit of measure,** in this case, mL.

PROBLEM

Refer to the Amoxil® label in Figure 6-15, and calculate the dosages.

1. The order is for amoxicillin susp. 250 mg. _____

2. Amoxil 125 mg has been ordered. _____

3. amoxicillin 375 mg has been ordered. _____

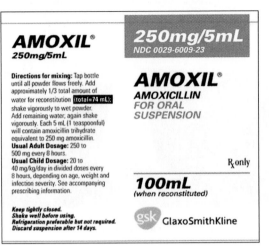

Figure 6-15

ANSWERS **1.** 5 mL **2.** 2.5 mL **3.** 7.5 mL **Note:** Your answers are incorrect unless they include mL as the unit of volume measure.

PROBLEM

Refer to the solution labels in Figures 6-16 and 6-17 and calculate the dosages.

1. Prozac® soln. 10 mg _____

2. cefaclor susp. 187 mg _____

3. Augmentin® susp. 125 mg _____

4. fluoxetine HCl soln. 30 mg _____

5. Prozac® soln. 40 mg _____

6. fluoxetine HCl soln. 20 mg _____

ANSWERS **1.** 2.5 mL **2.** 5 mL **3.** 10 mL **4.** 7.5 mL **5.** 10 mL **6.** 5 mL

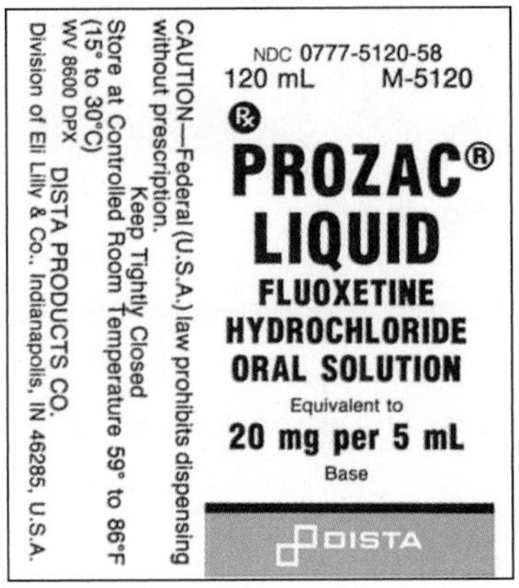

Figure 6-16

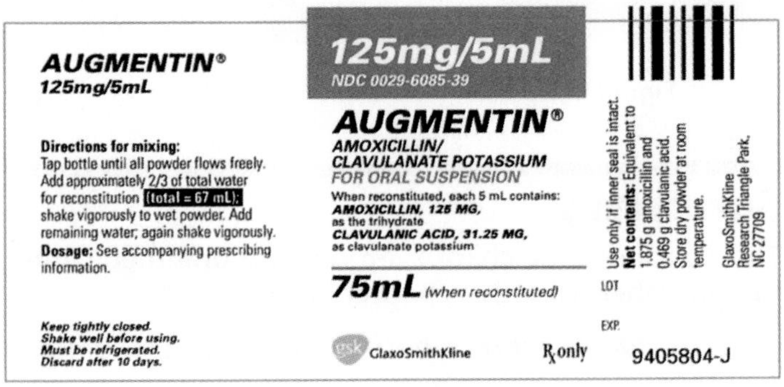

Figure 6-17

Measurement of Oral Solutions

Oral solutions can be measured using a **calibrated medicine cup** such as the one shown in Figure 6-18, which contains calibrations in mL, and sometimes in the older and now obsolete apothecary and household measures. To pour accurately, hold the cup at eye level, then line up the measure you need and pour until the medication is level with the desired dosage. Be extremely careful not to confuse the various calibrations on the cup if it still contains the older units of measure.

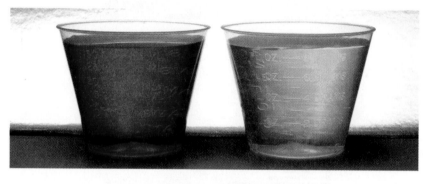

Figure 6-18

Solutions can also be measured using specially calibrated **oral syringes** such as those illustrated in Figures 6-19 and 6-20. Oral syringes have safety features built into their design to prevent their being mistaken for hypodermic syringes. One of these features is **color**, as illustrated in Figure 6-19 (hypodermic syringes are not colored, although their packaging and needle covers may be to aid in identification). A second feature is the syringe tip, which is a **different size** and **shape**, and is often **off center** (termed **eccentric**). Figure 6-20 illustrates an eccentric oral syringe tip. Notice that both oral syringes still contain household teaspoon (tsp) calibrations. Be careful not to confuse these with the metric mL calibrations. Hypodermic syringes (without a needle) can also be used to measure and administer oral dosages. The main concern with correct syringe identification is that oral syringes, which are **not sterile**, not be confused and used for hypodermic medications, which **are sterile**. This mistake has been made, in spite of the fact that hypodermic needles do not fit correctly on oral syringes. The precaution, therefore, does need to be stressed.

Oral solutions may also be ordered as drops, and when this is the case the dropper is integral to the bottle stopper. It is increasingly common for medicine droppers to be calibrated, for example in mL, or by actual dosage, 125 mg, etc. (see Figure 19-2 on page 274).

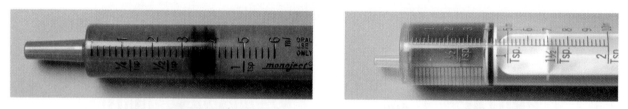

Figure 6-19

Figure 6-20

Summary

This concludes the chapter on reading oral medication labels. The important points to remember from this chapter are:

Most labels contain both generic and trade names.

Dosages are clearly printed on the label, except for preparations containing multiple drugs, which will list the name and dosage of each drug.

- Multiple dosage medications will be ordered by trade name and by the number of tablets or capsules to be given.

- The letters U.S.P. (United States Pharmacopeia) and N.F. (National Formulary) on drug labels identify their official generic listings.

- Additional letters following a drug name are used to identify additional drugs in the preparation or a special action of the drug.

- Most dosages of oral medications will involve giving ½ to 3 tablets or 1–3 capsules, which cannot be broken in half.

- Check drug expiration dates before use.

- When a medicine cup is used, pour and measure oral solutions at eye level.

- Liquid oral medications can be measured and administered using an oral medication syringe or hypodermic syringe (without the needle).

- Care must be taken not to use oral syringes for hypodermic medication preparation because these are not sterile.

Summary Self-Test

Locate the appropriate label for each drug order, and indicate the number of tablets or capsules and mL that will be required to administer them. Assume that all tablets are scored and can be broken in half.

PART I

1. Glucotrol® 15 mg _____

2. dexamethasone 4 mg _____

3. ciprofloxacin HCl 375 mg _____

4. Trental® 0.2 g _____

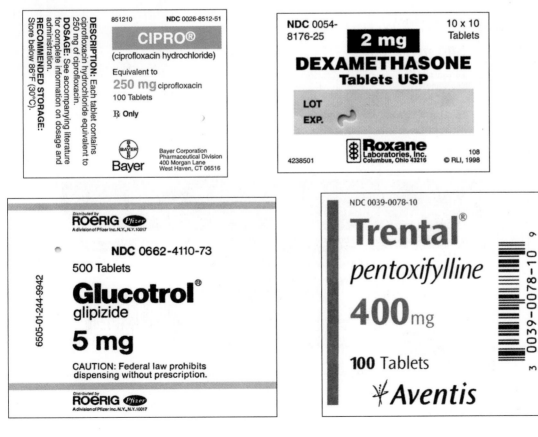

PART II

5. piroxicam 20 mg _____

6. amoxicillin susp. 250 mg _____

7. Lortab® 5/500 2 tab _____

8. Calan® SR 240 mg _____

9. alprazolam 750 mcg _____

10. gabapentin 0.2 g _____

11. Procanbid® 1 g _____

12. lithium 0.3 g _____

13. timolol maleate 30 mg _____

14. triazolam 500 mcg _____

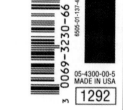

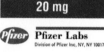

Store below 86°F (30°C)

Dispense in tight, light-resistant containers (USP).

DOSAGE AND USE
See accompanying prescribing information. One capsule per day.

Each capsule contains 20 mg piroxicam.

IMPORTANT: This closure is not child-resistant.

CAUTION: Federal law prohibits dispensing without prescription.

NDC 0069-3230-66
100 Capsules
Feldene®
(piroxicam) 20
20 mg
Pfizer **Pfizer Labs**
Division of Pfizer Inc, NY, NY 10017

6505-01-137-4628
0069-3230-66
05-4300-00-5
MADE IN USA
1292

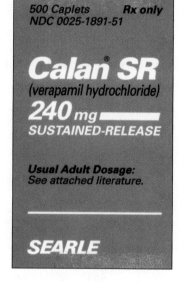

500 Caplets   **Rx only**
NDC 0025-1891-51

Calan® SR
(verapamil hydrochloride)
240 mg
SUSTAINED-RELEASE

Usual Adult Dosage:
See attached literature.

SEARLE

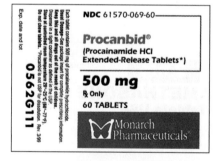

Exp. date and lot

Each tablet contains 500 mg of procainamide hydrochloride. Usual Dosage—See package insert for complete prescribing information. Keep this and all drugs out of the reach of children. Dispense in a tight container as defined in the USP. Store at controlled room temperature 20-25°C (68-77°F). Do not store tablets. "Procanbid is not USP for dissolution. Rev. 3/99

0562G111

NDC 61570-069-60
Procanbid®
(Procainamide HCl
Extended-Release Tablets*)
500 mg
℞ Only
60 TABLETS
Monarch Pharmaceuticals

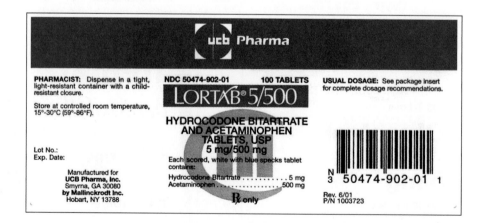

ucb Pharma

PHARMACIST: Dispense in a tight, light-resistant container with a child-resistant closure.

Store at controlled room temperature, 15°-30°C (59°-86°F).

Lot No.:
Exp. Date:

Manufactured for
UCB Pharma, Inc.
Smyrna, GA 30080
by Mallinckrodt Inc.
Hobart, NY 13788

NDC 50474-902-01   **100 TABLETS**
LORTAB® 5/500
**HYDROCODONE BITARTRATE
AND ACETAMINOPHEN
TABLETS, USP**
5 mg/500 mg
Each scored, white with blue specks tablet contains:
Hydrocodone Bitartrate . . . . 5 mg
Acetaminophen . . . . .500 mg
℞ only

USUAL DOSAGE: See package insert for complete dosage recommendations.

N
3 50474-902-01 1

Rev. 6/01
P/N 1003723

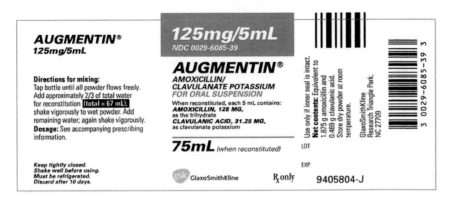

AUGMENTIN®
125mg/5mL

125mg/5mL
NDC 0029-6085-39

AUGMENTIN®
AMOXICILLIN/
CLAVULANATE POTASSIUM
FOR ORAL SUSPENSION

When reconstituted, each 5 mL contains:
AMOXICILLIN, 125 MG,
as the trihydrate
CLAVULANIC ACID, 31.25 MG,
as clavulanate potassium

75mL (when reconstituted)

Directions for mixing:
Tap bottle until all powder flows freely.
Add approximately 2/3 of total water
for reconstitution (total = 67 mL);
shake vigorously to wet powder. Add
remaining water; again shake vigorously.
Dosage: See accompanying prescribing
information.

Keep tightly closed.
Shake well before using.
Must be refrigerated.
Discard after 10 days.

Use only if inner seal is intact.
Net contents: Equivalent to
1.875 g amoxicillin and
0.469 g clavulanic acid.
Store dry powder at room
temperature.

GlaxoSmithKline
Research Triangle Park,
NC 27709

LOT

EXP.

gsk GlaxoSmithKline   R only   9405804-J

3 0029-6085-39 3

6

Blocadren® 20 mg
(Timolol Maleate)

Dist. by
MERCK & CO., INC.
Whitehouse Station, NJ 08889, USA

Store at controlled room temperature,
15-30°C (59-86°F). Keep container tightly
closed. Protect from light. Dispense in a
well-closed, light-resistant container.

100 Tablets   (BLOCADREN)

Lot

R only   NDC 0009-0017-59

**Pharmacist: Dispense in
this container with
patient leaflet attached.**

See package insert for
complete product
information.

Keep container tightly
closed.

Store at controlled room
temperature 20° to 25°C
(68° to 77°F) [see USP].

U.S. Patent No. 3,987,052

Pharmacia & Upjohn
Company
A subsidiary of
Pharmacia Corporation
Kalamazoo, MI 49001, USA

Halcion® C IV

triazolam
tablets, USP

0.25 mg

10 Tablets

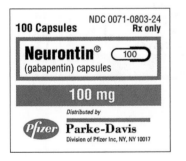

100 Capsules   NDC 0071-0803-24
Rx only

Neurontin® (100)

(gabapentin) capsules

100 mg

Distributed by

Pfizer **Parke-Davis**
Division of Pfizer Inc, NY, NY 10017

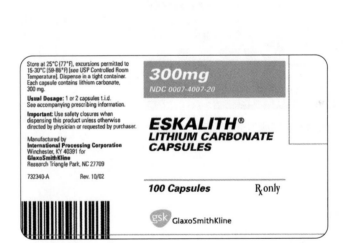

Store at 25°C (77°F), excursions permitted to
15-30°C (59-86°F) [see USP Controlled Room
Temperature]. Dispense in a tight container.
Each capsule contains lithium carbonate,
300 mg.

Usual Dosage: 1 or 2 capsules t.i.d.
See accompanying prescribing information.

Important: Use safety closures when
dispensing this product unless otherwise
directed by physician or requested by purchaser.

Manufactured by
International Processing Corporation
Winchester, KY 40391 for
GlaxoSmithKline
Research Triangle Park, NC 27709

732340-A   Rev. 10/02

300mg
NDC 0007-4007-20

ESKALITH®
LITHIUM CARBONATE
CAPSULES

100 Capsules   R only

gsk GlaxoSmithKline

R only   NDC 0009-0029-01
6505-01-143-9269

See package insert for
complete product
information.

Keep container tightly
closed.

Dispense in tight, light-
resistant container.

Store at controlled room
temperature 20° to 25° C
(68° to 77° F) [see USP].

Pharmacia & Upjohn
Company
A subsidiary of
Pharmacia Corporation
Kalamazoo, MI 49001, USA

Xanax® C IV

alprazolam tablets,
USP

0.25 mg

100 Tablets

PART III

15. acetaminophen 650 mg   _____

16. Aldactone® 75 mg   _____

17. meclizine HCl 50 mg   _____

18. Sinemet® 10-100 1 tab   _____

19. ciprofloxacin HCl 0.375 g   _____

20. metoprolol tartrate 0.15 g   _____

21. nifedipine 10 mg   _____

22. furosemide 10 mg   _____

23. Lasix® 30 mg   _____

24. dexamethasone 3 mg   _____

25. Librium® 75 mg   _____

26. terbutaline sulfate 5 mg   _____

27. Toprol-XL® 0.1 g   _____

28. Synthroid® 225 mcg   _____

29. DiaBeta® 5000 mcg   _____

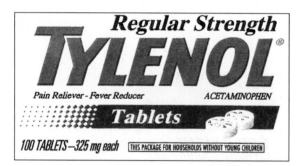

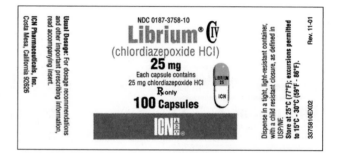

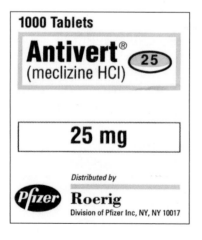

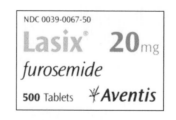

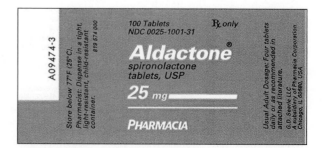

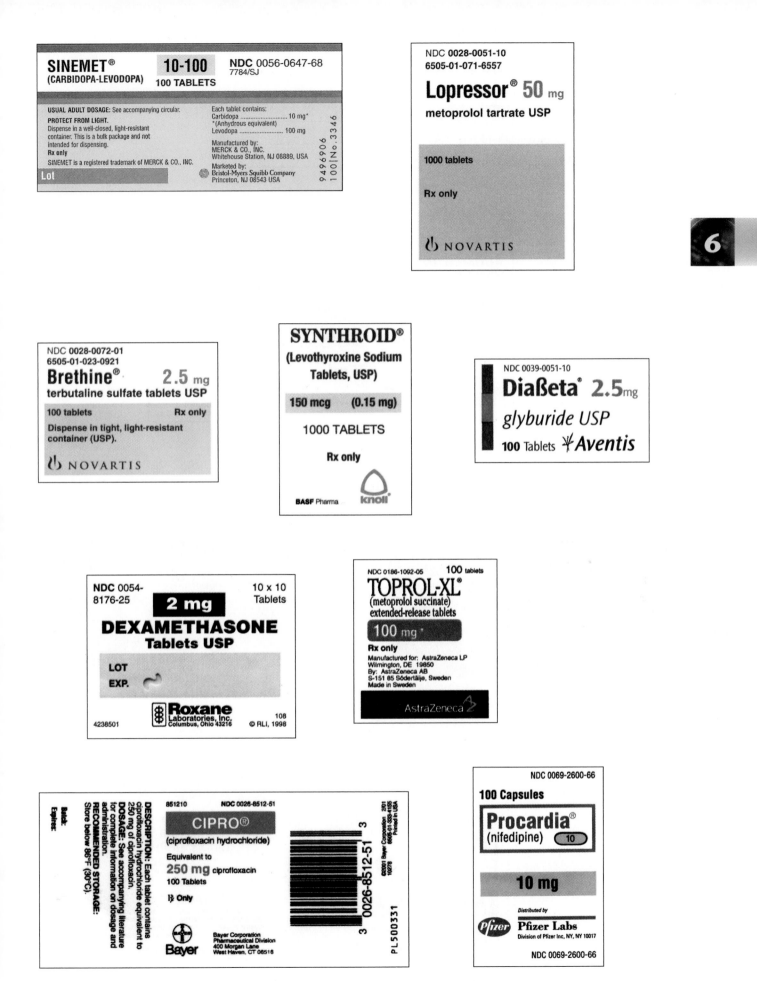

SINEMET® 10-100 | NDC 0056-0647-68
(CARBIDOPA-LEVODOPA) | 7784/SJ
100 TABLETS

USUAL ADULT DOSAGE: See accompanying circular.
PROTECT FROM LIGHT.
Dispense in a well-closed, light-resistant container. This is a bulk package and not intended for dispensing.
Rx only
SINEMET is a registered trademark of MERCK & CO., INC.

Lot

Each tablet contains:
Carbidopa .... 10 mg*
*(Anhydrous equivalent)
Levodopa .... 100 mg
Manufactured by:
MERCK & CO., INC.
Whitehouse Station, NJ 08889, USA
Marketed by:
Bristol-Myers Squibb Company
Princeton, NJ 08543 USA

949690 6
100|No.3346

NDC 0028-0051-10
6505-01-071-6557

Lopressor® 50 mg
metoprolol tartrate USP

1000 tablets

Rx only

Ͼ NOVARTIS

6

NDC 0028-0072-01
6505-01-023-0921
Brethine® 2.5 mg
terbutaline sulfate tablets USP

100 tablets | Rx only

Dispense in tight, light-resistant container (USP).

Ͼ NOVARTIS

SYNTHROID®
(Levothyroxine Sodium Tablets, USP)

150 mcg (0.15 mg)

1000 TABLETS

Rx only

BASF Pharma | knoll

NDC 0039-0051-10
Diaßeta® 2.5 mg
glyburide USP
100 Tablets ⚕ Aventis

NDC 0054-8176-25 | 10 x 10 Tablets
2 mg
DEXAMETHASONE
Tablets USP

LOT
EXP.

⚕ **Roxane**
Laboratories, Inc.
Columbus, Ohio 43216
© RLI, 1998

4238501 | 108

NDC 0186-1092-05 | 100 tablets
TOPROL-XL®
(metoprolol succinate)
extended-release tablets
100 mg*

Rx only
Manufactured for: AstraZeneca LP
Wilmington, DE 19850
By: AstraZeneca AB
S-151 85 Södertälje, Sweden
Made in Sweden

AstraZeneca

Batch:
Expires:

DESCRIPTION: Each tablet contains ciprofloxacin hydrochloride equivalent to 250 mg of ciprofloxacin.
DOSAGE: See accompanying literature for complete information on dosage and administration.
RECOMMENDED STORAGE:
Store below 86°F (30°C).

851210 | NDC 0026-8512-51

CIPRO®
(ciprofloxacin hydrochloride)

Equivalent to
250 mg ciprofloxacin
100 Tablets

℞ Only

Ⓑ **Bayer**

Bayer Corporation
Pharmaceutical Division
400 Morgan Lane
West Haven, CT 06516

©2001 Bayer Corporation 2801
10278 6505-01-353-4155
Printed in USA

3 0026-8512-51 3

PL500331

NDC 0069-2600-66
100 Capsules

Procardia®
(nifedipine) 10

10 mg

Distributed by
𝑃𝑓𝑖𝑧𝑒𝑟 **Pfizer Labs**
Division of Pfizer Inc, NY, NY 10017

NDC 0069-2600-66

PART IV

30. amoxicillin susp. 0.25 g   _____

31. Percocet® 2 tab   _____

32. metronidazole 0.75 g   _____

33. piroxicam 40 mg   _____

34. Lopid® 300 mg   _____

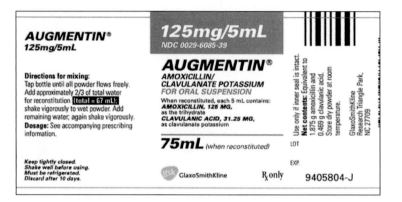

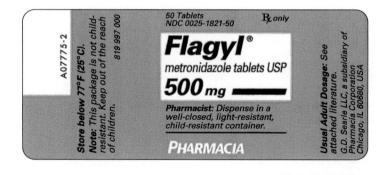

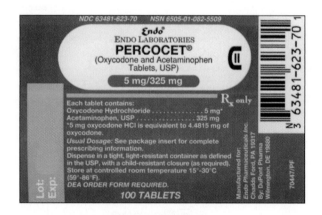

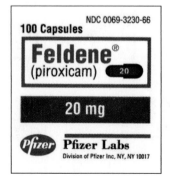

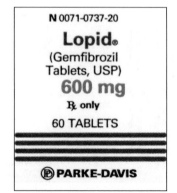

PART V

35. fluoxetine HCl 10 mg   _____

36. spironolactone 0.1 g   _____

37. cefpodoxime proxetil 0.2 g   _____

38. cimetidine 450 mg   _____

39. potassium chloride 40 mEq   _____

40. penicillin V potassium 600,000 units   _____

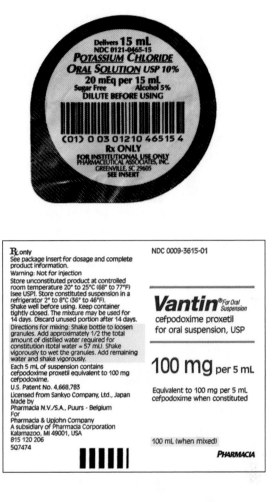

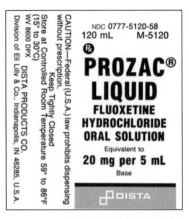

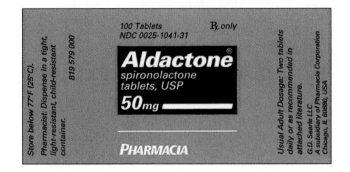

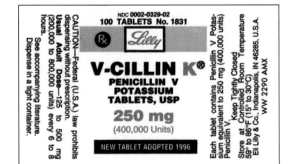

ANSWERS

1. 3 tab	**9.** 3 tab	**17.** 2 tab	**25.** 3 cap	**33.** 2 cap
2. 2½ tab	**10.** 2 cap	**18.** 1 tab	**26.** 2 tab	**34.** ½ tab
3. 1½ tab	**11.** 2 tab	**19.** 1½ tab	**27.** 1 tab	**35.** 10 mL
4. ½ tab	**12.** 1 cap	**20.** 3 tab	**28.** 1½ tab	**36.** 2 tab
5. 1 cap	**13.** 1½ tab	**21.** 1 cap	**29.** 2 tab	**37.** 10 mL
6. 10 mL	**14.** 2 tab	**22.** ½ tab	**30.** 10 mL	**38.** 1½ tab
7. 2 tab	**15.** 2 tab	**23.** 1½ tab	**31.** 2 tab	**39.** 30 mL
8. 1 cap	**16.** 3 tab	**24.** 1½ tab	**32.** 1½ tab	**40.** 1½ tab

7

Hypodermic Syringe Measurement

OBJECTIVES

The learner will measure parenteral solutions using:
1. a standard 3 mL syringe
2. a tuberculin syringe
3. 5, 6, 10, and 12 mL syringes
4. a 20 mL syringe

A variety of hypodermic syringes are in common clinical use. This chapter focuses on the frequently used 3 mL syringe. However, larger volume syringes are used on occasion, so it is necessary that you learn the **differences**, as well as the **similarities**, of all syringes in use.

Regardless of a syringe's volume or capacity—0.5, 1, 3, 5, 6, 10, 20, or 50 mL—all except specialized insulin syringes **are calibrated in mL**. However, these various capacity syringes contain **calibrations that differ from each other**. Recognizing the difference in syringe calibrations is the chief safety concern of this chapter.

The calibrations on different volume syringes differ from each other, requiring particular care in dosage measurement.

Standard 3 mL Syringe

The most commonly used hypodermic syringe is the 3 mL size illustrated in Figure 7-1. Notice that this syringe contains only one set of calibrations, for the metric mL scale. However, a limited number of 3 mL syringes still contain a second set of smaller calibrations, for the now obsolete apothecary minim (m) scale. If a syringe contains two calibrated scales be particularly careful not to mistake the minum calibrations for metric mL calibrations.

If a syringe contains a minim (m) calibration scale, care must be taken not to mistake it for the metric mL scale.

Notice that **longer calibrations** identify zero (0) and each ½ and full mL measure on the 3 mL syringe's calibrated scale. These longer calibrations are numbered: ½, 1, 1½, 2, 2½, and 3.

Next notice the **number of calibrations in each mL**, which is **10**, indicating that on this syringe each mL is **calibrated in tenths**. Tenths of a mL are written as **decimal fractions**, for example 1.2 mL, 2.5 mL, or 0.4 mL. Notice the arrow on this syringe, which identifies a 0.8 mL dosage.

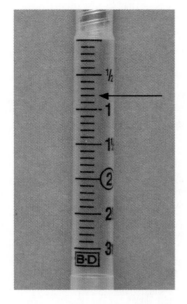

A 3 mL syringe.
Product courtesy of BD © 2006, Becton Dickinson, and Company.

Figure 7-1

PROBLEM

Use decimal numbers, for example, 2.2 mL, to identify the measurements indicated by the arrows on the standard 3 mL syringes.

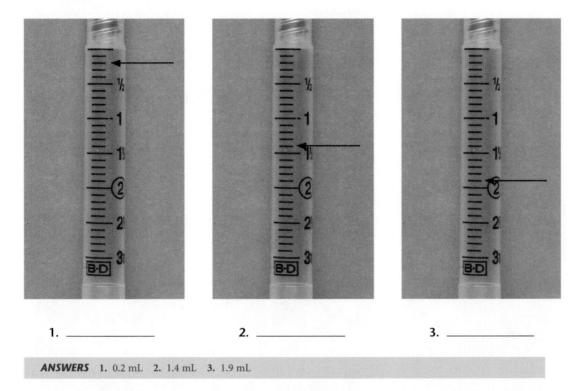

1. _____   2. _____   3. _____

ANSWERS   1. 0.2 mL   2. 1.4 mL   3. 1.9 mL

Did you have difficulty with the 0.2 mL calibration in problem 1? Remember that **the first long calibration on all syringes is zero**. It is slightly longer than the 0.1 mL and subsequent one-tenth calibrations. Be careful not to mistakenly count it as 0.1 mL.

You have just been looking at photos of syringe barrels only. In assembled syringes the colored suction tip of the plunger has two widened areas in contact with the barrel that look like two distinct rings. **Calibrations are read from the front, or top, ring**. Do not become confused by the second (bottom) ring, or by the raised middle section of the suction tip.

PROBLEM

What dosages are measured by the assembled syringes?

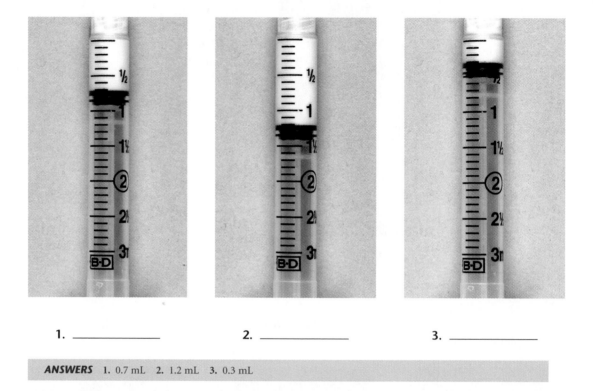

1. _____   2. _____   3. _____

ANSWERS   **1.** 0.7 mL   **2.** 1.2 mL   **3.** 0.3 mL

PROBLEM

Draw an arrow or shade in the syringe barrels to indicate the required dosages. Have your instructor check your accuracy.

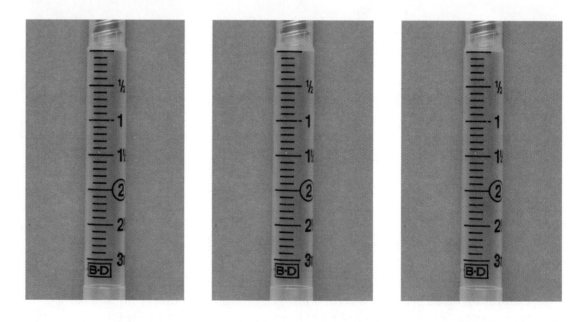

1. 1.3 mL   **2.** 2.4 mL   **3.** 0.9 mL

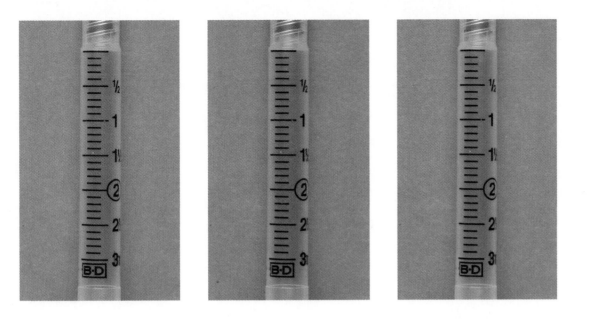

4. 2.5 mL   **5.** 1.7 mL   **6.** 2.1 mL

PROBLEM

Identify the dosages measured on the 3 mL syringes.

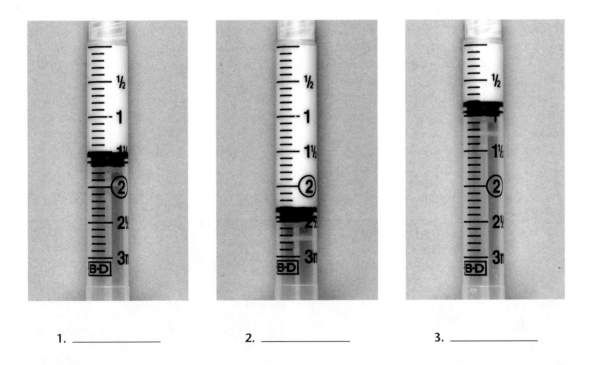

1. _____   2. _____   3. _____

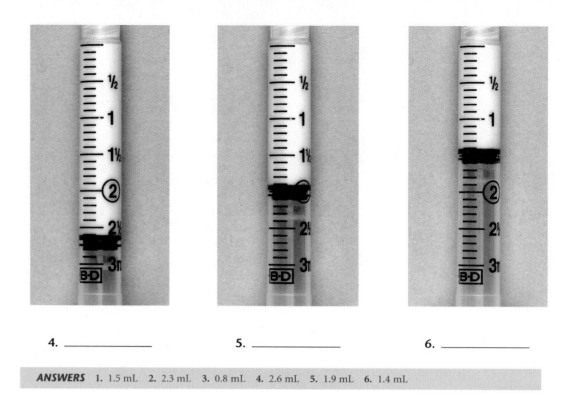

4. _____   5. _____   6. _____

Safety Syringes

A number of safety syringes have been developed in recent years to reduce the danger of accidental needle stick injuries. Several of these syringes are illustrated in the following photos. Take a few minutes to become familiar with them, because you will probably be using them in the clinical setting.

Refer first to the photos in Figure 7-2, which show two B-D SafetyGlide™ syringes. Each of these syringes contains a protective needle guard that can be activated by a single finger to cover and seal the needle after injection. The syringe shown in Figure 7-3, the VanishPoint™, has a needle that automatically retracts into the barrel after injection.

SafetyGlide™ syringes. *Product courtesy of BD © 2006, Becton, Dickinson and Company.*

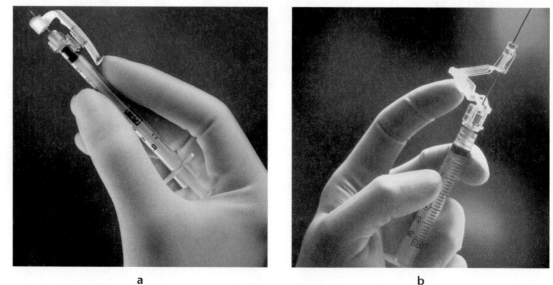

a   b

Figure 7-2 a and b

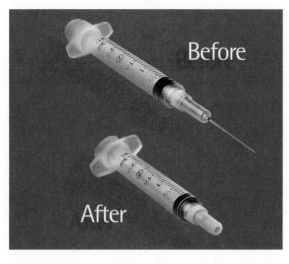

Retractable Technologies VanishPoint™ needle automatically retracts into the syringe barrel after injection.
Courtesy of Retractable Technologies.

Figure 7-3

A third type of safety syringe in common use is the Monoject® Safety Syringe (Figure 7-4). This syringe contains a protective sheath that can be used to protect the needle's sterility during transport. The protective sheath can be pulled forward and locked into place to provide a permanent needle shield for disposal following injection.

Notice that the Monoject Safety Syringe in Figure 7-4 contains two calibrated scales. The larger is the 3 mL metric scale with which you are already familiar. The smaller scale in the foreground, labeled "30 m," is the apothecary minim scale, which is scheduled to be phased out.

Kendall "Monoject® Safety Syringe." *Copyright 2005 Tyco Healthcare Group LP. All rights reserved. Reprinted with permission. Monoject is a trademark of Tyco Healthcare LP or its affiliate.*

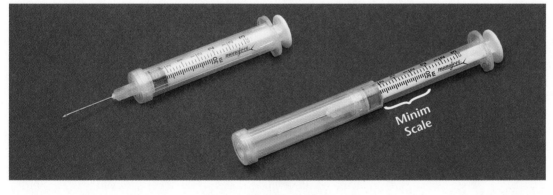

Figure 7-4

 The minim scale has been a common source of injection dosage errors. If your clinical facility still uses syringes that contain the minim scale, be extremely careful not to confuse it with the metric calibrations.

Tuberculin (TB) Syringe

When very small dosages are required they are measured in special tuberculin (TB) **0.5 or 1 mL syringes calibrated in hundredths**. Originally designed for the small dosages required for tuberculin skin testing, these syringes are also widely used in a variety of sensitivity and allergy tests. Pediatric dosages frequently require measurement in hundredths, as does heparin, an anticoagulant drug.

Refer to the 0.5 mL TB syringe in Figure 7-5, and take a careful look at its metric calibrated tenth and hundredth scale. Notice that slightly longer calibrations identify zero, 0.05, 0.1, 0.15, 0.2, and so on through the 0.5 mL measure. Shorter hundredth calibrations lie between these measures. Each tenth mL, .1, .2, .3, .4, and .5 is numbered on this particular TB syringe. Take a moment to study the dosage measured by the arrow in Figure 7-5, which is 0.43 mL.

The closeness and small size of TB syringe calibrations mandate particular care and an unhurried approach in TB syringe dosage measurement.

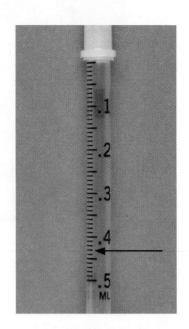

Figure 7-5

PROBLEM

Identify the measurements on the six tuberculin syringes.

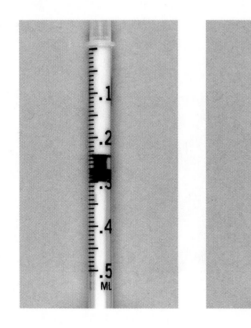

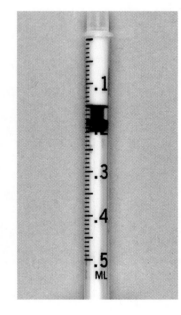

1. _____   2. _____   3. _____

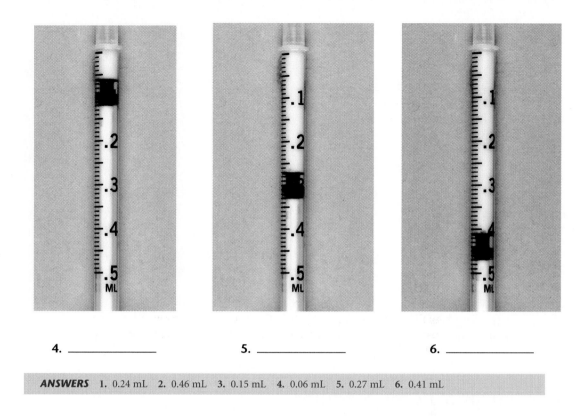

4. _____   5. _____   6. _____

PROBLEM

Draw an arrow or shade in the barrel to identify the dosages indicated on the TB syringes. Have your instructor check your answers.

1. 0.28 mL   **2.** 0.32 mL   **3.** 0.45 mL

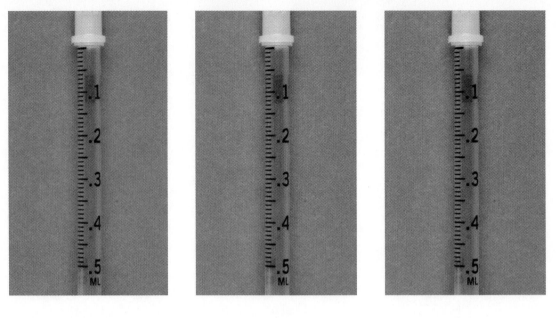

4. 0.12 mL   **5.** 0.27 mL   **6.** 0.30 mL

5, 6, 10, and 12 mL Syringes

When volumes larger than 3 mL are required, a 5, 6, 10, or 12 mL syringe may be used. Notice on the larger syringes in Figure 7-6 that mL are still designated by the abbreviation cc, which is being phased out. Examine the calibrations between the numbered mLs to determine how these syringes are calibrated.

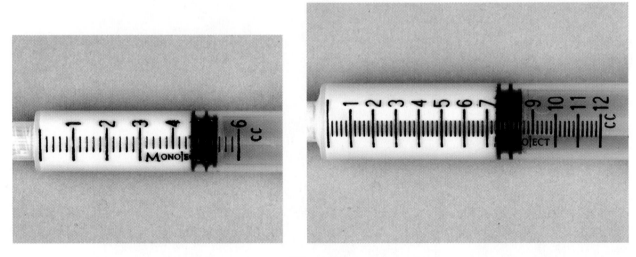

Figure 7-6

As you will discover, the calibrations divide each mL of these syringes into **five,** so that **each shorter calibration actually measures two-tenths, 0.2 mL**. The 6 mL syringe on the left measures 4.6 mL, and the 12 mL syringe on the right measures 7.4 mL. These syringes are most often used to measure whole rather than fractional mL, but in your practice readings we will include a full range of measurements.

PROBLEM

What mL dosages are measured on the syringes?

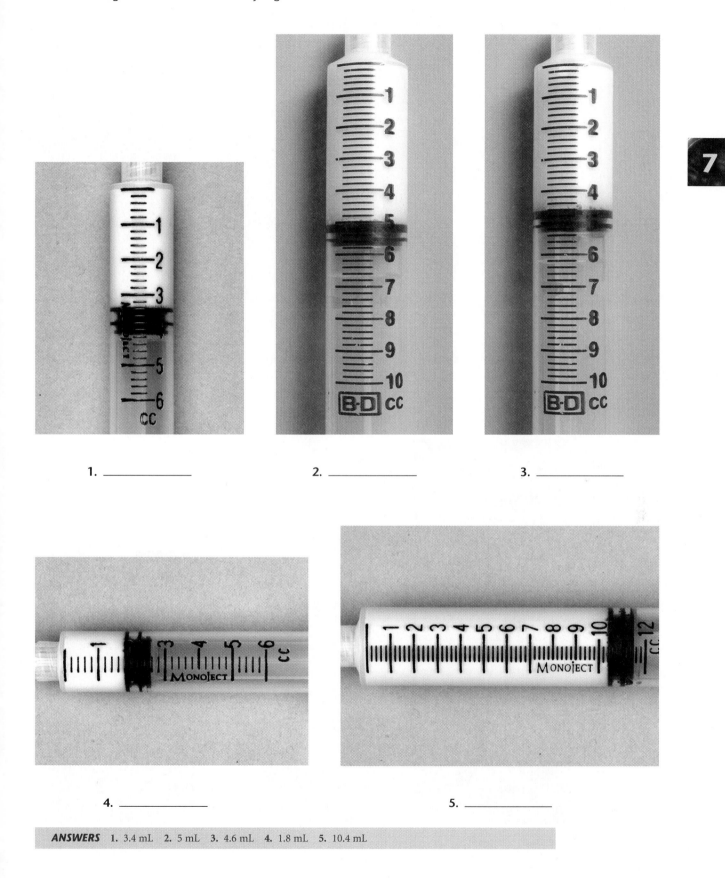

1. _____

2. _____

3. _____

4. _____

5. _____

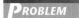

Measure the mL dosages indicated on the six syringes. Have an instructor check your accuracy.

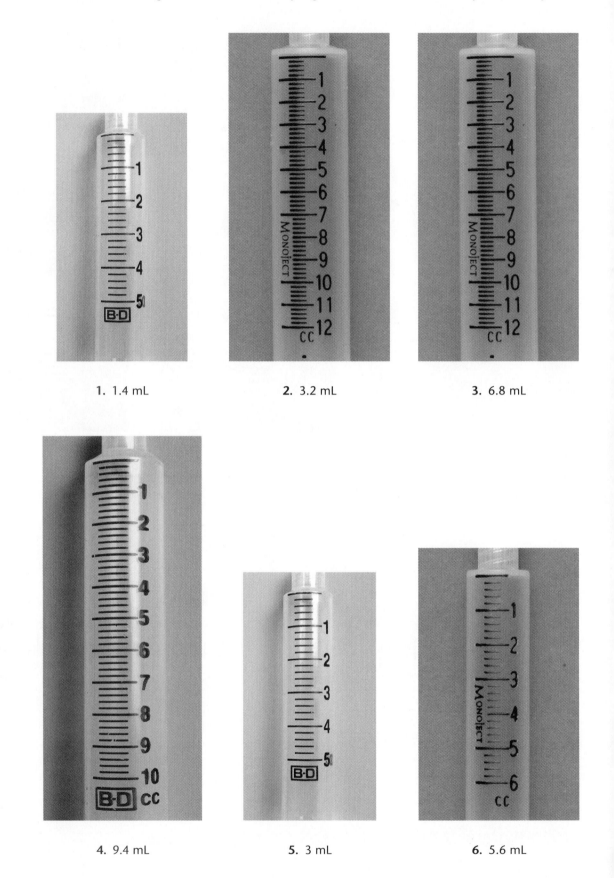

1. 1.4 mL

2. 3.2 mL

3. 6.8 mL

4. 9.4 mL

5. 3 mL

6. 5.6 mL

20 mL and Larger Syringes

Examine the 20 mL syringe in Figure 7-7 and determine how it is calibrated. Note that the soon to be replaced cc abbreviation is still used on this syringe.

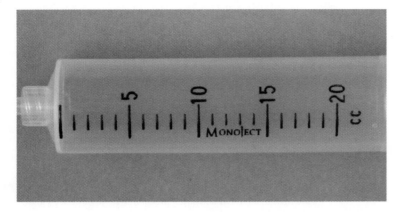

Figure 7-7

As you can see, this syringe is calibrated in **1 mL increments**, with longer calibrations identifying the 0, 5, 10, 15, and 20 mL volumes. Syringes with a 50 mL capacity are also calibrated in full mL measures. These syringes are used only for measurement of large full mL volumes.

PROBLEM

What mL dosages are measured on the following syringes?

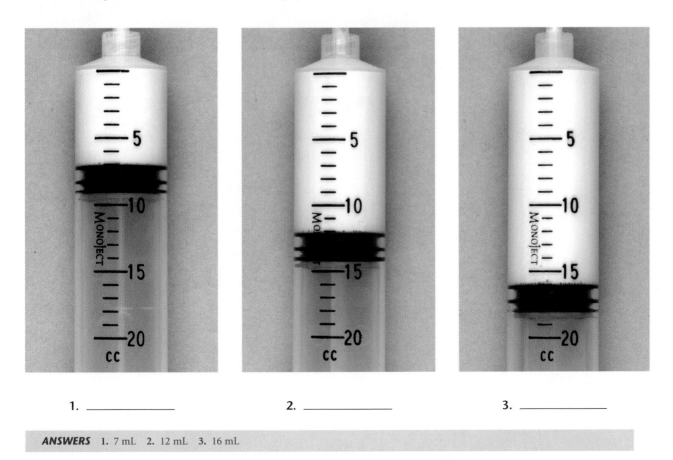

1. _____   2. _____   3. _____

ANSWERS   1. 7 mL   2. 12 mL   3. 16 mL

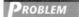

PROBLEM

Shade in or draw arrows on the three syringe barrels to identify the mL volumes listed. Have your answers checked by your instructor.

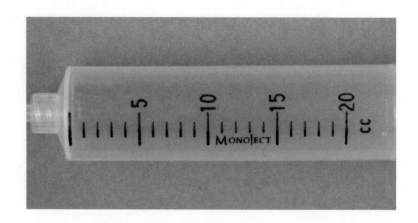

1. 11 mL

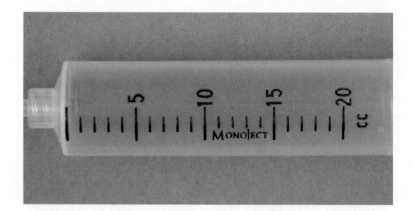

2. 18 mL

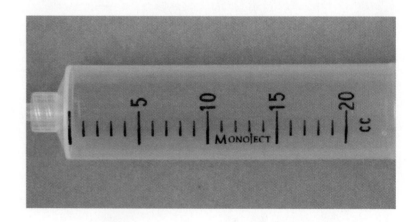

3. 9 mL

Summary

This concludes your introduction to syringe calibrations. The important points to remember from this chapter are:

- 3 mL syringes are calibrated in tenths.
- TB syringes are calibrated in hundredths.
- If a syringe still contains the apothecary now obsolete minim (m) scale, care must be taken not to mistake it for metric, mL, calibrations.
- 5, 6, 10, and 12 mL syringes are calibrated in fifths (two-tenths).
- Syringes larger than 12 mL are calibrated in full mL measures.
- The first long calibration on all syringes indicates zero.
- All syringe calibrations must be read from the top, or front, ring of the plunger's suction tip.

Summary Self-Test

Identify the mL dosages measured on the syringes.

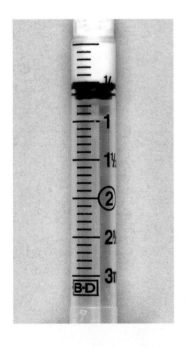

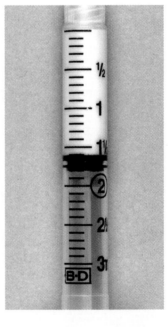

1. _____

2. _____

3. _____

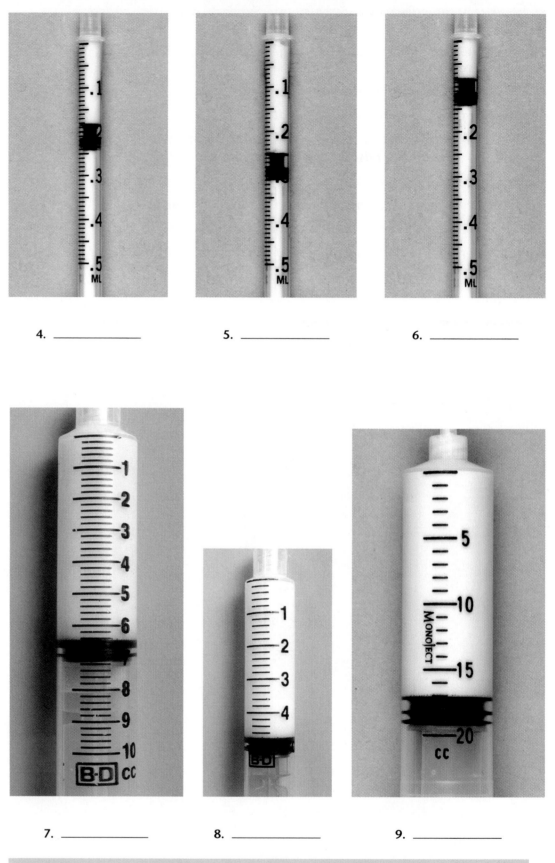

4. _____

5. _____

6. _____

7. _____

8. _____

9. _____

ANSWERS   **1.** 0.5 mL   **2.** 2.5 mL   **3.** 1.6 mL   **4.** 0.18 mL   **5.** 0.25 mL   **6.** 0.08 mL   **7.** 6.4 mL
8. 4.8 mL   **9.** 17 mL

Draw arrows on the syringes to measure the indicated mL dosages. Have your answers checked by your instructor.

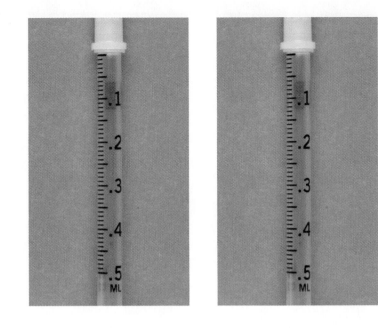

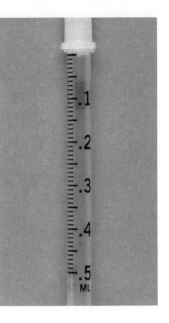

10. 0.42 mL   **11.** 0.31 mL   **12.** 0.44 mL

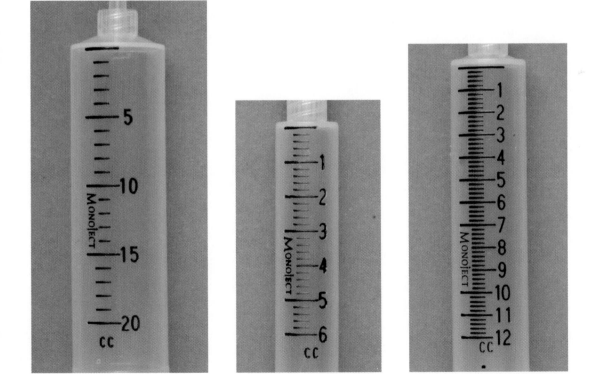

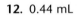

13. 13 mL   **14.** 1.2 mL   **15.** 7.6 mL

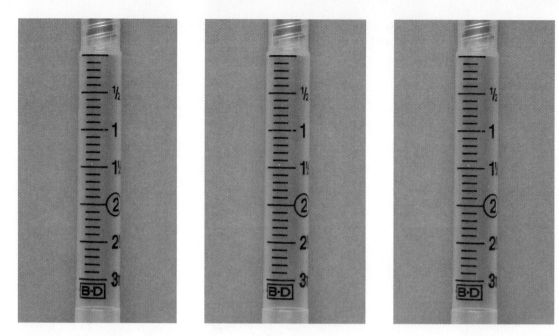

16. 1.7 mL   **17.** 2.2 mL   **18.** 0.9 mL

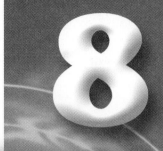

Reading Parenteral Medication Labels

Parenteral medications are administered by injection, with intravenous (IV), intramuscular (IM), and subcutaneous (subcut.) being the most frequently used routes. The labels of oral and parenteral solutions are very similar, but the size of the average parenteral dosage label is much smaller. Intramuscular and subcutaneous solutions, in particular, are manufactured so that the **average adult dosage will be contained in a volume of between 0.5 mL and 3 mL**. Volumes larger than 3 mL are difficult for a single injection site to absorb, and this 0.5–3 mL volume can be used as a guideline for accuracy of calculations in IM and subcutaneous dosages. Excessively larger or smaller volumes should be questioned, and calculations rechecked.

Intravenous medication administration is usually a two-step procedure: the dosage is prepared first, then it may be further diluted in IV fluids before administration. In this chapter we will be concerned only with the first step of IV drug preparation, which is accurate measurement of the prescribed dosage.

Parenteral drugs are packaged in a variety of single-use glass ampules, single- and multiple-use rubber-stoppered vials, and in premeasured syringes. See Figure 8-1.

OBJECTIVES

The learner will:

1. read parenteral solution labels and identify dosage strengths

2. measure parenteral dosages in metric, milliequivalent, unit, percentage, and ratio strengths using 3 mL, TB, 6, 12, and 20 mL syringes

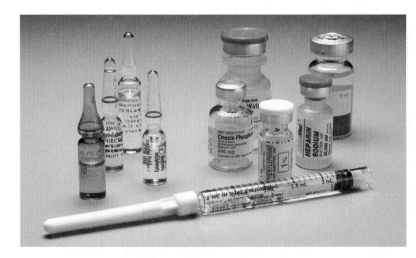

Ampules and vials.

Figure 8-1

Reading Metric/SI Solution Labels

We will begin by looking at parenteral solution labels with dosages in metric units of measure.

EXAMPLE 1

Refer to the Vistaril® label in Figure 8-2. The immediate difference you will notice between this and oral solution labels is the **size**. Ampules and vials are small and their labels are small, which requires that they be **read with particular care**. The information, however, is similar to oral labels. Vistaril is the trade name of the drug; hydroxyzine hydrochloride is the generic name. The dosage strength is 50 mg per mL (in the red rectangular area). The total vial contents are 10 mL (in black, center left). Calculating dosages is not usually complicated. For example, if a dosage of Vistaril 100 mg were ordered you would give 2 mL; if 50 mg are ordered give 1 mL; for 25 mg give 0.5 mL.

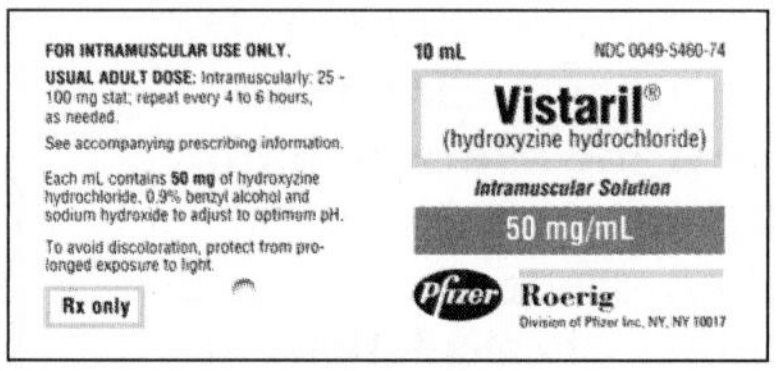

Figure 8-2

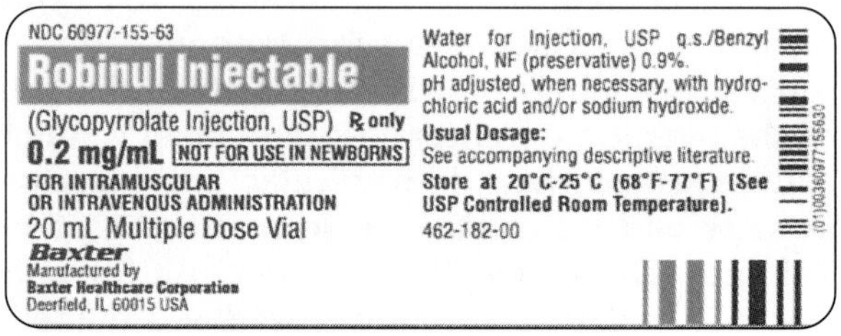

Figure 8-3

EXAMPLE 2

The Robinul® (glycopyrrolate) label in Figure 8-3 has a dosage strength of 0.2 mg/mL. To prepare a 0.2 mg dosage you would draw up 1 mL; to prepare a 0.4 mg dosage you would draw up 2 mL; a 0.3 mg dosage would require 1.5 mL.

EXAMPLE 3

The fentanyl citrate IV solution label in Figure 8-4 has dosage strengths expressed in both mcg and mg. To prepare a 0.25 mg (250 mcg) dosage you will need 5 mL; for a 0.125 mg dosage, 2.5 mL. Once again these simple dosages can be calculated mentally.

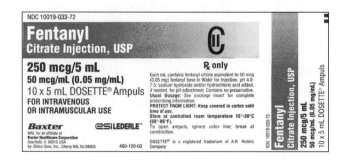

Figure 8-4

Refer to the gentamicin label in Figure 8-5 and answer the questions.

1. What is the total volume of this vial?   _____

2. What is the dosage strength?   _____

3. If gentamicin 80 mg were ordered, how many mL would this be?   _____

4. If gentamicin 60 mg were ordered, how many mL would this be?   _____

5. How many mL would you need to prepare a 20 mg dosage?   _____

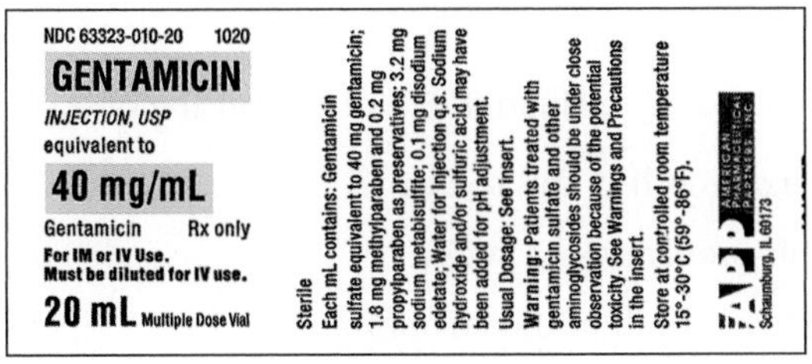

8

NDC 63323-010-20   1020
GENTAMICIN
INJECTION, USP
equivalent to
40 mg/mL
Gentamicin   Rx only
For IM or IV Use.
Must be diluted for IV use.
20 mL Multiple Dose Vial

Sterile
Each mL contains: Gentamicin sulfate equivalent to 40 mg gentamicin; 1.8 mg methylparaben and 0.2 mg propylparaben as preservatives; 3.2 mg sodium metabisulfite; 0.1 mg disodium edetate; Water for Injection q.s. Sodium hydroxide and/or sulfuric acid may have been added for pH adjustment.
Usual Dosage: See insert.
Warning: Patients treated with gentamicin sulfate and other aminoglycosides should be under close observation because of the potential toxicity. See Warnings and Precautions in the insert.
Store at controlled room temperature 15°-30°C (59°-86°F).

APP
AMERICAN PHARMACEUTICAL PARTNERS, INC.
Schaumburg, IL 60173

Figure 8-5

ANSWERS   1. 20 mL   2. 40 mg/mL   3. 2 mL   4. 1.5 mL   5. 0.5 mL

Percent (%) and Ratio Solution Labels

Drugs labeled as **percentage solutions** often express the drug strength in **metric measures in addition to percentage strength**. Refer to the lidocaine label in Figure 8-6. Notice that this is a 2% solution, and the vial that contains it has a total volume of 5 mL. Also notice that the dosage strength is listed in metric measures: 20 mg/mL. Lidocaine is most often ordered in mg; for example, 20 mg would require 1 mL, 10 mg would require 0.5 mL, and 30 mg would require 1.5 mL. However, lidocaine is also used as a local anesthetic and you may, for example, be asked to prepare 3 mL of 2% lidocaine, which requires no calculation at all, but simply locating the correct percentage strength and drawing up 3 mL.

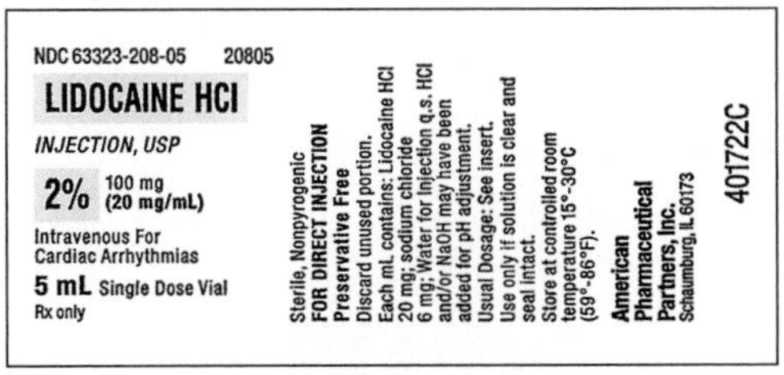

NDC 63323-208-05   20805
LIDOCAINE HCl
INJECTION, USP
2% 100 mg (20 mg/mL)
Intravenous For
Cardiac Arrhythmias
5 mL Single Dose Vial
Rx only

Sterile, Nonpyrogenic
FOR DIRECT INJECTION
Preservative Free
Discard unused portion.
Each mL contains: Lidocaine HCl 20 mg; sodium chloride 6 mg; Water for Injection q.s. HCl and/or NaOH may have been added for pH adjustment.
Usual Dosage: See insert.
Use only if solution is clear and seal intact.
Store at controlled room temperature 15°-30°C (59°-86°F).

American Pharmaceutical Partners, Inc.
Schaumburg, IL 60173

401722C

Figure 8-6

Refer to the lidocaine label in Figure 8-7 and answer the questions.

1. What is the percentage strength of this solution? _____

2. How many mL does the vial contain? _____

3. If you are asked to prepare 5 mL of solution, how much will you draw up in the syringe? _____

4. The dosage also appears on this label in metric measures. What is the metric dosage strength of this solution? _____

5. If you are asked to prepare 25 mg from this vial, what volume will you draw up? _____

Refer to the calcium gluconate label in Figure 8-8 and answer the questions.

6. What is the percentage strength of this solution? _____

7. How many mL does this preparation contain? _____

8. What is the mEq dosage strength of this solution? _____

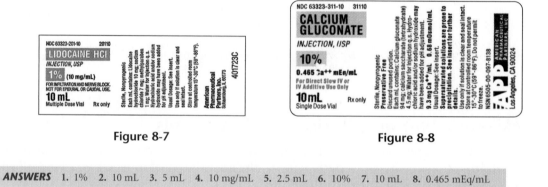

Figure 8-7   Figure 8-8

ANSWERS   1. 1%   2. 10 mL   3. 5 mL   4. 10 mg/mL   5. 2.5 mL   6. 10%   7. 10 mL   8. 0.465 mEq/mL

Parenteral medications expressed in **ratio strengths** are not common, and **when they are ordered it will be by number of mL**. Ratio labels may also contain dosages in metric weights.

Refer to the epinephrine label in Figure 8-9 and answer the questions.

1. What is the ratio strength of this solution? _____

2. What volume is this contained in? _____

3. What is the metric dosage strength of this solution? _____

Figure 8-9

ANSWERS   1. 1 : 1000   2. 1 mL   3. 1 mg/mL

Solutions Measured in International Units

A number of drugs are measured in **international units**. The labels shown below will introduce you to several examples.

PROBLEM

Refer to the heparin label in Figure 8-10 and answer the questions.

1. What is the total volume of this vial?   _____

2. What is the dosage strength?   _____

3. If a volume of 1.5 mL is prepared, how many units will this be?   _____

4. How many mL will you need to prepare a dosage of 5500 units?   _____

5. If 0.25 mL of this medication is prepared, what dosage will this be?   _____

Refer to the oxytocin label in Figure 8-11 and answer the questions.

6. What is the dosage strength of this solution?   _____

7. If a dosage of 10 units is ordered, what volume will you need?   _____

8. If a dosage of 5 units is ordered, what volume will you prepare?   _____

Refer to the Bicillin® C-R label in Figure 8-12 and answer the questions.

9. What is the dosage strength of this medication?   _____

10. If 600,000 units was ordered, how many mL would this require?   _____

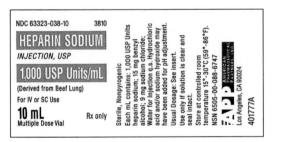

Figure 8-10

Figure 8-11

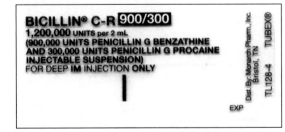

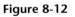

Figure 8-12

ANSWERS **1.** 10 mL   **2.** 1000 units/mL   **3.** 1500 units   **4.** 5.5 mL   **5.** 250 units   **6.** 10 units per mL
7. 1 mL   **8.** 0.5 mL   **9.** 1,200,000 units/2 mL   **10.** 1 mL

Solutions Measured as Milliequivalents (mEq)

The next four labels will introduce you to milliequivalent (mEq) dosages. Refer to the calcium gluconate label in Figure 8-13 and notice that in addition to its 10% strength, this label identifies a dosage strength of 0.465 mEq/mL. If a dosage of 0.465 mEq were ordered, you would draw up 1 mL in the syringe.

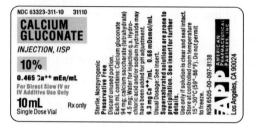

Figure 8-13

PROBLEM

Refer to the potassium chloride label in Figure 8-14 and answer the questions.

1. What are the total dosage and volume of this vial?   _____

2. What is the dosage in mEq per mL?   _____

3. If you were asked to prepare 15 mEq for addition to an IV, what volume would you draw up?   _____

Refer to the potassium chloride label in Figure 8-15 and answer the dosage questions.

4. What is the strength of this solution in mEq per mL?   _____

5. If you were asked to prepare 40 mEq for addition to an IV solution, what volume would you draw up in the syringe?   _____

6. What volume would you need for a dosage of 20 mEq?   _____

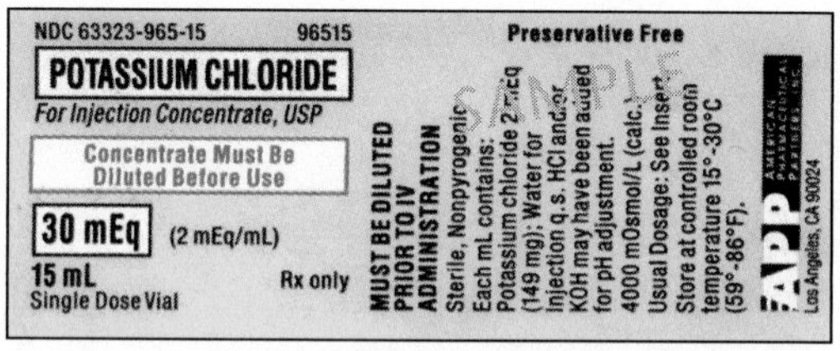

Figure 8-14

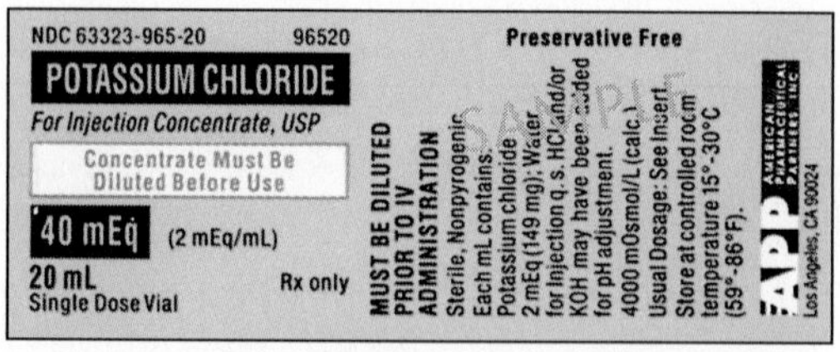

Figure 8-15

Refer to the sodium bicarbonate label in Figure 8-16. Notice that this solution lists the drug strength in mEq, percentage, and mg. Read the label very carefully and locate the answers to the questions.

7. What is the dosage strength expressed in mEq/mL?   _____

8. What is the total volume of the vial, and how many mEq does this volume contain?   _____

9. What is the strength per mL expressed as mg?   _____

10. If you were asked to prepare 10 mL of an 8.4% sodium bicarbonate solution, what volume would you draw up in a syringe?   _____

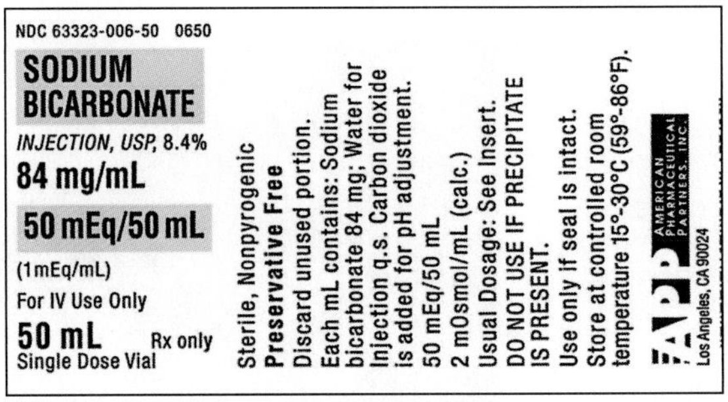

Figure 8-16

ANSWERS 1. 30 mEq; 15 mL   2. 2 mEq/mL   3. 7.5 mL   4. 2 mEq/mL   5. 20 mL   6. 10 mL
7. 1 mEq/mL   8. 50 mL; 50 mEq   9. 84 mg/mL   10. 10 mL

Summary

This concludes the introduction to parenteral solution labels. The important points to remember from this chapter are:

■ *The most commonly used parenteral administration routes are IV, IM, and subcutaneous.*

■ *The labels of most parenteral solutions are quite small and must be read with particular care.*

■ *The average IM and subcutaneous dosage will be contained in a volume of between 0.5 mL and 3 mL. This volume can be used as a guideline to accuracy of calculations.*

■ *IV medication preparation is usually a two-step procedure: measurement of the dosage, then dilution according to the manufacturer's recommendations or physician's order.*

■ *Parenteral drugs may be measured in metric, ratio, percentage, unit, or mEq dosages.*

■ *If dosages are ordered by percentage or ratio strength, they are usually specified in mL to be administered.*

■ *Most IM and subcutaneous dosages are prepared using a 3 mL or tuberculin (TB) syringe.*

Summary Self-Test

Read the parenteral drug labels provided to measure the following mL dosages. Then indicate on the syringe provided exactly how much solution you will draw up to obtain these dosages. Have your answers checked by your instructor to be sure you have measured the dosages correctly.

Dosage Ordered	mL Needed

1. Depo-Provera® 0.4 g _____

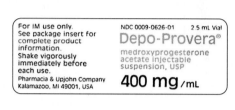

For IM use only.
See package insert for complete product information.
Shake vigorously immediately before each use.
Pharmacia & Upjohn Company
Kalamazoo, MI 49001, USA

NDC 0009-0626-01   2.5 mL Vial
Depo-Provera®
medroxyprogesterone acetate injectable suspension, USP
400 mg /mL

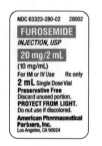

2. furosemide 10 mg _____

NDC 63323-280-02   28002
FUROSEMIDE
INJECTION, USP
20 mg/2 mL
(10 mg/mL)
For IM or IV Use   Rx only
2 mL Single Dose Vial
Preservative Free
Discard unused portion.
PROTECT FROM LIGHT.
Do not use if discolored.
American Pharmaceutical Partners, Inc.
Los Angeles, CA 90024

3. heparin 2500 units _____

NDC 63323-047-10   4710
HEPARIN SODIUM
INJECTION, USP
5,000 USP Units/mL
(Derived from Porcine Intestinal Mucosa)
For IV or SC Use
10 mL   Rx only
Multiple Dose Vial

Sterile, Nonpyrogenic
Each mL contains: 5,000 USP Units heparin sodium; 15 mg benzyl alcohol; 6 mg sodium chloride; Water for injection q.s. Hydrochloric acid and/or sodium hydroxide may have been added for pH adjustment.
Usual Dosage: See insert.
Use only if solution is clear and seal intact.
Store at controlled room temperature 15°-30°C (59°-86°F).
APP
Schaumburg, IL 60173
401796B

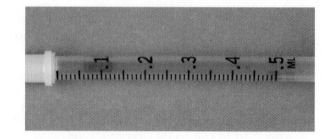

Dosage Ordered	mL Needed

4. Cleocin® 0.9 g _____

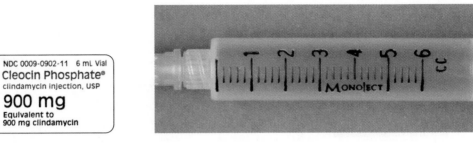

Single Dose Container.
See package insert for complete product information.
Store at controlled room temperature 20° to 25°C (68° to 77°F).
Do not refrigerate.
812 823 707
Pharmacia & Upjohn Company
Kalamazoo, MI 49001, USA

LOT/EXP

NDC 0009-0902-11   6 mL Vial
Cleocin Phosphate®
clindamycin injection, USP
900 mg
Equivalent to
900 mg clindamycin

5. atropine 0.2 mg _____

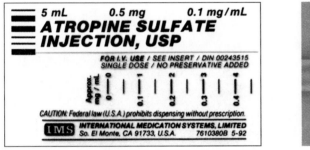

5 mL   0.5 mg   0.1 mg/mL
ATROPINE SULFATE
INJECTION, USP
FOR I.V. USE / SEE INSERT / DIN 00243515
SINGLE DOSE / NO PRESERVATIVE ADDED
Approx. mg/mL
CAUTION: Federal law (U.S.A.) prohibits dispensing without prescription.
IMS INTERNATIONAL MEDICATION SYSTEMS, LIMITED
So. El Monte, CA 91733, U.S.A.   7610380B 5-92

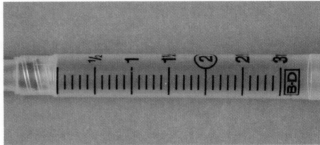

6. hydroxyzine HCl 25 mg _____

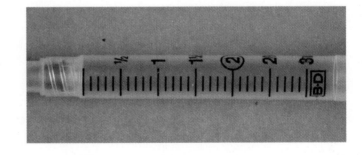

FOR INTRAMUSCULAR USE ONLY
USUAL ADULT DOSE: Intramuscularly: 25 -
100 mg stat; repeat every 4 to 6 hours, as
needed. See accompanying prescribing
information.
Each mL contains **25 mg** of hydroxyzine
hydrochloride, 0.9% benzyl alcohol and
sodium hydroxide to adjust to optimum pH.
To avoid discoloration, protect from prolonged exposure to light.
CAUTION: Federal law prohibits
dispensing without prescription.

10 mL   NDC 0049-5450-74
Vistaril®
(hydroxyzine hydrochloride)
Intramuscular Solution
25 mg/mL
Pfizer Roerig
Division of Pfizer Inc, NY, NY 10017

7. Robinul 100 mcg _____

NDC 60977-155-81
Robinul
Injectable
(Glycopyrrolate
Injection, USP)
0.2 mg/mL ℞ only
FOR IM OR IV USE
1 mL Single Dose Vial
Manufactured by
Baxter Healthcare Corp.
Deerfield, IL 60015 USA
462-176-00
(01)00360977155814

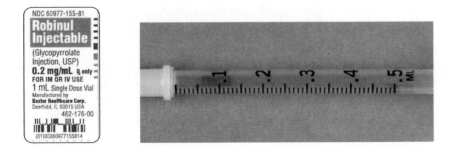

Dosage Ordered	mL Needed

8. Tigan® 0.2 g   _____

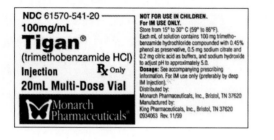

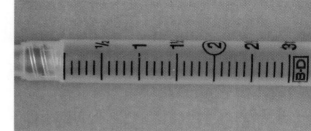

9. methotrexate 0.25 g   _____

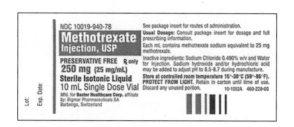

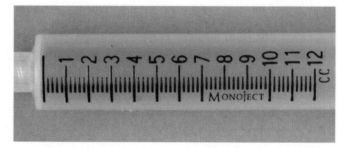

10. cyanocobalamin 1 mg   _____

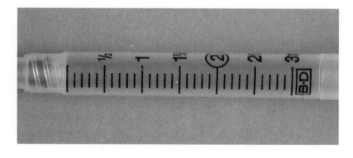

11. diazepam 5 mL   _____

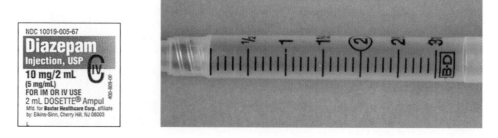

Dosage Ordered	mL Needed

12. epinephrine 2 mg _____

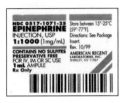

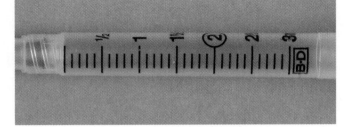

13. fentanyl citrate 0.25 mg _____

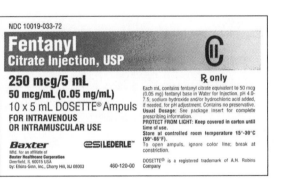

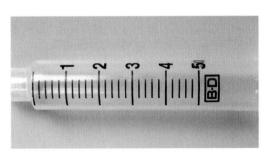

14. calcium gluconate 0.93 mEq _____

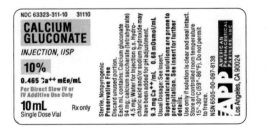

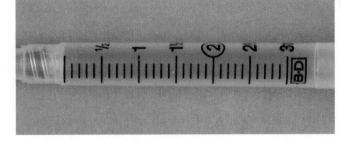

15. Haldol® 7.5 mg _____

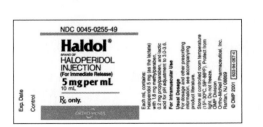

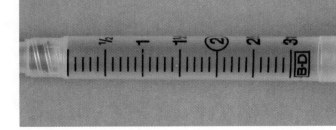

Dosage Ordered	mL Needed

16. heparin 500 units   _____

NDC 63323-038-10   3810

HEPARIN SODIUM

INJECTION, USP

1,000 USP Units/mL

(Derived from Beef Lung)

For IV or SC Use

10 mL   Rx only

Multiple Dose Vial

Sterile, Nonpyrogenic.
Each mL contains: 1,000 USP Units
heparin sodium; 15 mg benzyl
alcohol; 9 mg sodium chloride;
Water for Injection q.s. Hydrochloric
acid and/or sodium hydroxide may
have been added for pH adjustment.
Usual Dosage: See insert.
Use only if solution is clear and
seal intact.
Store at controlled room
temperature 15°–30°C (59°–86°F).
NSN 6505-00-088-6747

APP
AMERICAN PHARMACEUTICAL PARTNERS
Los Angeles, CA 90024

401777A

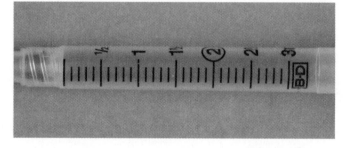

17. benztropine mesylate 500 mcg   _____

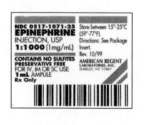

USUAL ADULT DOSAGE:
See accompanying circular.

NDC 0006-3275-01
2 mL INJECTION
COGENTIN®
(BENZTROPINE MESYLATE)
2 mg per 2 mL

Lot & Exp.

◆ MERCK & CO., INC.
Whitehouse Station, NJ 08889, USA

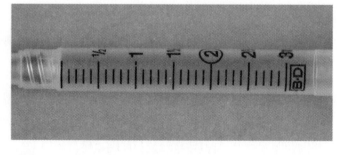

18. epinephrine 0.5 mg   _____

NDC 0517-1071-25
EPINEPHRINE
INJECTION, USP
1:1000 (1mg/mL)
CONTAINS NO SULFITES
PRESERVATIVE FREE
FOR IV, IM OR SC USE
1 mL AMPULE
Rx Only

Store between 15°–25°C
(59°–77°F).
Directions: See Package
Insert.
Rev. 10/99
AMERICAN REGENT
LABORATORIES, INC.
SHIRLEY, NY 11967

19. medroxyprogesterone 1 g   _____

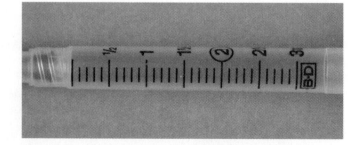

● For IM use only.
See package insert for
complete product
information.
Shake vigorously
immediately before
each use.
Pharmacia & Upjohn Company
Kalamazoo, MI 49001, USA

8122224806

NDC 0009-0626-01   2.5 mL Vial
Depo-Provera®
medroxyprogesterone
acetate injectable
suspension, USP
400 mg /mL

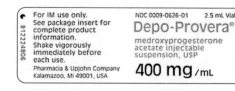

Dosage Ordered	mL Needed

20. gentamicin 60 mg _____

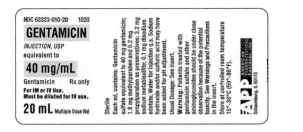

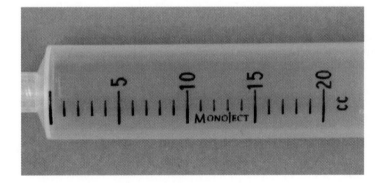

21. lidocaine HCl 50 mg _____

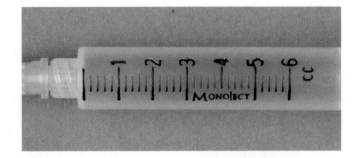

22. sodium chloride 40 mEq _____

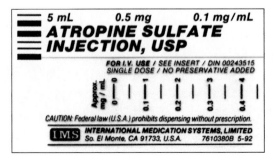

23. atropine 200 mcg _____

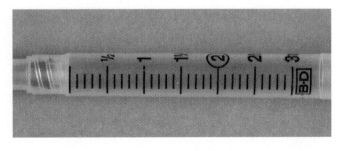

Dosage Ordered	**mL Needed**

24. meperidine 50 mg _____

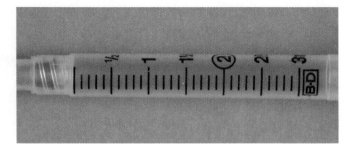

25. Tigan® 0.1 g _____

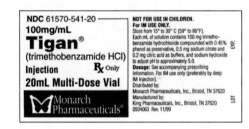

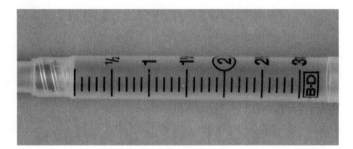

26. clindamycin 0.3 g _____

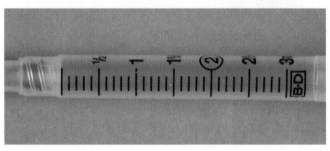

27. morphine sulfate 15 mg _____

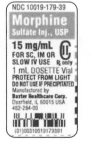

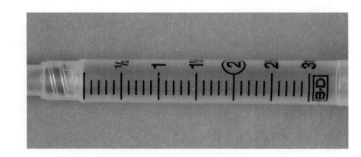

Dosage Ordered	mL Needed

28. Terramycin® 0.1 g _____

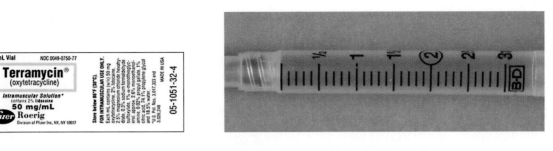

29. Thorazine® 50 mg _____

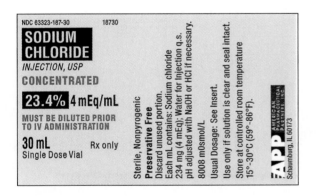

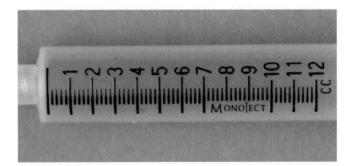

30. sodium chloride 20 mEq _____

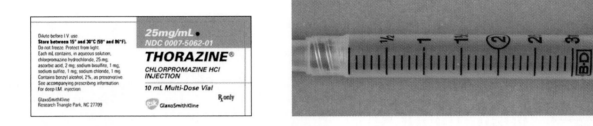

31. meperidine 50 mg _____

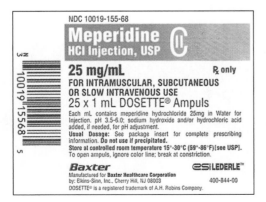

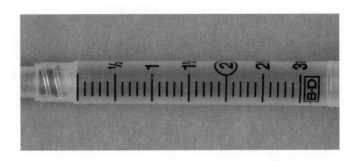

Dosage Ordered	mL Needed

32. furosemide 30 mg   _____

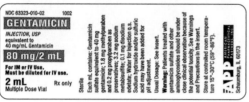

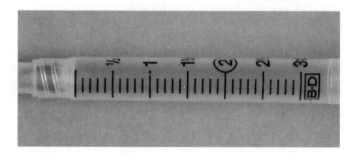

33. gentamicin 60 mg   _____

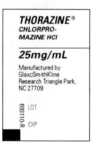

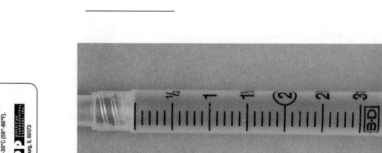

34. chlorpromazine HCl 50 mg   _____

THORAZINE®
CHLORPRO-
MAZINE HCI

25mg/mL

Manufactured by
GlaxoSmithKline
Research Triangle Park,
NC 27709

LOT

EXP

35. dexamethasone 2 mg   _____

NDC 63323-165-01   16501

**DEXAMETHASONE
SODIUM PHOSPHATE**

INJECTION, USP
equivalent to

4 mg/mL

Dexamethasone Phosphate
For IM or IV Use, See Insert
For Other Routes
1 mL
Sterile, Nonpyrogenic
Usual Dosage: See Insert.
Rx only
**American Pharmaceutical
Partners, Inc.**
Los Angeles, CA 90024

401779A

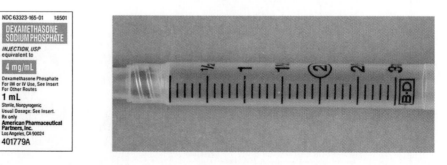

Dosage Ordered	mL Needed

36. chlorpromazine 75 mg _____

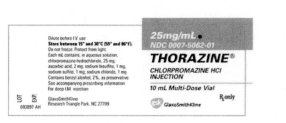
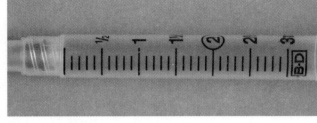

37. fentanyl 0.05 mg _____

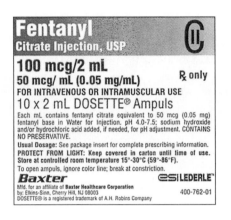
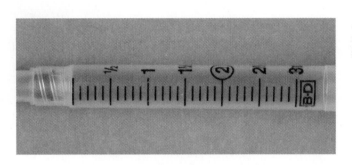

38. Pitocin® 15 units _____

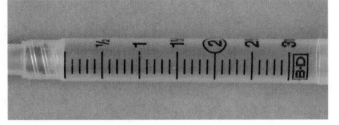
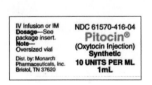

39. morphine 15 mg _____

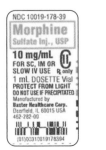
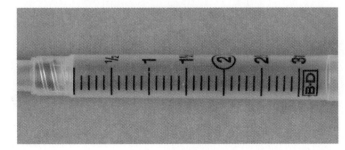

Dosage Ordered	mL Needed

40. cyanocobalamin 1 mg

_____

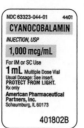

NDC 63323-044-01   4401
CYANOCOBALAMIN
INJECTION, USP
1,000 mcg/mL
For IM or SC Use
1 mL Multiple Dose Vial
Usual Dosage: See insert.
PROTECT FROM LIGHT.
Rx only
American Pharmaceutical
Partners, Inc.
Schaumburg, IL 60173
401802B

41. Cogentin® 1000 mcg

_____

USUAL ADULT DOSAGE:
See accompanying circular.

NDC 0006-3275-01
2 mL INJECTION
COGENTIN®
(BENZTROPINE MESYLATE)
2 mg per 2 mL
Lot & Exp.
⚕ **MERCK & CO., INC.**
Whitehouse Station, NJ 08889, USA
9113908

42. medroxyprogesterone acetate
1000 mg

_____

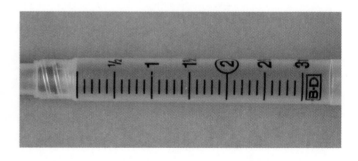

LOT/EXP
812224806

● For IM use only.
See package insert for
complete product
information.
Shake vigorously
immediately before
each use.
Pharmacia & Upjohn Company
Kalamazoo, MI 49001, USA

NDC 0009-0626-01   2.5 mL Vial
Depo-Provera®
medroxyprogesterone
acetate injectable
suspension, USP
400 mg /mL

ANSWERS

1. 1 mL	**10.** 1 mL	**19.** 2.5 mL	**28.** 2 mL	**37.** 1 mL
2. 1 mL	**11.** 1 mL	**20.** 1.5 mL	**29.** 2 mL	**38.** 1.5 mL
3. 0.5 mL	**12.** 2 mL	**21.** 5 mL	**30.** 5 mL	**39.** 1.5 mL
4. 6 mL	**13.** 5 mL	**22.** 10 mL	**31.** 2 mL	**40.** 1 mL
5. 2 mL	**14.** 2 mL	**23.** 2 mL	**32.** 3 mL	**41.** 1 mL
6. 1 mL	**15.** 1.5 mL	**24.** 0.5 mL	**33.** 1.5 mL	**42.** 2.5 mL
7. 0.5 mL	**16.** 0.5 mL	**25.** 1 mL	**34.** 2 mL	
8. 2 mL	**17.** 0.5 mL	**26.** 2 mL	**35.** 0.5 mL	
9. 10 mL	**18.** 0.5 mL	**27.** 1 mL	**36.** 3 mL	

Reconstitution of Powdered Drugs

9

OBJECTIVES

The learner will:
1. prepare solutions from powdered drugs using directions printed on vial labels
2. prepare solutions from powdered drugs using drug literature or inserts
3. determine expiration dates and times for reconstituted drugs
4. calculate simple dosages from reconstituted drugs

A number of drugs are shipped in powdered form because they **retain their potency only a short time in solution**. Reconstitution of these drugs is usually the responsibility of hospital pharmacies, but you will need to know how to read and follow reconstitution directions, and how to label drugs with an expiration date and time once they have been reconstituted. The drug label, or instructional package insert, will give specific directions for reconstitution of the drug. Reading these requires care, and this chapter will take you through the entire process step by step.

Reconstitution of a Single Strength Solution

Let's start with the simplest type of reconstitution instructions, for a single strength solution. Examine the label for the Solu-Medrol® 500 mg vial in Figure 9-1.

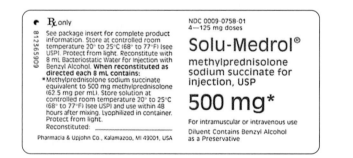

R only

See package insert for complete product information. Store at controlled room temperature 20° to 25°C (68° to 77°F) [see USP]. Protect from light. Reconstitute with 8 mL Bacteriostatic Water for Injection with Benzyl Alcohol. **When reconstituted as directed each 8 mL contains:**
*Methylprednisolone sodium succinate equivalent to 500 mg methylprednisolone (62.5 mg per mL). Store solution at controlled room temperature 20° to 25°C (68° to 77°F) [see USP] and use within 48 hours after mixing. Lyophilized in container. Protect from light.
Reconstituted: _____

Pharmacia & Upjohn Co., Kalamazoo, MI 49001, USA

NDC 0009-0758-01
4 — 125 mg doses

Solu-Medrol®
methylprednisolone sodium succinate for injection, USP

500 mg*

For intramuscular or intravenous use
Diluent Contains Benzyl Alcohol as a Preservative

Figure 9-1

The first step in reconstitution is to locate the directions. They are on the left side of this label. Locate the "Reconstitute with 8 mL Bacteriostatic Water for Injection with Benzyl Alcohol" instructions. Water, or any other solution specified for reconstitution, is called the **diluent**. The **type of diluent** specified will be **different for different drugs**. The **volume of diluent will also vary**. Therefore, reading the label carefully to identify both the type and the volume of diluent to be used is mandatory.

Once the type of diluent is identified, the next step is to use a **sterile syringe and aseptic technique** to draw up the 8 mL volume required. Inject it slowly into the vial **above the medication level**, because air bubbles can distort drug dosages. If the diluent volume is large, as in this case, be aware that the syringe plunger will be forced out to expel air to re-equalize the internal vial pressure as you inject. Very large volumes of diluent will have to be injected in divided amounts to keep the internal vial pressure equalized. When all the diluent has been injected, the vial must be rotated and upended until all the medication has been dissolved. **Do not shake**, because this also can add air bubbles to the medication and distort dosages.

After reconstitution, locate the information that relates to the **length of time** the reconstituted solution may be stored and **how it must be stored**. Look again at the directions and locate this information. You will find that this solution of Solu-Medrol can be stored at room temperature, it must be used within 48 hours of reconstitution, and it must be protected from light.

The next step is to print your initials on the label as the person who reconstituted the drug, in case any questions subsequently arise concerning the preparation. Next add the expiration date and time to the label. Let's assume you reconstituted this Solu-Medrol solution at **2 p.m. on January 3**. What expiration (EXP) date and time will you print on the label? The reconstituted drug lasts only 48 hours at room temperature, so you would print, "**Exp. Jan. 5, 2 p.m.**," which is 48 hours (2 days) from the time you reconstituted it.

 The person who reconstitutes a drug is responsible for labeling it with the date and time of expiration and with her/his name or initials.

Next look near the top right of the label and locate the dosage strength: "4–125 mg doses." Because you injected 8 mL of diluent, this will be approximately 2 mL for each 125 mL dose. However, **the reconstituted volume does not always equal the volume of diluent injected.** The powdered medication itself has a volume and makes the total volume somewhat larger than the diluent volume injected. So, be prepared to see variations in the reconstituted volumes of other medications.

Refer to the dosage strength again. If a 250 mg dosage is needed, what volume will you draw up? The dosage strength is 125 mg per 2 mL, so for 250 mg you will need 4 mL. A 500 mg dosage will require the entire 8 mL vial contents, and a 125 mg dosage will require 2 mL.

Reconstituted medications are in the minority, and consequently their labels are difficult to obtain. The next two samples have been designed to provide practice in reconstitution.

Refer to the sample medication label in Figure 9-2 and answer the questions about this medication.

1. How much diluent is added to the vial for reconstitution? _____

2. What type of diluent is used? _____

3. What is the dosage strength per mL of the prepared solution? _____

4. If an order is for 80 mg, what volume must you give? _____

5. What is the dosage strength of the total vial? _____

6. How long will the drug retain its potency at room temperature? _____

7. If the drug is reconstituted at 8 a.m. on October 3 and stored at room temperature, what expiration date will you print on the label? _____

8. How long will the solution retain its potency if refrigerated? _____

9. What expiration date will you print on the label if the solution is reconstituted on June 10 at 9 a.m. and stored under refrigeration? _____

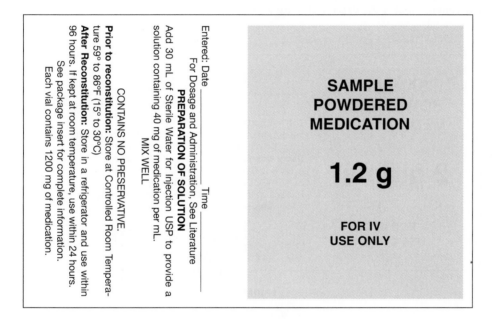

Figure 9-2

ANSWERS 1. 30 mL 2. sterile water 3. 40 mg per mL 4. 2 mL 5. 1.2 g 6. 24 hours
7. Exp 8 a.m. Oct 4 8. 96 hr (4 days) 9. Exp June 14 9 a.m.

Read the sample powdered medication label in Figure 9-3 and answer the questions.

1. What volume of diluent must be used to reconstitute this medication for IM use? _____

2. What kind of diluent is specified? _____

3. How long will the reconstituted solution retain its potency at room temperature? _____

4. If the medication is reconstituted at 11 a.m. February 25 and stored at room temperature, what expiration date and time will you print on the label? _____

5. What else will you print on the label? _____

6. What will be the dosage strength per mL of this reconstituted solution? _____

7. If a dosage of 500 mg is ordered, how much solution will you prepare? _____

8. What is the usual adult dose? _____

9. If reconstituted at 9:20 a.m. on December 18 and stored under refrigeration, what is the expiration date and time? _____

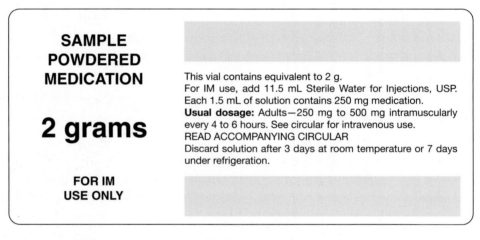

SAMPLE POWDERED MEDICATION

2 grams

FOR IM USE ONLY

This vial contains equivalent to 2 g.
For IM use, add 11.5 mL Sterile Water for Injections, USP.
Each 1.5 mL of solution contains 250 mg medication.
Usual dosage: Adults—250 mg to 500 mg intramuscularly every 4 to 6 hours. See circular for intravenous use.
READ ACCOMPANYING CIRCULAR
Discard solution after 3 days at room temperature or 7 days under refrigeration.

Figure 9-3

ANSWERS 1. 11.5 mL 2. Sterile Water for Injection 3. 3 days 4. Exp 11 a.m. Feb. 28 5. your initials or name 6. 250 mg per 1.5 mL 7. 3 mL 8. 250–500 mg IM every 4–6 hr 9. 9:20 a.m. Dec. 25

Reconstitution of Multiple Strength Solutions

Some powdered drugs offer a choice of dosage strengths. When this is the case you must choose the strength most appropriate for the dosage ordered. For example, refer to the penicillin label in Figure 9-4. The dosage strengths that can be obtained are listed on the right.

Notice that three dosage strengths are listed: 250,000 units, 500,000 units, and 1,000,000 units per mL. If the dosage ordered is 500,000 units, the most appropriate strength to mix would be 500,000 units per mL. Read across from this strength, and determine how much diluent must be added to obtain it. The answer is 33 mL. If the dosage ordered is 1,000,000 units, what would be the most appropriate strength to prepare, and how much diluent would this require? The answer is 1,000,000 units/mL, and 11.5 mL.

Figure 9-4

SEE ACCOMPANYING PRESCRIBING INFORMATION.

RECOMMENDED STORAGE IN DRY FORM.

Store below 86°F (30°C).

Buffered with sodium citrate and citric acid to optimum pH.

AFTER RECONSTITUTION, SOLUTION SHOULD BE REFRIGERATED. DISCARD UNUSED SOLUTION AFTER 7 DAYS.

Rx only

MADE IN USA

7488

NDC 0049-0530-28

Buffered

Pfizerpen®
(penicillin G potassium)

For Injection

TWENTY MILLION UNITS 20

FOR INTRAVENOUS INFUSION ONLY

Pfizer **Roerig**
Division of Pfizer Inc, NY, NY 10017

USUAL DOSAGE
6 to 40 million units daily by intravenous infusion only.

mL diluent added	Approx. units per mL of solution
75 mL	250,000 u/mL
33 mL	500,000 u/mL
11.5 mL	1,000,000 u/mL

PATIENT_____

ROOM_____

DATE/_____
TIME
BY_____

05-4211-00-8

Notice that this label does not tell you what type of diluent to use. **When information is missing from the label, look for it on the package information insert that comes with the drug.** Don't start guessing. All the information you need is in print somewhere; just take your time and locate it.

A multiple strength solution such as the one in Figure 9-4 requires that you add one additional piece of information to the label after you reconstitute it: the dosage strength you have just mixed.

PROBLEM

Refer to the Pfizerpen® label in Figure 9-4 to answer these questions.

1. If you add 75 mL of diluent to prepare a solution of penicillin, what dosage strength will you print on the label?   _____

2. Does this prepared solution require refrigeration?   _____

3. If you reconstitute it on June 1 at 2 p.m., what expiration time and date will you print on the label?   _____

4. What is the total dosage strength of this vial?   _____

Refer to the sample label in Figure 9-5 and answer the questions.

5. What is the total strength of medication in this vial? __________

6. What kind of diluent is recommended for reconstitution? __________

7. If you wish to prepare a 1 g/10 mL strength, how much diluent will you add to the vial? __________

8. How much diluent will you add for a 1 g/5 mL strength? __________

9. How must these large diluent volumes be added? __________

10. What is the expiration time for this drug if it is stored at room temperature? __________

11. If you reconstitute this drug at 0915 on April 17 and store it under refrigeration, what will you print on the label? __________

12. By what route is this drug to be administered? __________

13. What is the usual adult dose? __________

6 grams

SAMPLE POWDERED MEDICATION

FOR IV USE ONLY

Prescription only.
Store at Controlled Room Temperature
20° to 25°C (68° to 77°F)
Primarily for institutional use.
IMPORTANT: This vial is under reduced pressure. Addition of diluent generates a positive pressure. Before reconstituting, see Instructions for Reconstitution.
Usual Adult Dosage: 1 gram every 8 to 12 hours. In severe, refractory or life-threatening infections, 2 grams every 8 hours. See accompanying prescribing information.
In two stages, add Sodium Chloride Injection, Sterile Water for Injection or Bacteriostatic Water for Injection according to table below. See accompanying prescribing information. SHAKE WELL.
Use promptly. (Discard vial within 4 hours after initial entry.)

Approx. Concentration	Amount of Diluent
1 gram/5 mL	26 mL
1 gram/10 mL	56 mL

Properly reconstituted solutions are stable for 24 hours at room temperature or 7 days if refrigerated.

Figure 9-5

ANSWERS **1.** 250,000 units/mL **2.** Yes **3.** Exp 2 p.m. June 8 **4.** twenty million units **5.** 6 grams **6.** Sodium Chloride; Sterile Water; Bacteriostatic Water **7.** 56 mL **8.** 26 mL **9.** in two stages (steps) **10.** 24 hours **11.** Exp 0915 April 24 **12.** IV **13.** 1 g every 8–12 hours; in severe infections 2 g every hour

Reconstitution from Package Insert Directions

If the label does not contain reconstitution directions you must obtain these from the information insert that accompanies the vial. The drug Vancocin® HCl falls into this category. Refer to the Vancocin label and its reconstitution directions in Figures 9-6 and 9-7.

Refer to the Vancocin HCl label and insert in Figures 9-6 and 9-7 and answer the questions.

1. How much diluent must be added to this 500 mg vial for IV reconstitution? _____

2. What kind of diluent must be used? _____

3. If you reconstitute the drug at 3 p.m. on May 4 and the solution is refrigerated, what expiration information will you print on the label? _____

4. What is the concentration per mL of this solution? _____

5. What is the total dosage of the vial? _____

6. What additional minimum dilution will be required for IV administration? _____

9

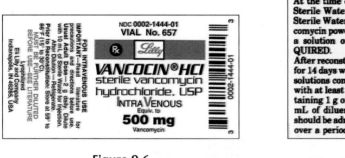

NDC 0002-1444-01
VIAL No. 657

℞ *Lilly*

VANCOCIN®HCl
sterile vancomycin
hydrochloride, USP
INTRA**V**ENOUS
Equiv. to
500 mg
Vancomycin

FOR INTRAVENOUS USE
IMPORTANT—Read literature for precautions and directions before use.
Usual Adult Dose—2 g daily. Dilute with 10 mL of Sterile Water for Injection. After Dilution—Refrigerate.
Prior to Reconstitution: Store at 59° to 86°F (15° to 30°C).
MUST BE FURTHER DILUTED BEFORE USE—SEE LITERATURE
Eli Lilly and Company
Indianapolis, IN 46285, USA

0002-1444-01

Figure 9-6

PREPARATION AND STABILITY
At the time of use, reconstitute by adding either 10 mL of Sterile Water for Injection to the 500-mg vial or 20 mL of Sterile Water for Injection to the 1-g vial of dry, sterile vancomycin powder. Vials reconstituted in this manner will give a solution of 50 mg/mL. FURTHER DILUTION IS REQUIRED.
After reconstitution, the vials may be stored in a refrigerator for 14 days without significant loss of potency. Reconstituted solutions containing 500 mg of vancomycin must be diluted with at least 100 mL of diluent. Reconstituted solutions containing 1 g of vancomycin must be diluted with at least 200 mL of diluent. The desired dose, diluted in this manner, should be administered by intermittent intravenous infusion over a period of at least 60 minutes.

Figure 9-7

ANSWERS 1. 10 mL 2. Sterile Water 3. Exp 3 p.m. May 18 4. 50 mg/mL 5. 500 mg 6. 100 mL

Summary

This concludes the chapter on reconstitution of powdered drugs. The important points to remember from this chapter are:

- *If the vial label does not contain reconstitution directions, they can be found on the vial package insert.*

- *The type and amount of diluent to be used for reconstitution must be exactly as specified in the instructions.*

- *If directions are given for both IM and IV reconstitution, be careful to read the correct set for the solution you are preparing.*

- *The person who reconstitutes a powdered drug must initial the vial and print the expiration time and date on the label unless all the drug is used immediately.*

- *If a multiple strength solution is prepared, the strength of the reconstituted drug also must be printed on the label.*

Summary Self-Test

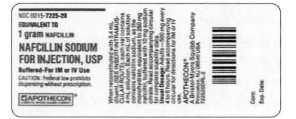

Figure 9-8

Refer to the nafcillin sodium label in Figure 9-8 and answer the questions about reconstitution.

1. What is the total dosage of this vial? _____

2. What volume of diluent must be used for reconstitution? _____

3. What will be the dosage strength of 1 mL of reconstituted solution? _____

Figure 9-9

Refer to the Velosef® label in Figure 9-9 and answer the questions.

4. What is the dosage strength of this vial? _____

5. What volume of diluent must you add to prepare the solution for IM use? _____

6. For IV use? _____

7. How long will this reconstituted cephradine retain its potency at room temperature? _____

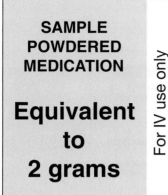

SAMPLE POWDERED MEDICATION

Equivalent to 2 grams

For IV use only

See package insert for Dosage and Administration.

Before constitution, store between 15° and 30°C (59° and 86°F) and protect from light. IMPORTANT: The vial is under reduced pressure. Addition of diluent generates a positive pressure.

Before constituting see Instructions for Constitution.

To prepare IV infusion, add 100 mL sterile sodium chloride for injection in two stages.

After constitution, solutions maintain potency for 24 hours at room temperature (not exceeding 25°C [77°F]), or for 7 days under refrigeration.

Figure 9-10

Refer to the medication label in Figure 9-10 and answer the questions.

8. How much and what type of diluent is used to reconstitute this IV solution? _____

9. What is the total strength of the vial? _____

10. How long will the solution retain its potency at room temperature? _____

11. If refrigerated? _____

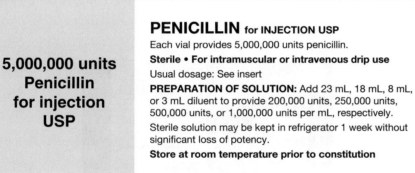

5,000,000 units Penicillin for injection USP

PENICILLIN for INJECTION USP
Each vial provides 5,000,000 units penicillin.
Sterile • For intramuscular or intravenous drip use
Usual dosage: See insert
PREPARATION OF SOLUTION: Add 23 mL, 18 mL, 8 mL, or 3 mL diluent to provide 200,000 units, 250,000 units, 500,000 units, or 1,000,000 units per mL, respectively.
Sterile solution may be kept in refrigerator 1 week without significant loss of potency.
Store at room temperature prior to constitution

Figure 9-11

Refer to the penicillin label in Figure 9-11 and answer the questions.

12. How much diluent must be added to obtain a 250,000 units/mL concentration? _____

13. To obtain a 1,000,000 units/mL concentration? _____

14. The type of diluent is not specified. Where would you find this information? _____

15. If this solution is reconstituted at 8:10 p.m. November 30, and stored under refrigeration, what expiration information will you print on the label? _____

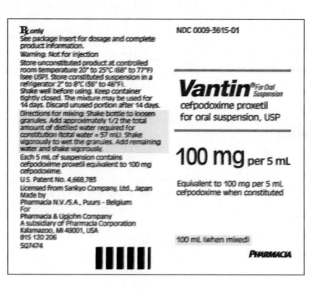

Figure 9-12

Refer to the Vantin® Oral Suspension label in Figure 9-12 and answer the questions.

16. How much diluent will be required to reconstitute this medication?   _____

17. What type of diluent is listed for reconstitution?   _____

18. How is this diluent to be added?   _____

19. What is the reconstituted dosage strength?   _____

20. How long will the reconstituted Vantin solution retain its potency?   _____

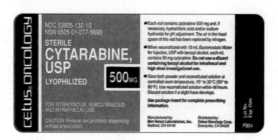

Figure 9-13

Refer to the cytarabine label in Figure 9-13 and answer the questions.

21. What is the total strength of this medication?   _____

22. What diluent must be used for reconstitution?   _____

23. How much?   _____

24. There is a special precaution on the label about a diluent not to be used. What is it?   _____

25. How long does the reconstituted cytarabine solution retain its potency at room temperature?   _____

SAMPLE ANTIBIOTIC POWDER 6 grams FOR IM USE ONLY	**Prescription only.** **Store at Controlled Room Temperature** **20° to 25°C (68° to 77°F)** **Primarily for institutional use.** **IMPORTANT:** This vial is under reduced pressure. Addition of diluent generates a positive pressure. Before reconstituting, see Instructions for Reconstitution. **Usual Adult Dosage:** 1 gram every 8 to 12 hours. In severe, refractory or life-threatening infections, 2 grams every 8 hours. See accompanying prescribing information. In two stages, add Sodium Chloride Injection, Sterile Water for Injection or Bacteriostatic Water for Injection according to table below. See accompanying prescribing information. SHAKE WELL. **Use promptly.**

Approx. Concentration	Amount of Diluent
1 gram/5 mL	26 mL
1 gram/10 mL	56 mL

Properly reconstituted solutions are stable for 24 hours at room temperature or 7 days if refrigerated. Slight yellowing does not affect potency.
Each vial contains equivalent to 6 grams of antibiotic.

Figure 9-14

Refer to the sample label in Figure 9-14 and answer the questions for preparation of a 1 g/5 mL solution.

26. What type of diluent is recommended for reconstitution? _____

27. How much diluent must be added? _____

28. If this drug is reconstituted at 0200 on March 23 and stored at room temperature, what expiration information will you print on the label? _____

29. If it is stored under refrigeration, what date and time will you print? _____

30. What is the total dosage strength of this vial? _____

31. What must you print on the label in addition to the expiration date? _____

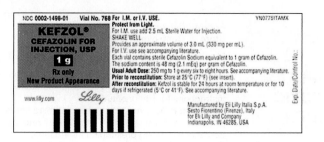

Figure 9-15

Refer to the Kefzol® label in Figure 9-15 and answer the questions.

32. What is the generic name for Kefzol? _____

33. What is the total dosage strength of this vial? _____

34. What volume of diluent must be added for IM use? _____

35. What type of diluent is specified? _____

36. What will the reconstituted volume of medication be? _____

37. Why is this volume larger than the amount of diluent added? _____

38. What is the reconstituted dosage strength? _____

39. What volume of solution will be required for a dosage of cefazolin 660 mg? _____

40. How long will Kefzol retain its potency at room temperature? _____

41. If you reconstitute the solution at 2:44 p.m. on Saturday, August 17 and refrigerate it, what must you print on the label? _____

42. What else must you print on the label? _____

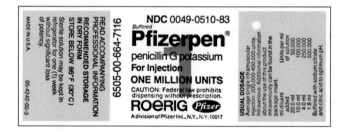

Figure 9-16

Refer to the penicillin G potassium label in Figure 9-16 and answer the questions.

43. What is the total dosage strength of this vial? _____

44. How much diluent must be added to prepare a 100,000 units/mL strength? _____

45. How much diluent must be added to prepare a 500,000 units/mL strength? _____

46. How much diluent must be added to prepare a 50,000 units/mL strength? _____

47. This label does not specify the type of diluent to use. Where will you find this information? _____

48. Penicillin is a suspension that tends to trap air bubbles, which could distort the dosage. List two critical steps in the reconstitution process designed to prevent air bubbles. _____

49. How must this solution be stored? _____

50. If reconstituted at 1:10 a.m. on December 18, what must you print on the label? _____

51. What else must you print on the label? _____

52. Why print? _____

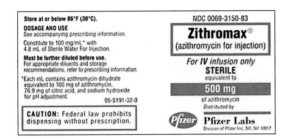

Figure 9-17

Refer to the Zithromax® label in Figure 9-17 and answer the questions.

53. What is the generic name for Zithromax? _____

54. What is the dosage strength of this vial? _____

55. What diluent is specified for reconstitution? _____

56. How much diluent is required? _____

57. What is the reconstituted dosage strength? _____

ANSWERS

1. 1 g	**18.** add half and shake, add remainder and shake	**28.** Exp 0200 March 24	**45.** 1.8 mL
2. 3.4 mL		**29.** Exp 0200 March 30	**46.** 20 mL
3. 250 mg		**30.** 6 grams	**47.** package insert
4. 250 mg	**19.** 100 mg per 5 mL	**31.** your name or initials	**48.** inject diluent above the medication; rotate and upend the vial to mix rather than shake
5. 1.2 mL	**20.** 14 days	**32.** cefazolin	
6. 5 mL	**21.** 500 mg	**33.** 1 g	
7. 2 hours	**22.** Bacteriostatic Water with benzyl alcohol	**34.** 2.5 mL	
8. 100 mL; Sterile Sodium Chloride		**35.** Sterile Water	**49.** refrigerate
	23. 10 mL	**36.** 3 mL	**50.** Exp 1:10 a.m. December 25
9. 2 g	**24.** no diluents containing benzyl alcohol if for intrathecal or high investigational use	**37.** drug also occupies space	
10. 24 hours		**38.** 330 mg/mL	**51.** your name or initials
11. 7 days		**39.** 2 mL	**52.** handwriting may be difficult to read
12. 18 mL		**40.** 24 hours	
13. 3 mL	**25.** 48 hours	**41.** Exp 2:44 p.m. August 27	**53.** azithromycin
14. package insert information sheet	**26.** Sodium Chloride; Sterile Water; Bacteriostatic Water	**42.** your name or initials	**54.** 500 mg
15. Exp 8:10 p.m. Dec 7		**43.** one million units	**55.** Sterile Water for Injection
16. 57 mL		**44.** 10 mL	**56.** 4.8 mL
17. distilled water	**27.** 26 mL, in 2 stages		**57.** 100 mg/mL

10

Measuring Insulin Dosages

Insulin dosages are measured in units, with the 100 units per mL strength being used almost exclusively. Dosages are measured using **special insulin syringes** that are **calibrated to match the dosage strength of insulin being used**. For example, 100 units syringes are used to prepare 100 units strength dosages. This chapter will show you a variety of 100 units syringes to illustrate how to measure dosages. However, let's begin with an introduction to the types of insulin in use. Note that many of the labels contain a U-100 designation, which represents the 100 units/mL strength.

Types of Insulin

Insulins are classified by **origin** (animal or human) and by **action** (rapid-, intermediate-, or long-acting). The origin or source of insulins is printed on every label, and it is important to know where to locate this information because physicians may specify origin when writing insulin orders. Notice the small print on the Regular insulin label in Figure 10-1, which identifies its animal (pork) origin, and the Regular insulin label in Figure 10-2, which identifies its human (recombinant DNA) origin. Also notice how similar these labels are, making careful reading of labels essential for correct identification. Insulins prepared in multiple-use vials are routinely labeled with each patient's name. However, this does not eliminate the need to read the label carefully prior to

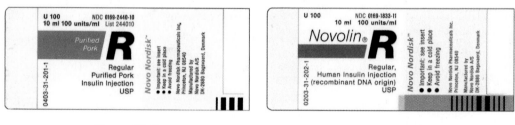

Figure 10-1   Figure 10-2

dosage preparation. Next look at the labels in Figures 10-3 and 10-4. Both of these insulins are of human origin and use the trade name Humulin®. Then notice the initials that follow the trade name: L (Lente®) and U (Ultralente®). These identify the type of insulin by action time. There are four basic action times of insulins. The most rapid-acting insulins, with an action starting in 5–10 minutes, peaking in 1–1½ hr, and ending in 3–5 hr, are insulin lispro (Humalog®) and insulin aspart (Novolog®). Regular and Semilente® also have a rapid action, beginning in ½ hr, peaking in 2½–5 hr, and ending in 8 hr. In the intermediate range are the Lente® and NPH insulins, beginning in 1½–2½ hr, peaking in 4–15 hr, and ending in 16–24 hr. Among the long-acting insulins are the Ultralente® and glargine, whose action is spread over a 24–36 hr range.

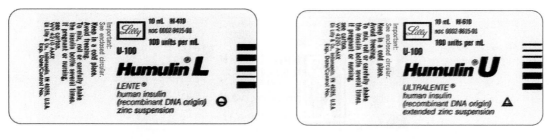

Figure 10-3   Figure 10-4

Combined rapid- and medium-action insulins are also in use. Two examples are the 70/30 illustrated in Figure 10-5, and the 50/50 combination illustrated in Figure 10-6.

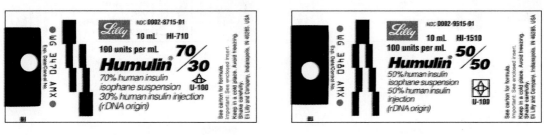

Figure 10-5   Figure 10-6

PROBLEM

Identify the type and origin of each of the insulins in the labels (Figures 10-7 through 10-11).

Type of Insulin   Origin

1. _____   _____

2. _____   _____

3. _____   _____

4. _____   _____

5. _____   _____

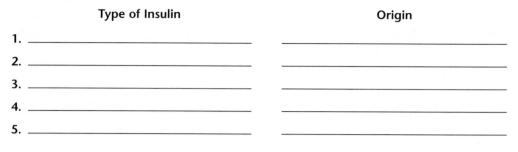

1.   **Figure 10-7**

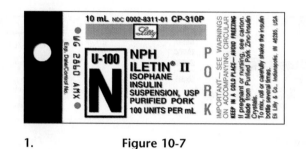

2.   **Figure 10-8**   3.   **Figure 10-9**

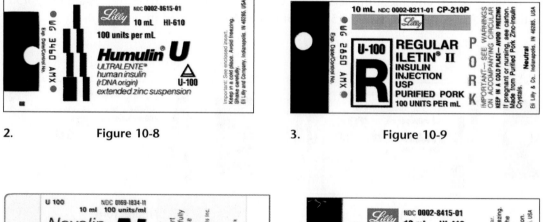

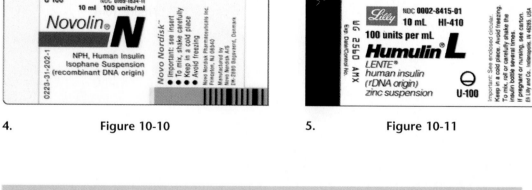

4.   **Figure 10-10**   5.   **Figure 10-11**

100 unit/mL Insulin and Syringes

Refer back to each of the labels you have just read and you will notice that **all have a 100 units per mL** (U-100) strength.

 To prepare U-100 insulin dosages you must use a 100 units/mL calibrated syringe.

Refer to the 100 units/mL (U-100) syringe pictured in Figure 10-12 and you will notice that it is very small. In order to read the calibrations and number of units it is necessary to **rotate insulin syringes from side to side**. To make it possible for you to practice measuring insulin dosages in this chapter, the calibrations for this syringe have been flattened out. These are the identical calibrations that appear on the syringes, so your dosage practice will be authentic.

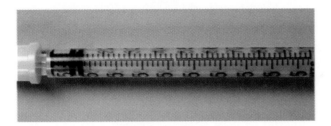

Figure 10-12

Although insulin syringes are calibrated to the 100 units/mL dosage, they do not all have a 1 mL capacity. There are actually several sizes (capacities) of U-100 syringes in use. The easiest of these to read and use are the Lo-Dose® syringes.

Lo-Dose® Syringes

Lo-Dose syringes have a capacity of 30 or 50 units. Lo-Dose insulin syringes do exactly what their name implies: they **measure low dosages, but on an enlarged and easier to read scale**. This larger scale is an important safety feature for diabetic patients, who frequently have vision problems, as well as for ease of use by medical personnel.

Refer to the calibrations for 50 units Lo-Dose capacity syringes in the problems that follow. Notice that **each calibration measures 1 unit**, and that **each 5 units increment is numbered**.

PROBLEM

Refer to the syringe calibrations for the 50 units Lo-Dose syringes below and identify the dosages indicated by the shaded areas.

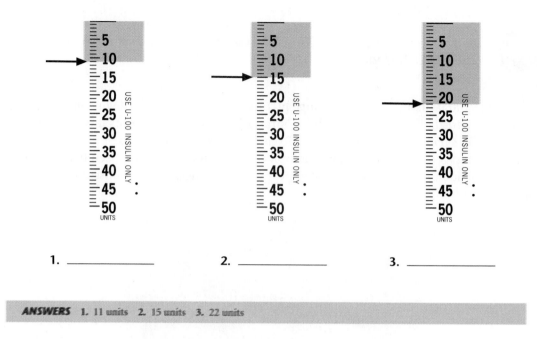

1. _____

2. _____

3. _____

PROBLEM

Use the Lo-Dose calibrations below to shade in the indicated dosages. Have your instructor check your accuracy.

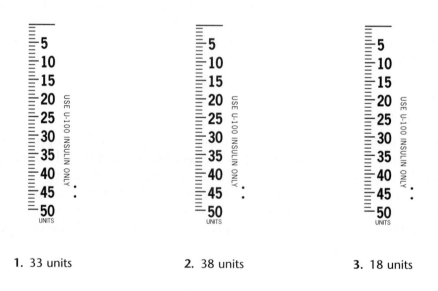

1. 33 units

2. 38 units

3. 18 units

100 Unit Capacity Syringes

There are two different 100 units insulin syringes in common use. Refer to the first of these syringe calibrations below. Notice the 100 units capacity, and that, in contrast to the Lo-Dose syringes, only **each 10 units increment is numbered**: 10, 20, 30, etc. Next notice the number of calibrations in each 10 units increment, which is five, indicating that **this syringe is calibrated in 2 units increments. Odd numbered units cannot be measured accurately using this syringe.**

PROBLEM

Identify the dosages indicated by the shading on the following 100 units capacity syringes.

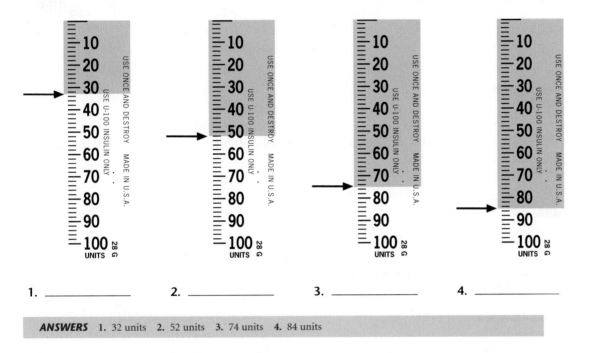

1. _____   2. _____   3. _____   4. _____

ANSWERS   1. 32 units   2. 52 units   3. 74 units   4. 84 units

PROBLEM

Shade in the following syringes to measure the dosages indicated. Have your instructor check your accuracy.

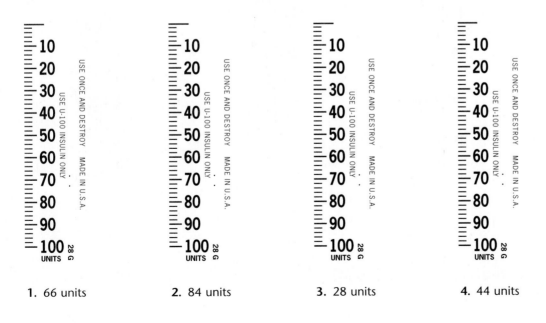

1. 66 units   2. 84 units   3. 28 units   4. 44 units

The second type of 100 units capacity syringe is illustrated in Figure 10-13. Notice that this syringe has a **double scale: the odd numbers are on the left, and the even are on the right**. Each 5 units increment is numbered, but on **opposite sides** of the syringe. This syringe does have a calibration for each 1 unit increment, but in order to count every one to measure a dosage the syringe would have to be rotated back and forth, which could cause confusion. There is a safer way to read the calibrations. **To measure odd numbered dosages,** for example, 7, 13, 27, etc., **use the odd (left) scale only; for even numbered dosages** such as 6, 10, 56, etc., **use the even (right) scale only. Count each calibration (on one side only) as 2 units, because that is what it is measuring.**

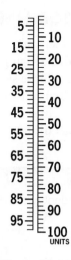

Figure 10-13

EXAMPLE 1

To prepare an 89 units dosage, start at 85 units on the uneven left scale, count the first calibration above this as 87 units, the next as 89 units (**each calibration on the same side measures 2 units**).

EXAMPLE 2

To measure a 26 units dosage, use the even numbered, right side calibrations. Start at 20 units, move up one calibration to 22 units, another to 24 units, and one more to 26 units (**each calibration is 2 units**).

PROBLEM

Identify the dosages measured on the 100 units capacity syringes provided.

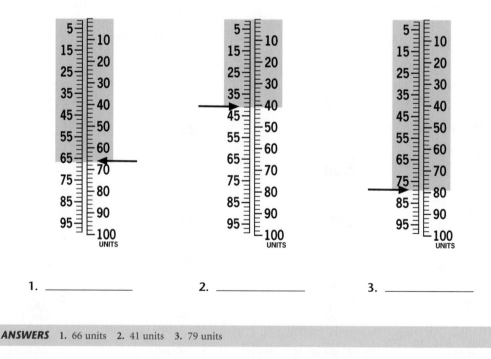

1. _____   2. _____   3. _____

ANSWERS 1. 66 units   2. 41 units   3. 79 units

Shade in each syringe provided to identify the indicated dosages.

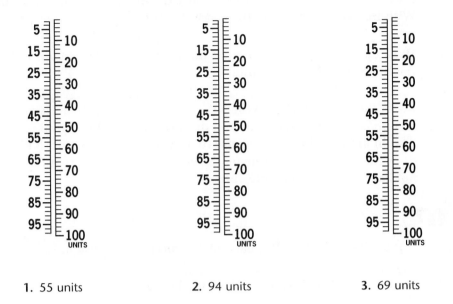

1. 55 units   **2.** 94 units   **3.** 69 units

Combining Insulin Dosages

Insulin-dependent individuals must have at least one, and sometimes several, subcutaneous injections of insulin per day. In order to reduce the number of injections as much as possible, it is common to combine two insulins in a single syringe, for example, a short-acting with either an intermediate- or long-acting insulin.

> *When two insulins are combined in the same syringe, the regular (shortest-acting) insulin is drawn up first.*

Both insulins will be withdrawn from sealed 10 mL vials, which requires that an amount of air equal to the insulin to be withdrawn be injected into each vial as a preliminary step. This keeps the pressure inside the vials equalized. An additional step concerns preparation of the insulin itself. Regular insulin does not need to be mixed prior to withdrawal, but intermediate- and long-acting insulins precipitate (settle) out. They need to be rotated and mixed immediately before withdrawal from the vial. **The smallest capacity syringe possible should be selected to prepare the dosage**, because the enlarged scale is easier to read and therefore more accurate.

The actual step-by-step procedure for combining insulins is as follows:

EXAMPLE 1

A dosage of 10 units of Regular and 48 units of NPH insulin has been ordered.

STEP 1 **Locate the correct insulins and rotate and upend the NPH until it is thoroughly mixed.**

STEP 2 **Use an alcohol wipe to cleanse both vial tops.**

STEP 3 The combined dosage (10 units + 48 units = 58 units) requires the use of a 100 units capacity syringe. Draw up 48 units of air and insert the needle into the NPH vial. Keep the needle tip above the insulin and inject the air. Withdraw the needle from the vial.

STEP 4 Draw up 10 units of air and inject this into the Regular insulin vial. Draw up the 10 units of Regular insulin.

STEP 5 Insert the needle back into the NPH vial and draw up 48 units of NPH insulin. This will require that you draw the plunger back until the total insulin in the syringe is 58 units (10 units Regular + 48 units NPH). Withdraw the needle and administer the insulin promptly so that the NPH does not have time to precipitate out.

EXAMPLE 2

The order is to give 16 units of Regular and 33 units of Lente insulin.

STEP 1 Locate the correct insulins and rotate the Lente to mix it.

STEP 2 Cleanse both vial tops.

STEP 3 Use a 50 unit capacity syringe (16 units + 22 units = 38 units). Draw up 22 units of air. Insert the needle in the Lente vial. Keep the needle tip above the insulin as you inject the air into the vial. Withdraw the needle.

STEP 4 Draw up 16 units of air and inject it into the Regular insulin vial. Draw up the 16 units of Regular insulin.

STEP 5 Insert the needle back into the Lente vial and draw up Lente insulin until the syringe capacity is 38 units (16 units Regular + 22 units Lente). Administer the dosage promptly.

PROBLEM

For each of the combined insulin dosages, indicate the total volume of the combined dosage and the smallest capacity syringe you can use to prepare it (30 units, 50 units, and 100 units capacity syringes are available).

	Total Volume	Syringe Size
1. 28 units Regular, 64 units NPH	_____	_____
2. 16 units Ultralente, 6 units Regular	_____	_____
3. 33 units Regular, 41 units Lente	_____	_____
4. 21 units Regular, 52 units NPH	_____	_____
5. 13 units Regular, 27 units Ultralente	_____	_____

ANSWERS **1.** 92 units; 100 units   **2.** 22 units; 30 units   **3.** 74 units; 100 units   **4.** 73 units; 100 units   **5.** 40 units; 50 units

Summary

This concludes the chapter on measuring insulin dosages. The important points to remember from this chapter are:

- *Insulin labels must be read very carefully because they look very similar.*

- *100 units/mL strength insulins are measured using specially calibrated insulin syringes.*

- *The smallest capacity syringe possible is used to increase accuracy of dosage preparation.*

- *Calibrations on 30 units and 50 units syringes are in 1 unit increments.*

- *Calibrations on 100 units syringes may be in 1 unit or 2 units increments.*

- *When insulin dosages are combined, the fastest-action insulin is drawn up first.*

- *Intermediate- and long-acting insulins precipitate out and must be thoroughly mixed immediately before measurement, and administered promptly after preparation.*

10

Summary Self-Test

Use the syringe calibrations provided to measure the following dosages. For combined insulin dosages, use arrows to indicate the exact calibration to be used for each insulin ordered. Have your instructor check your answers.

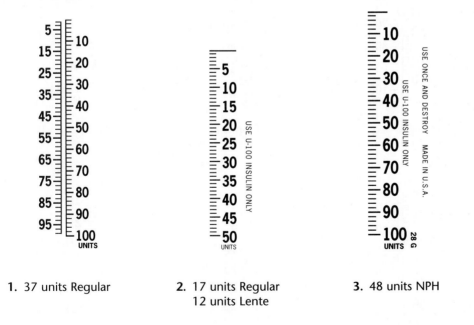

1. 37 units Regular

2. 17 units Regular
   12 units Lente

3. 48 units NPH

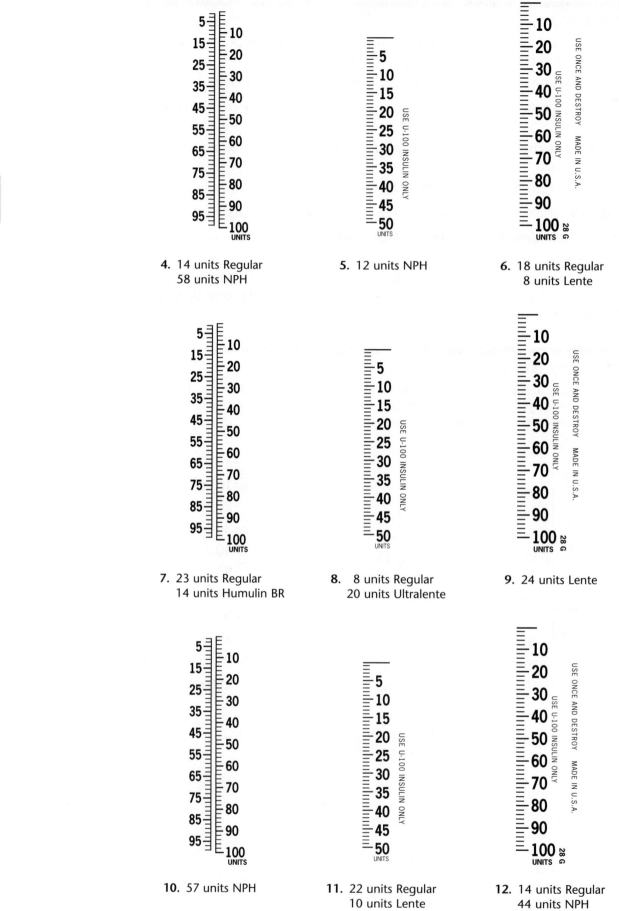

4. 14 units Regular
58 units NPH

5. 12 units NPH

6. 18 units Regular
8 units Lente

7. 23 units Regular
14 units Humulin BR

8. 8 units Regular
20 units Ultralente

9. 24 units Lente

10. 57 units NPH

11. 22 units Regular
10 units Lente

12. 14 units Regular
44 units NPH

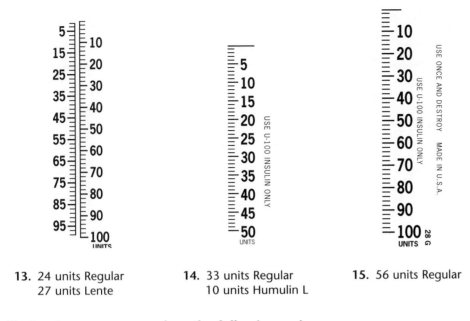

13. 24 units Regular
27 units Lente

14. 33 units Regular
10 units Humulin L

15. 56 units Regular

Identify the dosages measured on the following syringes.

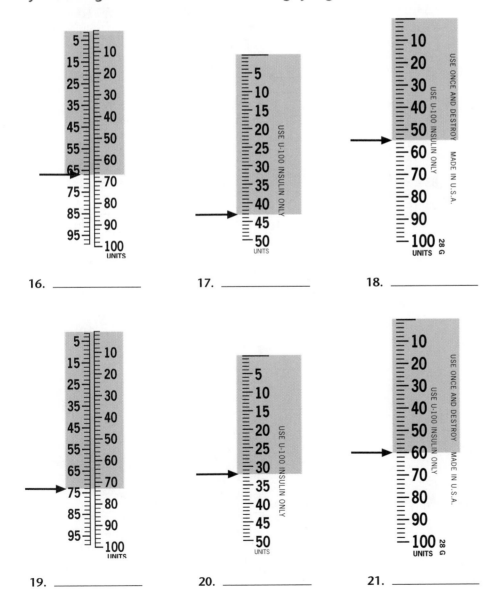

16. _____

17. _____

18. _____

19. _____

20. _____

21. _____

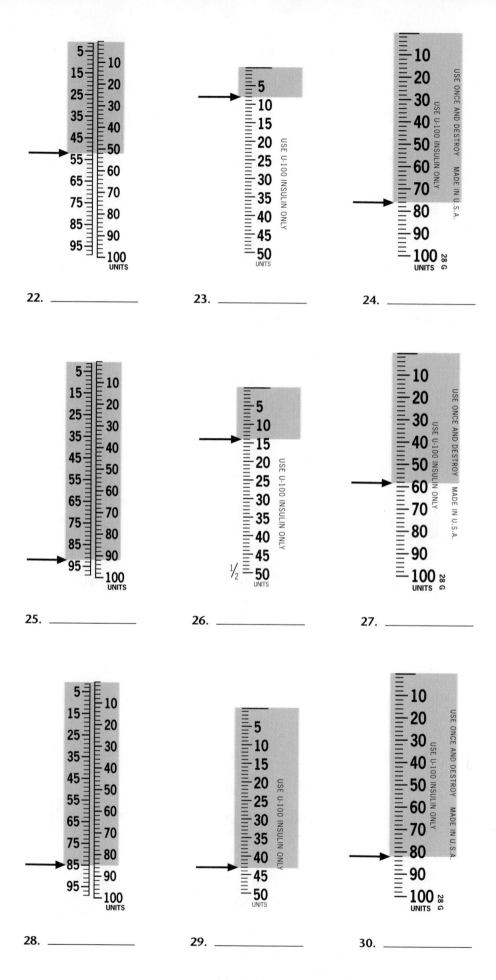

22. _____

23. _____

24. _____

25. _____

26. _____

27. _____

28. _____

29. _____

30. _____

10

SECTION FOUR

Dosage Calculation Using Dimensional Analysis

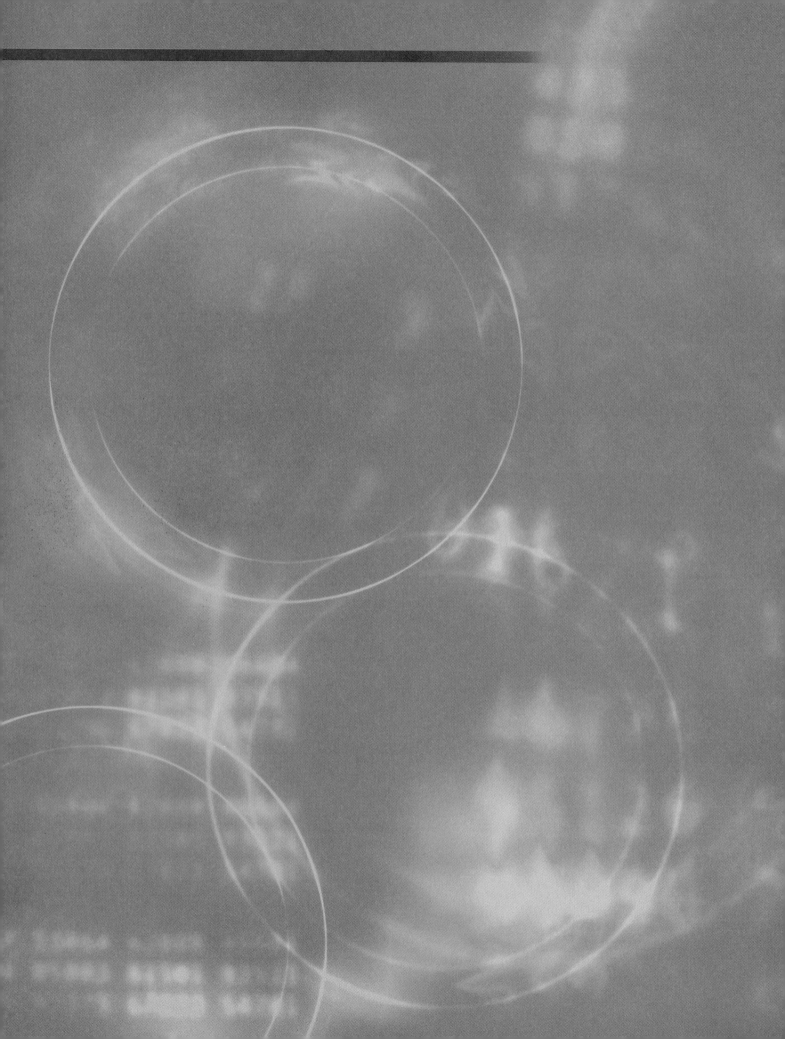

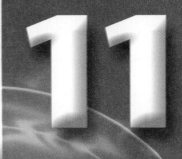

Dosage Calculation Using Dimensional Analysis

OBJECTIVES
The learner will:
1. use dimensional analysis to calculate dosages

PREREQUISITES
Chapters 1–8

Dimensional analysis (DA) is the name most commonly used in nursing and allied health for a **centuries' old calculation method** known as **units conversion**. You may already be familiar with units conversion from some of your physical science classes such as chemistry or physics, where it is widely used.

The tremendous advantage of DA is that it reduces the multiple steps required by most clinical calculations to **a single easy-to-solve equation**. DA is not difficult to learn, and once learned, its simplicity makes it virtually impossible to forget.

The Basic DA Equation

The best way to learn DA calculations is by doing them. Read each step of the following examples very carefully. Notice that color is used in the first few examples to help you follow the sequence of clinical ratio entry in the equation. Have scratch paper, pencil or pen, and your calculator ready to check the math in all examples.

EXAMPLE 1

The available dosage strength is **750 mg in 2.5 mL**, from which you must prepare a **600 mg** dosage.

The **first step** in setting up a DA equation is to **identify the unit of measure being calculated**. In **parenteral dosages** the unit being calculated **is always mL**. Enter the mL unit of measure being calculated **to the left of the equation, followed by an equal sign**.

$$mL =$$

There are two important reasons for identifying the unit of measure being calculated first: it eliminates any confusion over exactly **which** measure is being calculated, and it dictates how the first or "starting" clinical ratio, sometimes called a factor, is entered in the equation.

In a DA equation the unit of measure being calculated is written first to the left of the equation, followed by an equal sign.

When the mL unit of measure being calculated has been written, go back to the problem and **identify the complete clinical ratio that contains mL**. This is provided by the **dosage strength available**, which is **750 mg in 2.5 mL**. Enter this as a common fraction so that **the numerator entry matches the mL unit of measure being calculated: 2.5 mL** becomes the **numerator**, and **750 mg** becomes the **denominator**.

$$mL = \frac{2.5 \text{ mL}}{750 \text{ mg}}$$

In a DA equation the unit of measure being calculated must be matched in the numerator of the first clinical ratio entered.

From now on all additional ratios are entered so that **each denominator is matched in its successive numerator**. The **denominator in the first ratio is mg**, so the **next numerator must be mg**. Go back to the problem and you'll discover that this is provided by the **600 mg** dosage to be given. Enter this now as the next numerator to complete this single-step equation.

$$mL = \frac{2.5 \text{ mL}}{750 \text{ mg}} \times \frac{600 \text{ mg}}{}$$

The unit of measure in each denominator of a DA equation must be matched in the successive numerator entered.

All the pertinent clinical ratios have now been entered in this one-step DA equation. The next step is to **cancel the alternate denominator/numerator measurement units (but not their quantities) to be sure they match**. This check ensures that the clinical ratios were entered correctly. **After cancellation only the unit of measure being calculated should remain in the equation**. The denominator/numerator mg/mg units cancel, leaving only mL, the unit being calculated, remaining in the equation.

$$mL = \frac{2.5 \text{ mL}}{750 \text{ mg}} \times \frac{600 \text{ mg}}{}$$

Only the unit of measure being calculated should remain in the equation after the denominator and numerator units are cancelled.

Only mL, the unit being calculated, remains in the equation. The math can now be done.

$$mL = \frac{2.5 \text{ mL}}{750 \text{ mg}} \times \frac{600 \text{ mg}}{}$$

$$mL = \frac{2.5 \text{ mL}}{750 \text{ mg}} \times \frac{\overset{4}{600 \text{ mg}}}{5} \quad \text{divide by 150}$$

$$mL = \frac{\overset{2}{10}}{\underset{1}{5}} = 2 \text{ mL}$$

To obtain a dosage of 600 mg from an available dosage strength of 750 mg in 2.5 mL you would give 2 mL.

DA works exactly the same way for every calculation **regardless of the number of ratios entered**. As you can see, there are no complicated rules to memorize. In these simple steps you have already learned how to use DA for clinical calculations.

EXAMPLE 2

A dosage of **50,000 units** is ordered to be added to an IV solution. The strength available is **10,000 units/1.5 mL**. Calculate how many **mL** will contain this dosage.

Write the mL being calculated to the left of the equation followed by an equal sign.

$$mL =$$

The mL being calculated must be matched in the numerator of the first ratio entered. Look back at your problem and locate the complete ratio containing mL, the 10,000 units in 1.5 mL dosage strength available. Enter this ratio now with 1.5 mL as the numerator to match the mL numerator being calculated; 10,000 units becomes the denominator.

$$mL = \frac{1.5 \text{ mL}}{10,000 \text{ units}}$$

The units denominator of the first ratio must now be matched in the next numerator. This is provided by the 50,000 units ordered. Enter this now as the next numerator to complete this one-step equation.

$$mL = \frac{1.5 \text{ mL}}{10,000 \text{ units}} \times \frac{50,000 \text{ units}}{}$$

Cancel the alternate denominator/numerator units entries to double-check for correct ratio entry. Only the mL unit being calculated remains in the equation. Do the math.

$$mL = \frac{1.5 \text{ mL}}{10,000 \text{ units}} \times \frac{50,000 \text{ units}}{}$$

$$mL = \frac{15 \text{ mL}}{100,000 \text{ units}} \times \frac{\overset{1}{50,000} \text{ units}}{}_{2}$$

Eliminate the decimal point in 1.5, then reduce the numbers as much as possible; divide the final fraction

$$mL = \frac{15}{2} = 7.5 \text{ mL}$$

It will require a 7.5 mL volume of the 10,000 units/1.5 mL solution to prepare the 50,000 units ordered for this IV additive.

EXAMPLE 3

Tablet calculations are not common, but are done the same way using DA.

Scored (breakable) **tablets** with a strength of **0.5 mg** are available to prepare a dosage of **1.25 mg**. How many **tablets** must you give?

Enter the tab being calculated to the left of the equation followed by an equal sign.

$$tab =$$

The tab unit being calculated must be matched in the numerator of the first ratio entered. This is provided by the tab strength available, 0.5 mg in 1 tab. Enter this ratio with 1 tab as the numerator; 0.5 mg becomes the denominator.

$$\text{tab} = \frac{1 \text{ tab}}{0.5 \text{ mg}}$$

The mg denominator must now be matched in the next numerator. This is provided by the 1.25 mg ordered. Enter this now as the final numerator to complete the equation.

$$\text{tab} = \frac{1 \text{ tab}}{0.5 \text{ mg}} \times \frac{1.25 \text{ mg}}{}$$

Cancel the alternate denominator/numerator mg units to check that you have entered the ratios correctly. Only the tab being calculated remains. Do the math.

$$\text{tab} = \frac{1 \text{ tab}}{0.5 \;\cancel{\text{mg}}} \times \frac{1.25 \;\cancel{\text{mg}}}{}$$

$$\text{tab} = \frac{1 \text{ tab}}{\underset{2}{\cancel{50}} \;\cancel{\text{mg}}} \times \frac{\overset{5}{\cancel{125}} \;\cancel{\text{mg}}}{} \qquad \begin{array}{l}\text{Eliminate the decimal points.} \\ \text{Reduce the numbers}\end{array}$$

$$\text{tab} = \frac{5}{2} = \textbf{2.5 tab}$$

To obtain the 1.25 mg dosage ordered 2½ tab must be given.

Let's stop for a moment now and take a look at what happens if the ratios are incorrectly entered in a DA equation. We'll assume that the units of measure have not been entered with their quantities, and that the entries have been mixed up. The correct equation will be shown alongside for comparison.

EXAMPLE 4

A drug label reads **100 mg per 2 mL**. The medication order is for **130 mg**. How many **mL** must you prepare?

Correct	Incorrect
$\text{mL} = \dfrac{2 \text{ mL}}{100 \text{ mg}} \times \dfrac{130 \text{ mg}}{} = \textbf{2.6 mL}$	$\text{mL} = \dfrac{100}{2} \times \dfrac{130}{} = \textbf{6500 mL}$

In the incorrect equation the starting ratio is upside down, and since the units of measure were not entered with their quantities there is no way to catch this: the safety step of cancellation to check ratio entry cannot be done. But notice something else, the answer, 6500 mL, is impossible. If the entries in a DA equation are mixed up the numbers are often so outrageous that you will know instantly that you have made a mistake. **But mistakes are not always this obvious, so stick to the step-by-step calculation rules.** There is a reason for every one of them, and besides, they really are very simple. Let's look at a few more examples.

EXAMPLE 5

How many **mL** will you draw up to prepare a **1.2 g** dosage if the solution available is labeled **2 g in 3 mL?**

Write the mL unit being calculated to the left of the equation followed by an equal sign. Enter the starting ratio, 2 g in 3 mL, with mL as the numerator to match the mL being calculated; 2 g becomes the denominator.

$$\text{mL} = \frac{3 \text{ mL}}{2 \text{ g}}$$

Match the g denominator of the starting ratio in the next numerator with the 1.2 g ordered to complete the equation.

$$\text{mL} = \frac{3 \text{ mL}}{2 \text{ g}} \times \frac{1.2 \text{ g}}{}$$

Cancel the alternate denominator/numerator g units to double-check that the entries are correct. Only the mL being calculated remains.

$$\text{mL} = \frac{3 \text{ mL}}{2 \cancel{g}} \times \frac{1.2 \cancel{g}}{}$$

Do the math, expressing fractional answers to the nearest tenth.

$$\text{mL} = \frac{3 \text{ mL}}{2 \cancel{g}} \times \frac{1.2 \cancel{g}}{} = \textbf{1.8 mL}$$

The 1.2 g dosage ordered is contained in 1.8 mL of the 2 g/3 mL solution available.

EXAMPLE 6

Medication with a strength of **0.75 mg/mL** is available to prepare a dosage of **2 mg**. Calculate the mL this will require.

Write the mL being calculated to the left of the equation followed by an equal sign.

$$\text{mL} =$$

The mL being calculated must be matched with a numerator mL entry. This is provided by the 0.75 mg/mL ratio dosage strength available. Enter this with 1 mL as the numerator and 0.75 mg as the denominator.

$$\text{mL} = \frac{1 \text{ mL}}{0.75 \text{ mg}}$$

The mg denominator must now be matched. This is provided by the 2 mg dosage ordered. Enter this now as the final numerator to complete this one-step equation.

$$\text{mL} = \frac{1 \text{ mL}}{0.75 \text{ mg}} \times \frac{2 \text{ mg}}{}$$

Cancel the alternate denominator/numerator mg units of measure to check for correct ratio entry, then do the math.

$$\text{mL} = \frac{1 \text{ mL}}{0.75 \cancel{\text{ mg}}} \times \frac{2 \cancel{\text{ mg}}}{} = 2.67 = \textbf{2.7 mL}$$

It will require 2.7 mL of the 0.75 mg in 1 mL dosage available to administer the 2 mg ordered.

Calculate the following dosages using DA. Express mL answers to the nearest tenth.

1. A dosage of 0.3 g has been ordered. The strength available is 0.4 g/1.5 mL. _____

2. A dosage strength of 0.8 mg in 2 mL is to be used to prepare a 0.5 mg dosage. _____

3. Prepare a 1.8 mg dosage from a solution labeled 2 mg/3 mL. _____

4. The order is for 1500 mg. You have available a 1200 mg/mL solution. _____

5. A dosage strength of 0.2 mg in 1.5 mL is available. Give 0.15 mg. _____

6. The strength available is 1000 mg in 3.6 mL. Prepare a 600 mg dosage. _____

7. A 10,000 units dosage has been ordered. The strength available is 8000 units in 1 mL. _____

8. An IV additive has a dosage strength of 20 mEq per 20 mL. A dosage of 15 mEq has been ordered. _____

9. A 200,000 units dosage must be prepared from a 150,000 units/2 mL strength. _____

10. An IV additive order is for 400 mg. The solution available has a strength of 500 mg in 20 mL. _____

ANSWERS **1.** 1.1 mL **2.** 1.3 mL **3.** 2.7 mL **4.** 1.3 mL **5.** 1.1 mL **6.** 2.2 mL **7.** 1.3 mL **8.** 15 mL **9.** 2.7 mL **10.** 16 mL

You now know the basics of using DA in calculations. But **how do you know if the answer you obtain is correct?** The answer to this question is provided by the key points already covered:

if the unit being calculated is correctly identified to the left of the equation

if the starting ratio is entered so that its numerator matches the unit of measure being calculated

if the unit of measure in each denominator is matched in each successively entered numerator

if the only unit of measure remaining after cancellation is the same as the unit of measure being calculated

if the quantities have been correctly entered

if the math has been double-checked and is correct

then the answer will be correct.

A tall order? Not really. You are doing a clinical dosage calculation. All you must do is double-check each step and the answer will be correct.

In addition, **don't divorce your previous learning and reasoning from the calculation process.** You already know that most IM dosages are contained in a 0.5–3 mL volume, that IV additives may be contained in larger volumes, and that large numbers of tab/cap are unusual in dosages. **If you get an unreasonable answer to a calculation you must question it.** In time you will know the average dosages of all the drugs you give, and another safety component will be added to your repertoire, but that is beyond the scope of this text. For now, concentrate on the simple mechanics of calculation you have just been taught. Don't shortcut these steps, and you'll do just fine.

Equations Requiring Metric Conversions

The big advantage of DA is that it allows multiple ratios to be entered in a single equation, thus reducing calculation steps. This is especially useful when a drug is ordered in one unit of measure, for example mg, but is labeled in another, for example g or mcg.

There are two ways to handle a conversion. Sometimes it will be easier to do the conversion before setting up the equation. In other instances you may elect to incorporate the conversion into an equation. For practice purposes let's look at how **conversion ratios**, for example, **1 g = 1000 mg** or **1 mg = 1000 mcg**, are entered in a DA equation.

EXAMPLE 1

The IM dosage ordered is **275 mg**. The drug available is labeled **0.5 g per 2 mL**. How many **mL** must you give?

Enter the mL to be calculated to the left of the equation. Locate the ratio containing mL, the 0.5 g per 2 mL dosage strength, and enter it, with 2 mL as the numerator; 0.5 g becomes the denominator.

$$\text{mL} = \frac{2 \text{ mL}}{0.5 \text{ g}}$$

When you refer back to the problem you will not find a g measure to match the starting ratio g denominator. The dosage to be given is in mg. So a **conversion ratio** between g and mg is needed: 1 g = 1000 mg. Enter it now, with 1 g as the numerator to match the g of the previous denominator; 1000 mg becomes the new denominator.

$$\text{mL} = \frac{2 \text{ mL}}{0.5 \text{ g}} \times \frac{1 \text{ g}}{1000 \text{ mg}}$$

The final entry, the 275 mg dosage to be given, will automatically fall into its correct position as it is entered as the final numerator, to match the mg unit of the previous denominator. The equation is now complete.

$$\text{mL} = \frac{2 \text{ mL}}{0.5 \text{ g}} \times \frac{1 \text{ g}}{1000 \text{ mg}} \times \frac{275 \text{ mg}}{}$$

Cancel the alternate denominator/numerator g/g and mg/mg units to double-check ratio entry. Only the mL being calculated remains. Do the math.

$$\text{mL} = \frac{2 \text{ mL}}{0.5 \text{ g}} \times \frac{1 \text{ g}}{1000 \text{ mg}} \times \frac{275 \text{ mg}}{} = \textbf{1.1 mL}$$

To give a dosage of 275 mg you must prepare 1.1 mL of the 0.5 g/2 mL strength solution.

EXAMPLE 2

The drug label reads **800 mcg in 1.5 mL**. The IM order is for **0.6 mg**.

Enter the mL to be calculated and an equal sign to the left of the equation. Locate the ratio containing mL: 800 mcg/1.5 mL. Enter this with 1.5 mL as the numerator to match the mL being calculated; 800 mcg becomes the denominator.

$$\text{mL} = \frac{1.5 \text{ mL}}{800 \text{ mcg}}$$

There is no mcg measure in the problem, which is your cue to the necessity for a conversion ratio. Enter the 1000 mcg = 1 mg conversion ratio with 1000 mcg as the numerator to match the mcg of the previous denominator; 1 mg becomes the denominator.

$$\text{mL} = \frac{1.5 \text{ mL}}{800 \text{ mcg}} \times \frac{1000 \text{ mcg}}{1 \text{ mg}}$$

The mg denominator is now matched by entering the 0.6 mg dosage to be given and completes the equation.

$$\text{mL} = \frac{1.5 \text{ mL}}{800 \text{ mcg}} \times \frac{1000 \text{ mcg}}{1 \text{ mg}} \times \frac{0.6 \text{ mg}}{}$$

Cancel the alternate denominator/numerator mcg/mcg and mg/mg units of measure to check for correct ratio entry. Only the mL unit being calculated should remain in the equation. Do the math.

$$\text{mL} = \frac{1.5 \text{ mL}}{800 \text{ mcg}} \times \frac{1000 \text{ mcg}}{1 \text{ mg}} \times \frac{0.6 \text{ mg}}{} = 1.12 = \textbf{1.1 mL}$$

To give a dosage of 0.6 mg from the available 1.5 mL/800 mcg strength you must prepare 1.1 mL.

EXAMPLE 3

Prepare a **0.5 mg** dosage from an available strength of **200 mcg per mL**.

Enter the mL being calculated to the left of the equation followed by an equal sign. Enter the 1 mL/200 mcg dosage available as the starting ratio, with 1 mL as the numerator to match the mL being calculated; 200 mcg becomes the denominator.

$$\text{mL} = \frac{1 \text{ mL}}{200 \text{ mcg}}$$

A mcg to mg conversion ratio is needed. Enter this with 1000 mcg as the numerator to match the mcg in the previous denominator; 1 mg becomes the denominator.

$$\text{mL} = \frac{1 \text{ mL}}{200 \text{ mcg}} \times \frac{1000 \text{ mcg}}{1 \text{ mg}}$$

The mg denominator must now be matched. Enter the 0.5 mg dosage ordered as the final numerator to complete the equation.

$$\text{mL} = \frac{1 \text{ mL}}{200 \text{ mcg}} \times \frac{1000 \text{ mcg}}{1 \text{ mg}} \times \frac{0.5 \text{ mg}}{}$$

Cancel the alternate mcg/mcg and mg/mg measurement units to double-check for correct ratio entry. Only the mL unit being calculated remains in the equation. Do the math.

$$\text{mL} = \frac{1 \text{ mL}}{200 \text{ mcg}} \times \frac{1000 \text{ mcg}}{1 \text{ mg}} \times \frac{0.5 \text{ mg}}{} = \textbf{2.5 mL}$$

A 0.5 mg dosage requires a 2.5 mL volume of the 200 mcg/mL strength solution available.

EXAMPLE 4

The medication has a strength of **0.5 g/1.5 mL**. Prepare **750 mg**.

Enter the mL to be calculated to the left of the equation with its equal sign. Enter the starting ratio the 1.5 mL/0.5 g dosage available, with 1.5 mL as the numerator to match the mL being calculated; 0.5 g becomes the denominator.

$$mL = \frac{1.5 \text{ mL}}{0.5 \text{ g}}$$

There is no g dosage in the problem, which signals the need for a conversion ratio. Enter the 1 g = 1000 mg conversion ratio with 1 g as the numerator, to match the g in the denominator of the starting ratio; 1000 mg becomes the denominator.

$$mL = \frac{1.5 \text{ mL}}{0.5 \text{ g}} \times \frac{1 \text{ g}}{1000 \text{ mg}}$$

Enter the dosage ordered, 750 mg, as the final numerator to match the mg in the previous denominator. The equation is complete.

$$mL = \frac{1.5 \text{ mL}}{0.5 \text{ g}} \times \frac{1 \text{ g}}{1000 \text{ mg}} \times \frac{750 \text{ mg}}{}$$

Cancel the alternate g/g and mg/mg units to check the accuracy of ratio entry, then complete the math.

$$mL = \frac{1.5 \text{ mL}}{0.5 \text{ g}} \times \frac{1 \text{ g}}{1000 \text{ mg}} \times \frac{750 \text{ mg}}{} = 2.25 = \textbf{2.3 mL}$$

A 750 mg dosage requires 2.3 mL of the 0.5 g in 1.5 mL medication.

Calculate the dosages. Express mL answers to the nearest tenth.

1. Prepare 0.1 g of an IM medication from a strength of 200 mg/mL. _____

2. A drug label reads 0.1 g/2 mL. Prepare a 130 mg dosage. _____

3. An oral solution has a strength of 500 mg/5 mL. Prepare a 0.6 g dosage. _____

4. Prepare a 0.75 g dosage from a 250 mg/mL strength solution. _____

5. Prepare 500 mg for IM injection from an available strength of 1 g per 3 mL. _____

6. A dosage of 85 mg is ordered, and the drug available is labeled 0.1 g/1.5 mL. _____

7. The strength available is 500 mcg in 1.5 mL. Prepare a 0.75 mg dosage. _____

8. A dosage of 1500 mg has been ordered. Solution available is 0.5 g per mL. _____

9. The dosage strength available is 200 mcg per mL. A 0.5 mg dosage has been ordered. _____

10. The dosage ordered is 0.2 g. Tablets available are labeled 80 mg. _____

ANSWERS 1. 0.5 mL 2. 2.6 mL 3. 6 mL 4. 3 mL 5. 1.5 mL 6. 1.3 mL 7. 2.3 mL 8. 3 mL
9. 2.5 mL 10. 2½ tab

Summary

This ends your introduction to clinical calculations using DA (dimensional analysis). The important points to remember from this chapter are:

The unit of measure being calculated is written first to the left of the equation, followed by an equal sign.

*All ratios entered must include the quantity **and** the unit of measure.*

The numerator in the starting ratio must be in the same measurement unit as the unit of measure being calculated.

*The unit of measure in each denominator **must** be matched in the numerator of each successive ratio entered.*

Metric system conversions can be made by incorporating a conversion ratio directly into the DA equation.

The unit of measure in each alternate denominator and numerator must cancel, leaving only the unit of measure being calculated remaining in the equation.

The numerator of the starting ratio is never canceled.

Summary Self-Test

Use DA equations to calculate the dosages. Express mL answers to the nearest tenth (or hundredth where indicated) using the medication labels provided. Measure the dosages you calculate on the syringes provided. Have your answers checked by your instructor to be sure you have calculated and measured the dosages correctly.

Dosage Ordered   **mL Needed**

1. Depo-Provera® 0.3 g   _____

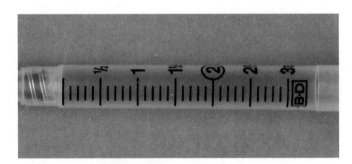

For IM use only.
See package insert for complete product information.
Shake vigorously immediately before each use.
Pharmacia & Upjohn Company
Kalamazoo, MI 49001, USA

NDC 0009-0626-01   2.5 mL Vial
Depo-Provera®
medroxyprogesterone acetate injectable suspension, USP
400 mg/mL

Dosage Ordered	mL Needed

2. furosemide 15 mg _____

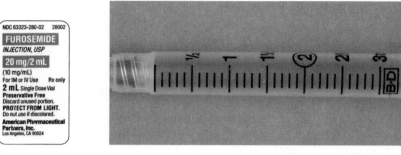

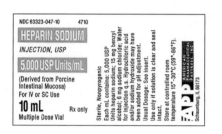

3. heparin 2000 units
(calculate to the nearest hundredth) _____

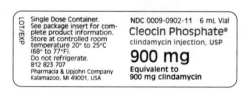

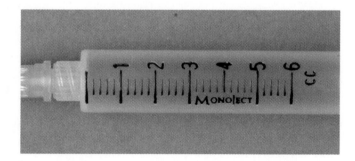

4. Cleocin® 0.75 g
for an IV additive _____

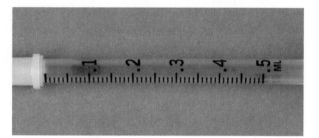

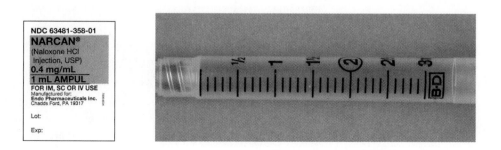

5. naloxone 350 mcg _____

Dosage Ordered	mL Needed

6. clindamycin 225 mg _____

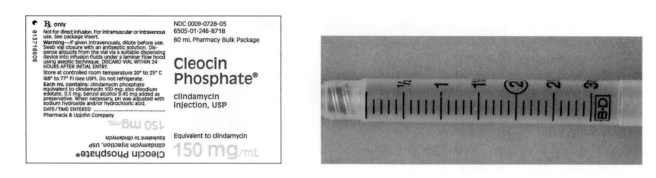

7. Robinul® 75 mcg
(calculate to the nearest
hundredth) _____

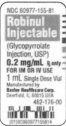

8. Tigan® 0.3 g _____

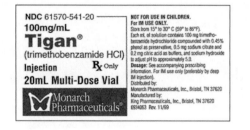

9. benztropine mesylate 2.4 mg _____

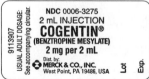

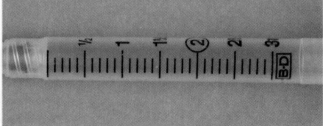

Dosage Ordered	mL Needed

10. cyanocobalamin 800 mcg   _____

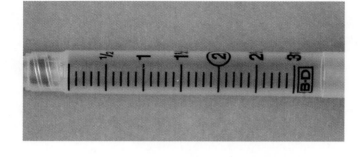

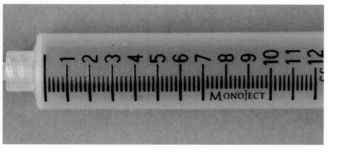

11. potassium chloride 16 mEq
for IV additive   _____

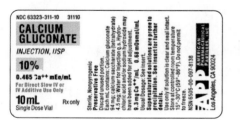

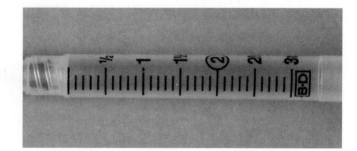

12. calcium gluconate 0.93 mEq
for an IV additive   _____

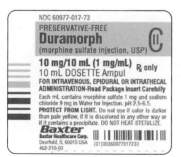

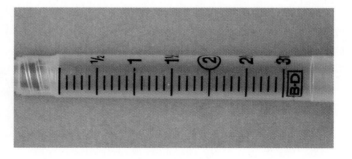

13. morphine sulfate 1.5 mg   _____

Dosage Ordered	mL Needed

14. heparin 450 units (calculate to the nearest hundredth)

_____

NDC 63323-038-10   3810

HEPARIN SODIUM

INJECTION, USP

1,000 USP Units/mL

(Derived from Beef Lung)

For IV or SC Use

10 mL   Rx only

Multiple Dose Vial

Sterile, Nonpyrogenic
Each mL contains: 1,000 USP Units heparin sodium; 15 mg benzyl alcohol; 9 mg sodium chloride; Water for Injection q.s. Hydrochloric acid and/or sodium hydroxide may have been added for pH adjustment.
Usual Dosage: See insert.
Use only if solution is clear and seal intact.
Store at controlled room temperature 15°-30°C (59°-86°F).
NSN 6505-00-088-6747

APP
PHARMACEUTICAL PARTNERS INC.
Los Angeles, CA 90024

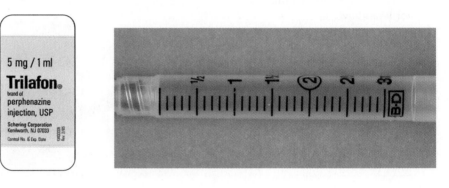

15. perphenazine 3 mg

_____

5 mg / 1 ml

Trilafon®

brand of
perphenazine
injection, USP

Schering Corporation
Kenilworth, NJ 07033

Control No. & Exp. Date

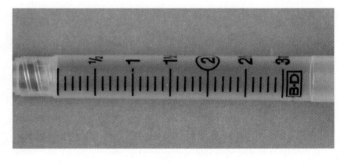

16. Dilantin® 0.1 g

_____

Dosage–See package insert.
Rx only

Manufactured by:
Parkedale Pharmaceuticals, Inc.
Rochester, MI 48307
For:
PARKE-DAVIS
Div of Warner-Lambert Co
Morris Plains, NJ 07950 USA

N 0071-4475-45
STERI-VIAL®
Dilantin®
(Phenytoin Sodium Injection, USP)
ready/mixed
250 mg in 5 mL
5 mL

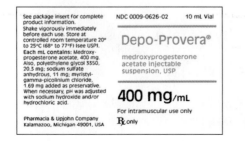

17. medroxyprogesterone 0.9 g

_____

See package insert for complete product information.
Shake vigorously immediately before each use. Store at controlled room temperature 20° to 25°C (68° to 77°F) [see USP].
Each mL contains: Medroxy-progesterone acetate, 400 mg. Also, polyethylene glycol 3350, 20.3 mg; sodium sulfate anhydrous, 11 mg; myristyl-gamma-picolinium chloride, 1.69 mg added as preservative. When necessary, pH was adjusted with sodium hydroxide and/or hydrochloric acid.

Pharmacia & Upjohn Company
Kalamazoo, Michigan 49001, USA

NDC 0009-0626-02   10 mL Vial

Depo-Provera®

medroxyprogesterone acetate injectable suspension, USP

400 mg/mL

For intramuscular use only
Rx only

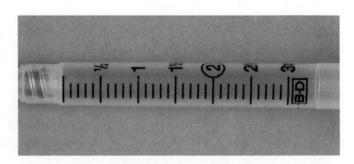

Dosage Ordered	mL Needed

18. gentamicin 70 mg _____

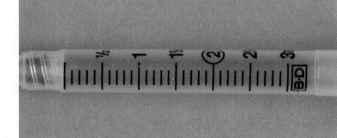

19. Vistaril® 120 mg _____

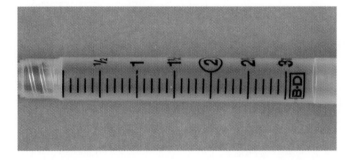

20. sodium chloride 60 mEq _____
for an IV additive

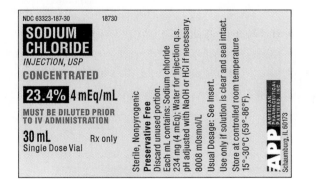
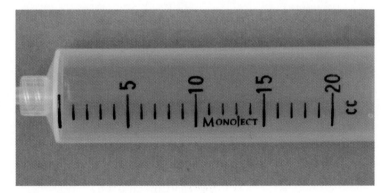

21. atropine 150 mcg   _____

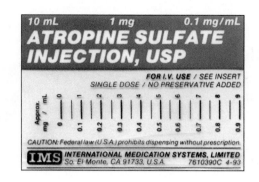

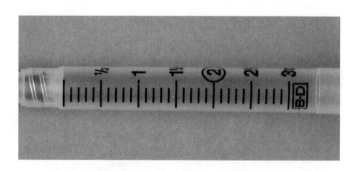

22. meperidine 75 mg   _____

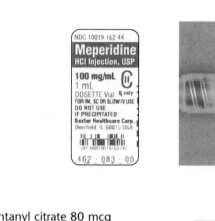

23. fentanyl citrate 80 mcg   _____

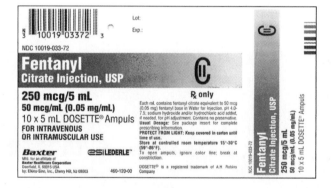

24. clindamycin 0.4 g   _____

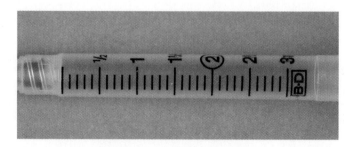

25. morphine sulfate 20 mg   _____

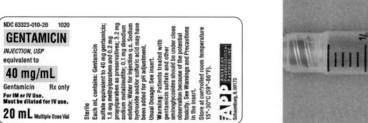

26. gentamicin 0.1 g   _____

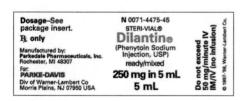

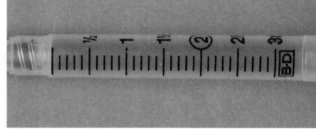

27. Dilantin® 0.15 g   _____

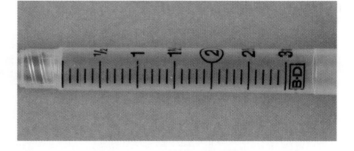

28. doxorubicin HCl 16 mg
for an IV additive   _____

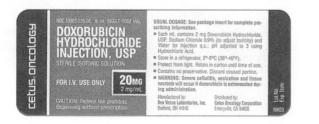

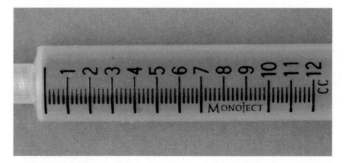

29. meperidine HCl 30 mg _____

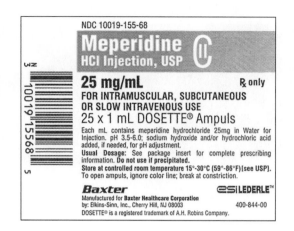

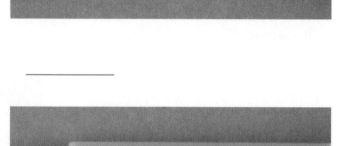

30. methotrexate 40 mg _____

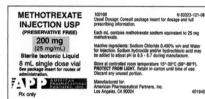

31. Celestone® 12 mg _____

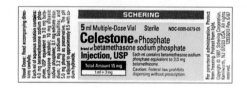

32. haloperidol decanoate 75 mg _____

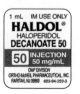

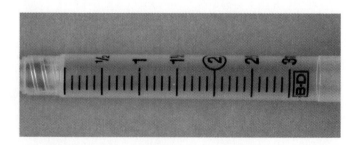

Dosage Ordered	mL Needed

33. dexamethasone 5 mg   _____

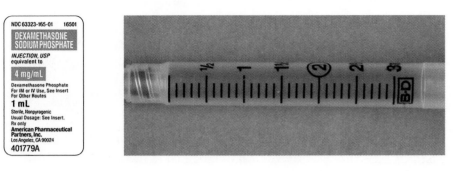

34. chlorpromazine HCl 40 mg   _____

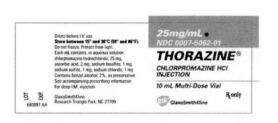

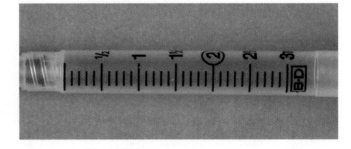

35. Pronestyl® 0.4 g   _____

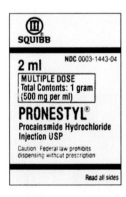

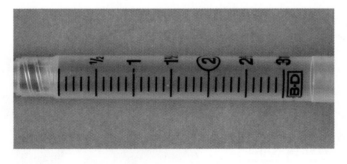

36. nalbuphine HCl 30 mg   _____

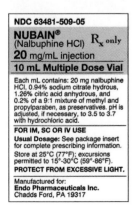

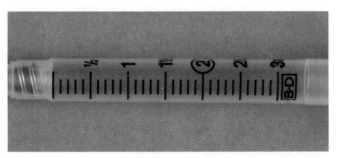

Dosage Ordered	mL Needed

37. morphine 15 mg _____

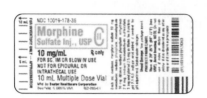

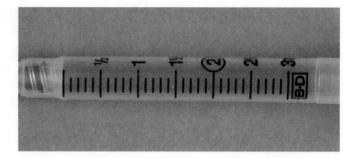

38. cyanocobalamin 750 mg _____

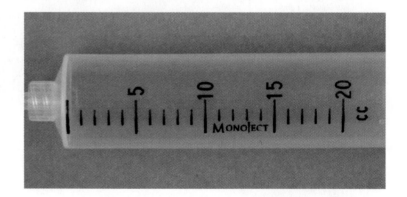

39. aminophylline 0.4 g
for an IV additive _____

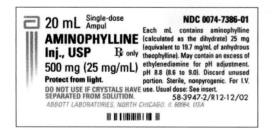

Dosage Ordered	mL Needed

40. naloxone HCl 0.5 mg _____

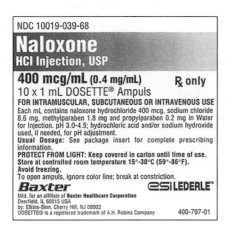

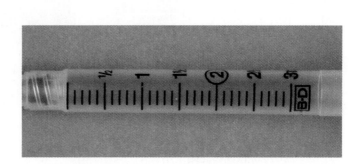

41. Cogentin® 1.5 mg _____

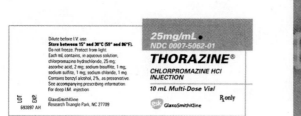

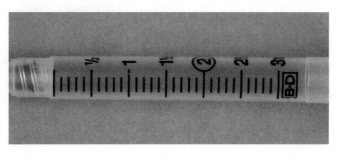

42. chlorpromazine 60 mg _____

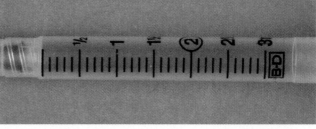

43. gentamicin 0.1 g _____

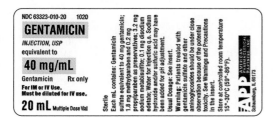

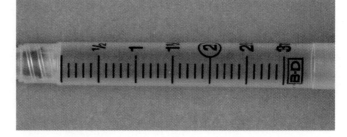

Dosage Ordered	mL Needed

44. Robinul® 180 mcg _____

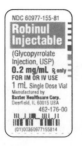

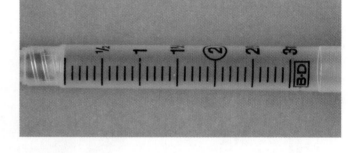

45. hydroxyzine HCl 70 mg _____

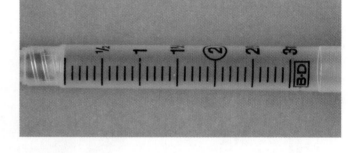

46. Bicillin® C-R 400,000 units _____

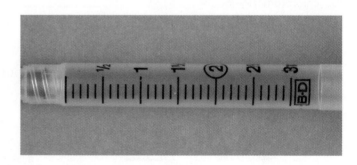

47. heparin sodium 2500 units _____
(calculate to the nearest hundredth)

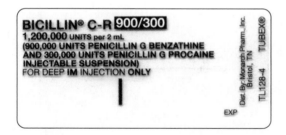

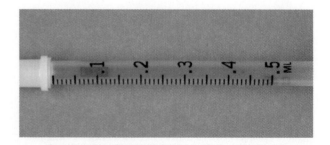

Dosage Ordered	mL Needed

48. potassium chloride 20 mEq
for an IV additive

_____

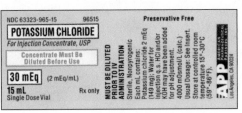

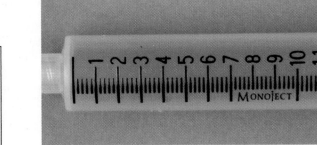

49. oxytocin 25 units

_____

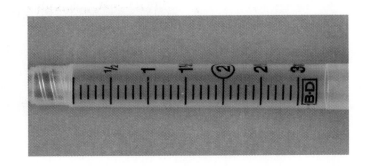

50. epinephrine 1.4 mg

_____

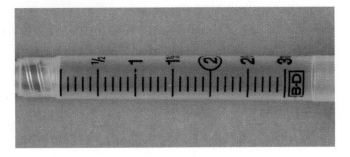

51. Depo-Provera® 0.45 g

_____

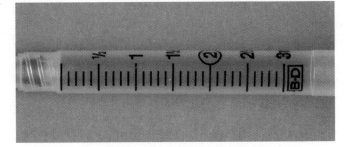

	Dosage Ordered	**mL Needed**

52. furosemide 15 mg _____

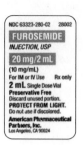

53. dexamethasone 6000 mcg _____

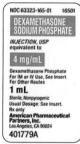

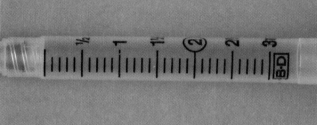

54. phenytoin Na 0.1 g _____

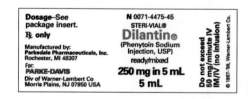

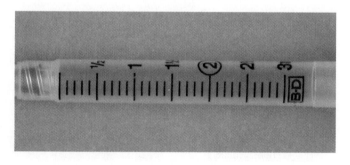

55. lidocaine HCl 15 mg _____

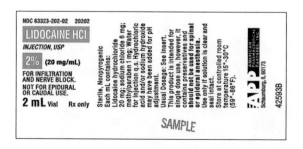

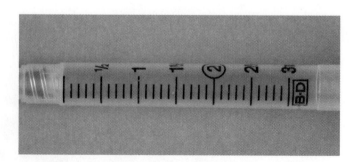

ANSWERS

1. 0.8 mL	12. 2 mL	23. 1.6 mL	34. 1.6 mL	45. 1.4 mL
2. 1.5 mL	13. 1.5 mL	24. 2.7 mL	35. 0.8 mL	46. 0.7 mL
3. 0.4 mL	14. 0.45 mL	25. 1.3 mL	36. 1.5 mL	47. 0.5 mL
4. 5 mL	15. 0.6 mL	26. 2.5 mL	37. 1.5 mL	48. 10 mL
5. 0.9 mL	16. 2 mL	27. 3 mL	38. 0.8 mL	49. 2.5 mL
6. 1.5 mL	17. 2.3 mL	28. 8 mL	39. 16 mL	50. 1.4 mL
7. 0.38 mL	18. 1.8 mL	29. 1.2 mL	40. 1.3 mL	51. 1.1 mL
8. 3 mL	19. 2.4 mL	30. 1.6 mL	41. 1.5 mL	52. 1.5 mL
9. 2.4 mL	20. 15 mL	31. 4 mL	42. 2.4 mL	53. 1.5 mL
10. 0.8 mL	21. 1.5 mL	32. 1.5 mL	43. 2.5 mL	54. 2 mL
11. 8 mL	22. 0.8 mL	33. 1.3 mL	44. 0.9 mL	55. 0.8 mL

Dosage Calculation from Body Weight and Body Surface Area

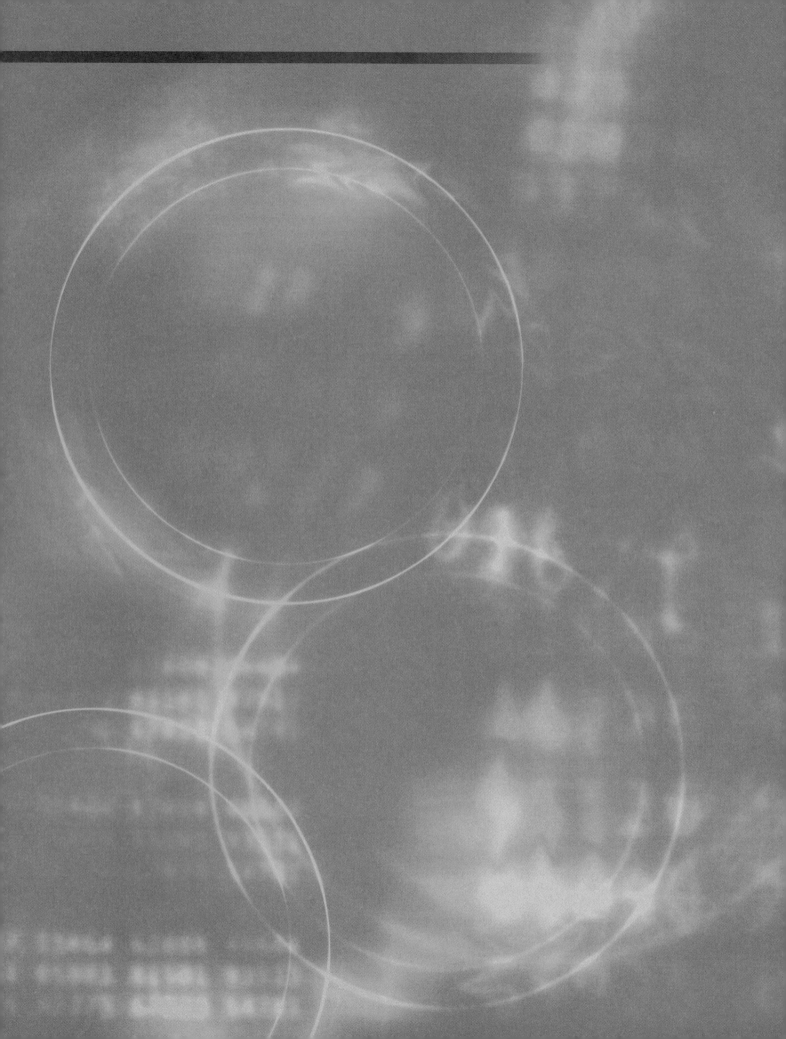

Adult and Pediatric Dosages Based on Body Weight

Body weight is a major factor in calculating drug dosages for both adults and children. It is the most important determiner of dosages for infants and neonates, whose ability to metabolize drugs is not fully developed. The dosage that will produce optimum therapeutic results for any particular individual, either child or adult, depends not only on dosage but on individual variables, including drug sensitivities and tolerance, age, weight, sex, and metabolic, pathologic, or psychologic conditions.

The physician will, of course, order the drug and dosage. However, it is a nursing responsibility to check each dosage to be sure the order is correct. Each drug label or drug package insert provides specific dosage details, but more complete information is readily available in drug formularies, the *PDR*, and other nursing and medical references. The hospital pharmacist is an excellent resource person who can also supply additional information.

Individualized dosages can be calculated in terms of mcg or mg per kg or lb, per day. The total daily dosage may be administered in divided (more than one) dosages, for example, q.6.h. (four doses), or t.i.d. (three doses).

Because body weight is critical in calculating infant and neonatal dosages, measurement is done using a scale calibrated in kg. Adult weights may be recorded in either kg or lb, and occasionally conversions between these two measures are necessary.

OBJECTIVES

The learner will:
1. convert body weight from lb to kg
2. convert body weight from kg to lb
3. calculate dosages using mg/kg, mcg/kg, and mg/lb
4. determine if dosages ordered are within the normal range

Converting lb to kg

If body weight is recorded in lb, but the drug literature lists dosage per kg, a conversion from lb to kg will be necessary. There are 2.2 lb in 1 kg. This means that kg body weights are smaller than lb weights, so **the conversion from lb to kg is made by dividing body weight by 2.2**. For ease of calculation, fractional lb, in adults only, may sometimes be converted to the nearest quarter lb, and written as decimal fractions instead of oz: ¼ lb (4 oz) as 0.25, ½ lb (8 oz) as 0.5, and ¾ lb (12 oz) as 0.75. No approximation is appropriate for infants or neonates.

EXAMPLE *1*　A child weighs 41 lb 12 oz. Convert to the nearest tenth kg.

41 lb 12 oz = 41.75 ÷ 2.2 = 18.97 = **19 kg**

The kg weight should be a smaller number than 41.75 because you are dividing, and it is, 19 kg.

EXAMPLE *2*　Convert the weight of a 144½ lb adult to the nearest tenth kg.

144½ = 144.5 ÷ 2.2 = 65.68 = **65.7 kg**

EXAMPLE *3*　Convert the weight of a 27¼ lb child to the nearest tenth kg.

27¼ lb = 27.25 ÷ 2.2 = 12.38 = **12.4 kg**

PROBLEM

Convert the body weights from lb to kg. Round weights to the nearest tenth kg.

1. 58¾ lb　=　_____ kg
2. 63½ lb　=　_____ kg
3. 163¼　=　_____ kg
4. 39¾　=　_____ kg
5. 100¼　=　_____ kg

6. 134½　=　_____ kg
7. 112¾　=　_____ kg
8. 73¼　=　_____ kg
9. 121½　=　_____ kg
10. 92¾　=　_____ kg

ANSWERS　1. 26.7 kg　2. 28.9 kg　3. 74.2 kg　4. 18.1 kg　5. 45.6 kg　6. 61.1 kg　7. 51.3 kg　8. 33.3 kg　9. 55.2 kg　10. 42.2 kg

Converting kg to lb

There are 2.2 lb in 1 kg. To convert from kg to lb, **multiply by 2.2**. Because you are multiplying, the answer in lb will be **larger** than the kg you started with. Express weight to the nearest tenth lb.

EXAMPLE *1*　A child weighs 23.3 kg. Convert to lb.

23.3 kg = 23.3 × 2.2 = 51.26 = **51.3 lb**

The answer must be larger because you are multiplying, and it is.

EXAMPLE *2*　Convert an adult weight of 73.4 kg to lb.

73.4 kg = 73.4 × 2.2 = 161.48 = **161.5 lb**

EXAMPLE *3*　Convert the weight of a 14.2 kg child to lb.

14.2 kg = 14.2 × 2.2 = 31.24 = **31.2 lb**

PROBLEM

Convert the body weights from kg to lb. Round weights to the nearest tenth lb.

1. 21.3 kg = _____ lb   6. 43.7 kg = _____ lb

2. 99.2 kg = _____ lb   7. 63.8 kg = _____ lb

3. 28.7 kg = _____ lb   8. 57.1 kg = _____ lb

4. 71.4 kg = _____ lb   9. 84.2 kg = _____ lb

5. 30.8 kg = _____ lb   10. 34.9 kg = _____ lb

ANSWERS   **1.** 46.9 lb   **2.** 218.2 lb   **3.** 63.1 lb   **4.** 157.1 lb   **5.** 67.8 lb   **6.** 96.1 lb   **7.** 140.4 lb   **8.** 125.6 lb   **9.** 185.2 lb   **10.** 76.8 lb

12

Calculating Dosages from Drug Label Information

The information you need to calculate dosages from body weight may be included on the actual drug label, which is common for pediatric oral liquid medications.

Calculating the dosage is a two-step procedure. First the **total daily dosage** is calculated, then it is **divided by the number of doses per day** to obtain the actual dose administered at one time.

Let's start by looking at some pediatric oral antibiotic labels that contain the mg/kg/day dosage guidelines.

EXAMPLE 1   Refer to the information written sideways on the left of the sample antibiotic label in Figure 12-1 for children's dosages. Notice that the average dosage is 20–40 mg/kg/day, or 40 mg/day for otitis media (ear infections). This dosage is to be given in three divided doses, or every 8 hours (24 hr ÷ 3 = 8 hr).

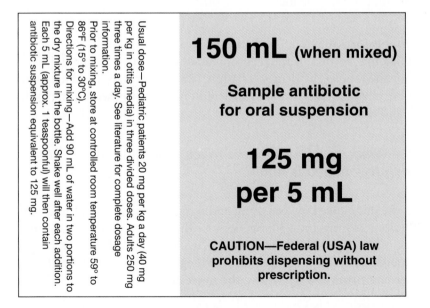

Figure 12-1

Once you have located the dosage information, you can move ahead and calculate the dosage. Let's assume you are checking the dosage ordered for an 18.2 kg child. Start by calculating the recommended 20–40 mg daily dosage range.

$$\textbf{Lower daily dosage} \ = \ 20 \ \text{mg/kg}$$

$$20 \ \text{mg} \ \times \ 18.2 \ \text{kg (weight of child)} \ = \ 364 \ \text{mg/day}$$

$$\textbf{Upper daily dosage} \ = \ 40 \ \text{mg/kg}$$

$$40 \ \text{mg} \ \times \ 18.2 \ \text{kg} \ = \ 728 \ \text{mg/day}$$

The recommended range for this 18.2 kg child is **364–728 mg/day**.

The drug is to be given in three divided doses.

$$\textbf{Lower dosage} \quad 364 \ \text{mg} \ \div \ 3 \ = \ \textbf{121 mg per dose}$$

$$\textbf{Upper dosage} \quad 728 \ \text{mg} \ \div \ 3 \ = \ \textbf{243 mg per dose}$$

The per dose dosage range is **121 mg to 243 mg per dose q.8.h.**

Now that you have the dosage range for this child, you are able to assess the accuracy of orders. Let's look at some orders and see how you can use the dosage range you just calculated.

1. **If the order is to give 125 mg q.8.h., is this within the recommended dosage range?**
   Yes, 125 mg q.8.h. is within the average range of 121–243 mg per dose.

2. **If the order is to give 375 mg q.8.h., is this within the recommended dosage range?**
   No, this is an overdosage. The maximum recommended dosage is 243 mg per dose. The 375 mg dose should not be given; the physician must be called and the order questioned.

3. **If the order is for 75 mg q.8.h., is this an accurate dosage?**
   The recommended lower limit for an 18.2 kg child is 121 mg. Although 75 mg might be safe, it will probably be ineffective. Notify the physician that the dosage appears to be too low.

4. **If the order is for 250 mg q.8.h., is this accurate?**
   Because 243 mg per dose is the recommended upper limit, 250 mg q.8.h. is essentially within normal range. The drug strength is 125 mg per 5 mL, and a 250 mg dosage is 10 mL. The physician has probably ordered this dosage based on the available dosage strength and ease of preparation.

 Discrepancies in dosages are much more significant if the quantity ordered is small.

For example, the difference between 4 mg and 6 mg is much more critical than the difference between 243 mg and 250 mg, because the drug potency is obviously greater. Additional factors that must be considered are age, weight, and medical condition. Although these factors cannot be dealt with at length, keep in mind that **the younger, the older, or more compromised by illness, the more critical a discrepancy is likely to be**.

5. **If the dosage ordered is 125 mg q.4.h., is this an accurate dosage?**
   In this order the frequency of administration, q.4.h., does not match the recommended q.8.h. The total daily dosage of 750 mg (125 mg × 6 doses = 750 mg) is slightly, but not significantly, higher than the 728 mg maximum. There may be a reason for the q.4.h. dosage, but call to verify the order.

To determine the safety of an ordered dosage, use the body weight to calculate the dosage range ordered, and compare this with the recommended dosage range. Assessment must also include the frequency of dosage ordered.

PROBLEM

Refer to the ampicillin (Principen®) label in Figure 12-2. Answer the questions for a 20 lb child.

1. What is the child's body weight in kg to the nearest tenth? _____

2. What is the recommended dosage in mg per day for this child? _____

3. How many doses will this be divided into? _____

4. How many mg will this be per dose? _____

5. The order is to give 250 mg q.6.h. Is this dosage appropriate? _____

6. How many mL would you need to administer a 250 mg dosage? _____

12

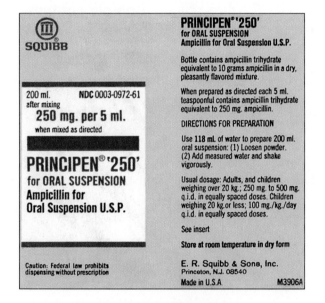

Figure 12-2

ANSWERS 1. 9.1 kg 2. 910 mg/day 3. 4 doses 4. 227.5 mg/dose 5. Yes 6. 5 mL

PROBLEM

Refer to the sample antibiotic label in Figure 12-3 and answer the questions.

1. What is the dosage strength of this suspension? _____

2. What will the mg per kg dosage be for a child with otitis media? _____

3. What will the daily dosage be for a child with otitis media weighing 10.4 kg? _____

4. The dosage is 187 mg every 4 hours for a child with a bronchial infection weighing 9.3 kg. Assess this dosage. _____

5. A child weighing 13.7 kg with a bronchial infection has an order for 187 mg every 8 hours. Assess this dosage. _____

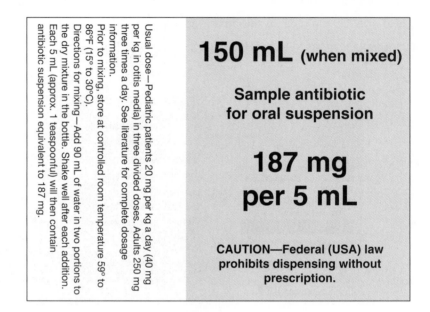

150 mL (when mixed)

Sample antibiotic for oral suspension

187 mg per 5 mL

CAUTION—Federal (USA) law prohibits dispensing without prescription.

Usual dose—Pediatric patients 20 mg per kg a day (40 mg per kg in otitis media) in three divided doses. Adults 250 mg three times a day. See literature for complete dosage information.

Prior to mixing, store at controlled room temperature 59° to 86°F (15° to 30°C).

Directions for mixing—Add 90 mL of water in two portions to the dry mixture in the bottle. Shake well after each addition. Each 5 mL (approx. 1 teaspoonful) will then contain antibiotic suspension equivalent to 187 mg.

Figure 12-3

ANSWERS   1. 187 mg per 5 mL   2. 40 mg per kg   3.   416 mg per day   4. The daily dosage should be 186 mg in two divided doses The dose is too high, and it is being given too often.   5. The daily dosage would be 274 mg to 548 mg divided into two dosages. The187 mg is ordered too frequently.

Calculating Dosages from Drug Literature

The labels you have just been reading were from oral syrups and suspensions, but the same calculation steps are necessary for dosages to be administered by the IV or IM route. Parenteral labels are much smaller in size and usually do not include dosage recommendations. To obtain these, you will have to refer to the drug package inserts, *PDR*, or similar references. These references will contain extensive details about each drug's chemistry, actions, adverse reactions, recommended administration, and so on, so it will be necessary for you to search for and select the information you need under the heading "Dosage and Administration." In the following exercises the searching has been done for you, and only those excerpts necessary for your calculations are shown.

Refer to the cefazolin (Kefzol®) insert in Figure 12-4 and locate the requested information for pediatric dosages.

1. What is the dosage range in mg/kg/day for mild to moderate infections?   _____

2. What is the dosage range for mild to moderate infections in mg/lb/day?   _____

3. The total dosage will be divided into how many doses per day?   _____

4. In severe infections, what is the maximum daily dosage recommended in mg/kg?   _____

   In mg/lb?   _____

12

KEFZOL®, STERILE CEFAZOLIN SODIUM, USP

ADMINISTRATION AND DOSAGE

In children, a total daily dosage of 25 to 50 mg/kg (approximately 10 to 20 mg/lb) of body weight, divided into 3 or 4 equal doses, is effective for most mild to moderately severe infections (Table 5). Total daily dosage may be increased to 100 mg/kg (45 mg/lb) of body weight for severe infections.

TABLE 5. PEDIATRIC DOSAGE GUIDE

Weight		25 mg/kg/Day Divided into 3 Doses		25 mg/kg/Day Divided into 4 Doses	
lb	kg	Approximate Single Dose (mg q8h)	Vol (mL) Needed with Dilution of 125 mg/mL	Approximate Single Dose (mg q6h)	Vol (mL) Needed with Dilution of 125 mg/mL
10	4.5	40 mg	0.35 mL	30 mg	0.25 mL
20	9	75 mg	0.6 mL	55 mg	0.45 mL
30	13.6	115 mg	0.9 mL	85 mg	0.7 mL
40	18.1	150 mg	1.2 mL	115 mg	0.9 mL
50	22.7	190 mg	1.5 mL	140 mg	1.1 mL

Weight		50 mg/kg/Day Divided into 3 Doses		50 mg/kg/Day Divided into 4 Doses	
lb	kg	Approximate Single Dose (mg q8h)	Vol (mL) Needed with Dilution of 225 mg/mL	Approximate Single Dose (mg q6h)	Vol (mL) Needed with Dilution of 225 mg/mL
10	4.5	75 mg	0.35 mL	55 mg	0.25 mL
20	9	150 mg	0.7 mL	110 mg	0.5 mL
30	13.6	225 mg	1 mL	170 mg	0.75 mL
40	18.1	300 mg	1.35 mL	225 mg	1 mL
50	22.7	375 mg	1.7 mL	285 mg	1.25 mL

Figure 12-4

ANSWERS   **1.** 25 mg–50 mg   **2.** 10 mg–20 mg   **3.** 3–4 doses per day   **4.** 100 mg/kg; 45 mg/lb

Notice that in this table sample dosages are provided for several kg and lb weights, for both the 25 mg and 50 mg dosage, and for both 3 and 4 doses per day. Tables such as this one can be helpful or harmful. They are helpful if they are easy to understand and the child whose dosage you are calculating fits one of the weights listed exactly; they can be harmful if they tend to confuse, which could easily happen if they are misread.

PROBLEM

Use the information you just obtained for Kefzol to do the calculations for a child who weighs 35 lb and has a moderately severe infection.

1. What is the lower daily dosage range? _____

2. What is the upper daily dosage range? _____

3. If the medication is given in four divided dosages, what will the per dosage range be? _____

4. If a dosage of 125 mg q.6.h. is ordered, will you need to question it? _____

12

ANSWERS 1. 350 mg/day   2. 700 mg/day   3. 87.5 mg to 175 mg per dose   4. No; it is within normal range

PROBLEM

Refer to the dosage information on Mezlin® in Figure 12-5 and answer the questions about adult IV dosages.

1. What is the recommended daily dosage range for serious infections? _____

2. How many divided doses, and at what intervals, should this dosage be given? _____

3. What is the maximum daily dosage? _____

4. Calculate the daily dosage range in g for a 176 lb adult. _____

5. If this dosage is to be given q.6.h., what will the individual dosage range be? _____

6. If a dosage of 2 g is ordered, what initial assessment would you make about it? _____

7. If a dosage of 10 g q.6.h. is ordered, what assessment would you make? _____

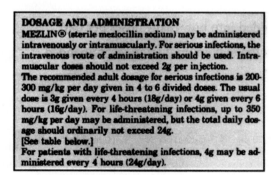

DOSAGE AND ADMINISTRATION
MEZLIN® (sterile mezlocillin sodium) may be administered intravenously or intramuscularly. For serious infections, the intravenous route of administration should be used. Intramuscular doses should not exceed 2g per injection.
The recommended adult dosage for serious infections is 200-300 mg/kg per day given in 4 to 6 divided doses. The usual dose is 3g given every 4 hours (18g/day) or 4g given every 6 hours (16g/day). For life-threatening infections, up to 350 mg/kg per day may be administered, but the total daily dosage should ordinarily not exceed 24g.
[See table below.]
For patients with life-threatening infections, 4g may be administered every 4 hours (24g/day).

Figure 12-5

ANSWERS 1. 200 mg/kg to 300 mg/kg   2. 4 to 6 doses; q.6.h. or q.4.h.   3. 24 g   4. 16 g–24 g   5. 4 g–6 g
6. The dosage is too low   7. The dosage is too high

PROBLEM

Refer to the dosage recommendations for Mithracin® in Figure 12-6 and answer the questions for treatment of testicular tumors in an adult weighing 240 lb.

1. What is the recommended daily dosage range in mcg/kg? _____

2. How often is this dosage to be given and for how long?

   _____ _____

3. What is the daily dosage range in mcg? in mg?
   (Calculate kg weight to the nearest tenth.) _____ _____

4. If a dosage of 3 mg IV q.a.m. is ordered, does this need to
   be questioned? _____

ANSWERS 1. 25–30 mcg/kg 2. 1× day; 8–10 days 3. 2728–3273 mcg/day; 2.7–3.3 mg/day 4. No; within normal range

---

MITHRACIN® ℞
(plicamycin)
FOR INTRAVENOUS USE

DOSAGE
The daily dose of Mithracin is based on the patient's body weight. If a patient has abnormal fluid retention such as edema, hydrothorax or ascites, the patient's ideal weight rather than actual body weight should be used to calculate the dose.
Treatment of Testicular Tumors: In the treatment of patients with testicular tumors the recommended daily dose of Mithracin (plicamycin) is 25 to 30 mcg (0.025–0.030 mg) per kilogram of body weight. Therapy should be continued for a period of 8 to 10 days unless significant side effects or toxicity occur during therapy. A course of therapy consisting of more than 10 daily doses is not recommended. Individual daily doses should not exceed 30 mcg (0.030 mg) per kilogram of body weight.

Figure 12-6

VELOSEF® for INJECTION
Cephradine for Injection USP

DOSAGE AND ADMINISTRATION

Infants and Children
The usual dosage range of VELOSEF is 50 to 100 mg/kg/day (approximately 23 to 45 mg/lb/day) in equally divided doses four times a day and should be regulated by age, weight of the patient and severity of the infection being treated.

PEDIATRIC DOSAGE GUIDE				
		50 mg/kg/day		100 mg/kg/day	
Weight		Approx. single dose mg q6h	Volume needed @ 208 mg/mL dilution	Approx. single dose mg q6h	Volume needed @ 227 mg/mL dilution
lbs	kg				
10	4.5	56 mg	0.27 mL	112 mg	0.5 mL
20	9.1	114 mg	0.55 mL	227 mg	1 mL
30	13.6	170 mg	0.82 mL	340 mg	1.5 mL
40	18.2	227 mg	1.1 mL	455 mg	2 mL
50	22.7	284 mg	1.4 mL	567 mg	2.5 mL

Figure 12-7

PROBLEM

Refer to the cephradine (Velosef®) literature in Figure 12-7 and answer the questions.

1. What is the daily dosage range in mg/kg/day? _____

2. What is the daily dosage range in mg/lb/day? _____

3. What is the recommended number of dosages per day? _____

4. What is the daily dosage range for a child weighing 12.6 kg? _____

5. What is the dosage range per dose for this child? _____

6. Is an order for cephradine 250 mg q.6.h. within the dosage range? _____

7. What is the daily dosage range for a child weighing 19½ lb? _____

8. What is the q.6.h. dose for this child? _____

9. Is 340 mg q.6.h. within the ordered range? _____

ANSWERS 1. 50–100 mg/kg/day 2. 23–45 mg/lb/day 3. 4 doses per day 4. 630–1260 mg/day 5. 158–315 mg/dose 6. Yes 7. 449–878 mg/day 8. 112–220 mg/dose 9. No, too high. Check with the physician.

Summary

This concludes the chapter on calculation and assessment of dosages based on body weight. The important points to remember from this chapter are:

Dosages are frequently ordered on the basis of weight, especially for children.

Dosages may be recommended based on mcg or mg per kg or lb per day, usually in divided doses.

Body weight may need to be converted from kg to lb, or from lb to kg, to correlate with dosage recommendations.

To convert lb to kg divide by 2.2; to convert kg to lb multiply by 2.2.

Calculating dosage is a two-step procedure: first calculate the total daily dosage for the weight; then divide this by the number of doses to be administered.

To check the accuracy of an order, calculate the correct dosage and compare it with the dosage ordered.

Dosage discrepancies are much more critical if the dosage range is low, for example, 2–5 mg, as opposed to high, for example, 250 mg.

Factors that make discrepancies particularly serious are low body weight, severity of medical condition, and age, the elderly and very young being particularly vulnerable.

If the drug label does not contain all the necessary information for safe administration, additional information can be obtained from drug package inserts, the PDR, drug formularies, or the hospital pharmacist.

Summary Self-Test

Read the dosage labels and literature provided to indicate if the dosages are within normal limits. If they are not, give the correct range. Express body weight conversions to the nearest tenth, and dosages to the nearest whole number in your calculations.

1. A 48 lb child has an order for antibiotic suspension 250 mg q.6.h. What is the daily recommended dosage for this child? What is the per dose dosage? Is the ordered dosage for this child correct? _____ _____ _____

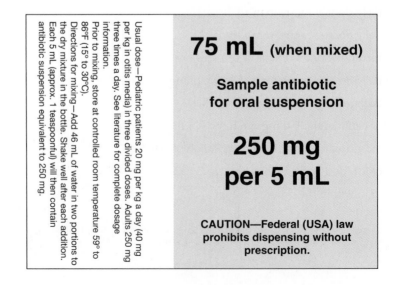

Usual dose—Pediatric patients 20 mg per kg a day (40 mg per kg in otitis media) in three divided doses. Adults 250 mg three times a day. See literature for complete dosage information.

Prior to mixing, store at controlled room temperature 59° to 86°F (15° to 30°C).

Directions for mixing—Add 46 mL of water in two portions to the dry mixture in the bottle. Shake well after each addition. Each 5 mL (approx. 1 teaspoonful) will then contain antibiotic suspension equivalent to 250 mg.

75 mL (when mixed)

Sample antibiotic for oral suspension

250 mg per 5 mL

CAUTION—Federal (USA) law prohibits dispensing without prescription.

2. Zinacef® (cefuroxime) 375 mg has been ordered IV q.8.h. for a child weighing 20.1 kg. Calculate the per day and q.8.h. per dose dosage ranges. Is the ordered dosage correct?

_____ _____ _____

3. Cefuroxime has been ordered for a child weighing 84 lb. If this medication is given q.6.h., what is the dosage range per day, and per dose?

_____ _____

4. A 140 lb adult has an order for IV methylprednisolone. Calculate the per dose dosage.

_____

5. A 7.9 kg infant has an order for Veetids® 125 mg q.8.h. Calculate the per dose dosage based on this infant's body weight. Is the dosage ordered correct?

_____ _____

ZINACEF®
[zin 'ah-sef]
(sterile cefuroxime sodium, Glaxo)

DOSAGE AND ADMINISTRATION

Infants and Children Above 3 Months of Age: Administration of 50 to 100 mg/kg/day in equally divided doses every six to eight hours has been successful for most infections susceptible to cefuroxime. The higher dose of 100 mg/kg/day (not to exceed the maximum adult dose) should be used for the more severe or serious infections.

In bone and joint infections, 150 mg/kg/day (not to exceed the maximum adult dose) is recommended in equally divided doses every eight hours. In clinical trials a course of oral antibiotics was administered to children following the completion of parenteral administration of ZINACEF.

In cases of bacterial meningitis, larger doses of ZINACEF are recommended, 200 to 240 mg/kg/day intravenously in divided doses every six to eight hours.

In children with renal insufficiency, the frequency of dosage should be modified consistent with the recommendations for adults.

SOLU–MEDROL®
brand of methylprednisolone sodium succinate sterile powder
(methylprednisolone sodium succinate for injection, USP)
For Intravenous or Intramuscular Administration

DOSAGE AND ADMINISTRATION

When high dose therapy is desired, the recommended dose of SOLU-MEDROL Sterile Powder (methylprednisolone sodium succinate) is 30 mg/kg administered intravenously over at least 30 minutes. This dose may be repeated every 4 to 6 hours for 48 hours.

Dosage may be reduced for infants and children but should be governed more by the severity of the condition and response of the patient than by age or size. It should not be less than 0.5 mg per kg every 24 hours.

SQUIBB

DO NOT USE IF CAKED

200 ml. after mixing   NDC 0003-0681-54

125 mg. (200,000 units) per 5 ml. when mixed as directed

VEETIDS®'125'
Penicillin V Potassium for Oral Solution U.S.P.
for ORAL SOLUTION

Caution: Federal law prohibits dispensing without prescription

Bottle contains penicillin V potassium equivalent to 5 grams penicillin V in a dry, pleasantly flavored, buffered mixture.

When prepared as directed each 5 ml. teaspoonful provides penicillin V potassium equivalent to 125 mg. (200,000 units) penicillin V.

DIRECTIONS FOR PREPARATION

Use 117 ml. of water to prepare 200 ml. oral solution: (1) Loosen powder. (2) Add measured water and shake vigorously.

Usual dosage: Adults and children — 1 to 2 teaspoonfuls 3 or 4 times daily. Infants — 15 to 56 mg./kg. daily in 3 to 6 divided doses.
See insert for detailed information
Store at room temperature in dry form

E. R. Squibb & Sons, Inc.
Princeton, N.J. 08540
Made in U.S.A.   M7823A

6. A 130 mg q.8.h. dosage of Vancocin® IV has been ordered for a child weighing 9.7 kg. Calculate the per dose dosage, and determine if this order is correct. _____ _____

7. Another child weighing 25.1 kg has an IV order for vancomycin. Calculate the per day and q.8.h. per dose dosages. _____ _____

8. Amoxil® oral suspension 125 mg q.8.h. has been ordered for an infant weighing 6.4 kg. Calculate the per dose dosage range. Is this a correct dosage? _____ _____

9. Calculate the q.8.h. dosage of amoxicillin suspension for a child weighing 41½ lb who has a severe infection. The Amoxil has a dosage strength of 250 mg/5 mL. What per dose dosage would you expect to be ordered from this available dosage strength? _____ _____

10. A child weighing 15.9 kg with a diagnosis of bacterial meningitis has an order for antibiotic "M" 850 mg q.6.h. IV. From the available information, calculate the per dose range and assess the dosage ordered. _____ _____

VANCOCIN® HCl
[văn 'kō-sĭn ăch 'sē-ĕl]
(vancomycin hydrochloride)
Sterile, USP
IntraVenous

DOSAGE AND ADMINISTRATION

Patients with Normal Renal Function
Adults —The usual daily intravenous dose is 2 g divided either as 500 mg every 6 hours or 1 g every 12 hours. Each dose should be administered over a period of at least 60 minutes. Other patient factors, such as age or obesity, may call for modification of the usual daily dose.
Children —The total daily intravenous dosage of Vancocin® HCl (vancomycin hydrochloride, Lilly), calculated on the basis of 40 mg/kg of body weight, can be divided and incorporated into the child's 24-hour fluid requirement. Each dose should be administered over a period of at least 60 minutes.
Infants and Neonates —In neonates and young infants, the total daily intravenous dosage may be lower. In both neonates and infants, an initial dose of 15 mg/kg is suggested, followed by 10 mg/kg every 12 hours for neonates in the first week of life and every 8 hours thereafter up to the age of 1 month. Close monitoring of serum concentrations of vancomycin may be warranted in these patients.

ANTIBIOTIC "M"

DOSAGE AND ADMINISTRATION

Infants and Children Above 3 Months of Age: Administration of 50 to 100 mg/kg/day in equally divided doses every 6 to 8 hours has been successful for most infections. The higher dose of 100 mg/kg/day (not to exceed the maximum adult dose) should be used for the more severe or serious infections.
In cases of bacerial meningitis, larger doses are recommended, initially 200 to 240 mg/kg/day intravenously in divided doses every six to eight hours.

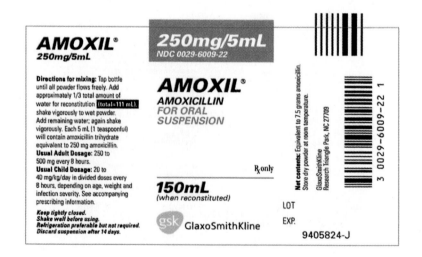

11. A child suffering from a genitourinary tract infection has an order
    of IV ampicillin sodium "N" 175 mg q.6.h. The child weighs
    30¼ lb. What is the recommended per dose dosage?
    Is the dosage ordered correct?   _____ _____

12. A 7.7 kg infant has ampicillin 62.5 mg ordered IV q.6.h.
    for a respiratory infection. Calculate the per dose dosage
    range, and determine if the dosage ordered is correct.   _____

13. A dosage of Ancef® 125 mg q.6.h. has been ordered for a child
    weighing 16 kg. Calculate the per dose dosage range for
    this child, and decide if it is within the normal range.   _____

Ampicillin Sodium "N"

For Parenteral Administration

Dosage (IM or IV)

Infection	Organisms	Adults	Children*
Respiratory tract	streptococci, pneumococci, nonpenicillinase-producing staphylococci, H. influenzae	250-500 mg q. 6 h.	25-50 mg/kg/day in equal doses q. 6 h.
Gastrointestinal tract	susceptible pathogens	500 mg q. 6 h.	50 mg/kg/day in equal doses q. 6 h.
Genitourinary tract	susceptible gram-negative or gram-positive pathogens	500 mg q. 6 h.	50 mg/kg/day in equal doses q. 6 h.
Urethritis (acute) in adult males	N. gonorrhoeae	500 mg b.i.d. for 1 day (IM)	
	(In complications such as prostatitis and epididymitis, prolonged and intensive therapy is recommended. Gonorrhea cases with suspected primary lesion of syphilis should have dark-field examinations before treatment. In any case suspected of concomitant syphilis, monthly serologic tests for at least 4 months are necessary.)		
Bacterial meningitis	N. meningitidis, H. influenzae	8-14 gram/day	100-200 mg/kg/day
	(Initial treatment is usually by IV drip, followed by frequent [q. 3-4 h.] IM injections.) S. viridans		

*Children's dosage recommendations are intended for those whose weight
will not result in a dosage higher than for the adult.

ANCEF®

brand of

sterile cefazolin sodium
and
cefazolin sodium
injection

Pediatric Dosage
In children, a total daily dosage of 25 to 50 mg per kg
(approximately 10 to 20 mg per pound) of body weight,
divided into three or four equal doses, is effective for most
mild to moderately severe infections. Total daily dosage
may be increased to 100 mg per kg (45 mg per pound) of
body weight for severe infections Since safety for use in
premature infants and in infants under one month has
not been established, the use of Ancef (sterile cefazolin
sodium) in these patients is not recommended

		25 mg/kg/Day Divided into 3 Doses		25 mg/kg/Day Divided into 4 Doses	
Weight					
			Vol. (mL) needed with dilution of 125 mg/mL		Vol. (mL) needed with dilution of 125 mg/mL
Lbs	Kg	Approximate Single Dose mg/q8h		Approximate Single Dose mg/q6h	
10	4.5	40 mg	0.35 mL	30 mg	0.25 mL
20	9.0	75 mg	0.60 mL	55 mg	0.45 mL
30	13.6	115 mg	0.90 mL	85 mg	0.70 mL
40	18 *	150 mg	1.20 mL	115 mg	0.90 mL
50	22.7	190 mg	1.50 mL	140 mg	1.10 mL

		50 mg/kg/Day Divided into 3 Doses		50 mg/kg/Day Divided into 4 Doses	
Weight					
			Vol. (mL) needed with dilution of 225 mg/mL		Vol. (mL) needed with dilution of 225 mg/mL
Lbs	Kg	Approximate Single Dose mg q8h		Approximate Single Dose mg/q6h	
10	4.5	75 mg	0.35 mL	55 mg	0.25 mL
20	9.0	150 mg	0.70 mL	110 mg	0.50 mL
30	13.6	225 mg	1.00 mL	170 mg	0.75 mL
40	18.1	300 mg	1.35 mL	225 mg	1.00 mL
50	22.7	375 mg	1.70 mL	285 mg	1.25 mL

14. A 198 lb adult is to be treated with IV Ticar® for bacterial septicemia. What is the daily dosage range in mg for this patient? _____

15. If the drug is administered q.4.h., what is the per dose in g? _____

16. Do you need to question a per dose dosage of 4 g? _____

17. An adult weighing 77.3 kg with good cardiorenal function who tolerated a test dose of Fungizone® is to receive this drug IV. What is the daily dosage? _____

18. Another adult who weighs 67.4 kg is also to receive amphotericin B for a severe, rapidly progressive fungal infection. What will the daily dosage be? _____

19. What would be the **maximum** daily Fungizone dosage for an adult weighing 80.3 kg? _____

12

TICAR ®

brand of

sterile ticarcillin disodium
for Intramuscular or Intravenous Administration

DOSAGE AND ADMINISTRATION
Clinical experience indicates that in serious urinary tract and systemic infections, intravenous therapy in the higher doses should be used. Intramuscular injections should not exceed 2 grams per injection.
Adults:

Bacterial septicemia Respiratory tract infections Skin and soft-tissue infections Intra-abdominal infections Infections of the female pelvis and genital tract	200 to 300 mg/kg/day by I.V. infusion in divided doses every 4 or 6 hours. (The usual dose is 3 grams given every 4 hours [18 grams/day] or 4 grams given every 6 hours [16 grams/day] depending on weight and the severity of the infection.)

Urinary tract infections
  Complicated:
 	
  Uncomplicated:
	150 to 200 mg/kg/day by I.V. infusion in divided doses every 4 or 6 hours.
	(Usual recommended dosage for average [70 kg] adults: 3 grams q.i.d.)
	1 gram I.M. or direct I.V. every 6 hours.

FUNGIZONE® INTRAVENOUS ℞
Amphotericin B For Injection USP

WARNING
This drug should be used *primarily* for treatment of patients with progressive and potentially life-threatening fungal infections; it should not be used to treat noninvasive forms of fungal disease such as oral thrush, vaginal candidasis and esophegeal candidiasis in patients with normal neutrophil counts.

DOSAGE AND ADMINISTRATION
CAUTION: Under no circumstances should a total daily dose of 1.5 mg/kg be exceeded. Amphotericin B overdoses can result in cardio-respiratory arrest (see OVERDOSAGE).
FUNGIZONE Intravenous should be administered by *slow* intravenous infusion. Intravenous infusion should be given over a period of approximately 2 to 6 hours (depending on the dose) observing the usual precautions for intravenous therapy (see PRECAUTIONS, General). The recommended concentration for intravenous infusion is 0.1 mg/mL (1 mg/10 mL).
Since patient tolerance varies greatly, the dosage of amphotericin B must be individualized and adjusted according to the patient's clinical status (e.g., site and severity of infection, etiologic agent, cardio-renal function, etc.).
A single intravenous test dose (1 mg in 20 mL of 5% dextrose solution) administered over 20–30 minutes may be preferred. The patient's temperature, pulse, respiration, and blood pressure should be recorded every 30 minutes for 2 to 4 hours.
In patients with good cardi-renal function and a well tolerated test dose, therapy is usually initiated with a daily dose of 0.25 mg/kg of body weight. However, in those patients having severe and rapidly progressive fungal infection, therapy may be initiated with a daily dose of 0.3 mg/kg of body weight. In patients with impaired cardio-renal function or a severe reaction to the test dose, therapy should be initiated with smaller daily doses (i.e., 5 to 10 mg).
Depending on the patient's cardio-renal status (see PRECAUTIONS, Laboratory Tests), doses may gradually be increased by 5 to 10 mg per day to final daily dosage of 0.5 to 0.7 mg/kg.

ANSWERS

1. 436 mg/day; 145 mg/dose. The 250 mg dosage is too high. Also the order is q.6.h., 4 times a day, not the usual q.8.h., which is 3 times a day
2. 1005–2010 mg/day; 335–670 mg/dose; 375 mg dosage ordered is correct
3. 1910–3820 mg/day; 478–955 mg/dose
4. 1908 mg/dose
5. Per dose range is 40–147 mg; the 125 mg order is correct
6. 129 mg/dose; the 130 mg ordered is correct
7. Per day dosage is 1004 mg; per dose dosage is 335 mg
8. Normal dose is 43–85 mg; the dosage ordered is too high
9. Per dose dosage range is 126–252 mg; 250 mg q.8.h. would be ordered
10. The q.6.h. per dosage range is 795–954 mg; the 850 mg dosage ordered is correct
11. 173 mg/dose; the 175 mg dosage ordered is correct
12. The 62.5 mg ordered is within the 48–96 mg per dose range
13. The 125 mg ordered is within the 100–200 mg per dose range
14. 18,000–27,000 mg/day
15. 3–4.5 g/dose
16. No
17. 19 mg/day
18. 20 mg/day
19. 120–121 mg/day

13

Adult and Pediatric Dosages Based on Body Surface Area

Body surface area (BSA or SA) is a major factor in calculating dosages for a number of drugs, because many of the body's physiologic processes are more closely related to body surface than they are to weight. Body surface is used extensively to calculate dosages of antineoplastic agents for cancer chemotherapy, and for patients with severe burns. However, an increasing number of other drugs also are calculated using BSA. The nursing responsibility for checking dosages based on BSA varies widely among hospitals; therefore, this chapter covers all three essentials: calculation of BSA, calculation of dosages based on BSA, and assessment of orders based on BSA.

Body surface is calculated in **square meters** (m²) using the **body weight and height**, a calculator that has square root ($\sqrt{}$) capabilities, and a simple formula. Two formulas are used, one for kg and cm metric measurements, and another for lb and in (inch) measurements.* We'll look at these separately.

Calculating BSA from kg and cm

The formula to calculate BSA from kg and cm measurements is very easy to use.

FORMULA

$$BSA = \sqrt{\frac{wt\ (kg) \times ht\ (cm)}{3600}}$$

EXAMPLE 1 Calculate the BSA of a man who weighs **104 kg** and whose height is **191 cm**. Express BSA to the nearest hundredth.

$$\sqrt{\frac{104\ (kg) \times 191\ (cm)}{3600}}$$

$$= \sqrt{5.517}$$

$$= 2.348 = \mathbf{2.35\ m^2}$$

*Taketomo, Carol K. *Pediatric Dosage Handbook*, 10th ed. Hudson, OH: Lexi-Comp, Inc. 2003.

Calculators may vary in the way square root must be obtained. Here is how the BSA was calculated in this example and throughout the chapter:

$$104. \times 191. \div 3600. = 5.517, \text{ then immediately enter } \sqrt{}$$

Practice with your own calculator to determine how it must be used to calculate a square root. Be careful to **insert periods after all whole numbers,** or you may obtain a wrong answer from preset decimal placement.

Only the final m² BSA is rounded to hundredths. Answers may vary slightly depending on how your calculator is set. Consider answers within 2–3 hundredths correct. Fractional weights and heights are also simple to calculate.

EXAMPLE 2   Calculate the BSA of an adolescent who weighs **59.1 kg** and is **157.5 cm** in height. Express BSA to the nearest hundredth.

$$\sqrt{\frac{59.1 \text{ (kg)} \times 157.5 \text{ (cm)}}{3600}}$$

$$= \sqrt{2.585}$$

$$= 1.607 = \textbf{1.61 m}^2$$

EXAMPLE 3   A child who is **96.2 cm** tall weighs **15.17 kg**. What is this child's BSA in m² to the nearest hundredth?

$$\sqrt{\frac{15.17 \text{ (kg)} \times 96.2 \text{ (cm)}}{3600}}$$

$$= \sqrt{0.4053}$$

$$= 0.636 = \textbf{0.64 m}^2$$

PROBLEM

Calculate the BSA in m². Express your answers to the nearest hundredth.

1. An adult weighing 59 kg whose height is 160 cm   _____
2. A child whose weight is 35.9 kg and whose height is 63.5 cm   _____
3. A child whose weight is 7.7 kg and whose height is 40 cm   _____
4. An adult whose weight is 92 kg and whose height is 178 cm   _____
5. A child whose weight is 46 kg and whose height is 102 cm   _____

ANSWERS   1. 1.62 m²   2. 0.8 m²   3. 0.29 m²   4. 2.13 m²   5. 1.14 m²

Calculating BSA from lb and in

The formula for calculating BSA from lb and in measurements is equally easy to use. **The only difference is the denominator, which is 3131.**

FORMULA

$$BSA = \sqrt{\frac{wt\ (lb)\ \times\ ht\ (in)}{3131}}$$

EXAMPLE 1 Calculate BSA to the nearest hundredth for a child who is **24 in** tall and weighing **34 lb**.

$$\sqrt{\frac{34\ (lb)\ \times\ 24\ (in)}{3131}}$$

$$= \sqrt{0.260}$$

$$= 0.510 = \mathbf{0.51\ m^2}$$

EXAMPLE 2 Calculate BSA to the nearest hundredth of an adult who is **61.3 in** tall and weighs **142.7 lb**.

$$\sqrt{\frac{142.7\ (lb)\ \times\ 61.3\ (in)}{3131}}$$

$$= \sqrt{2.793}$$

$$= 1.671 = \mathbf{1.67\ m^2}$$

EXAMPLE 3 A child weighs **105 lb** and is **51 in** tall. Calculate BSA to the nearest hundredth.

$$\sqrt{\frac{105\ (lb)\ \times\ 51\ (in)}{3131}}$$

$$= \sqrt{1.710}$$

$$= 1.307 = \mathbf{1.31\ m^2}$$

PROBLEM

Determine the BSA. Express your answers to the nearest hundredth.

1. A child weighing 92 lb who measures 35 in   _____

2. An adult who weighs 175 lb and who is 67 in tall   _____

3. An adult who is 70 in tall and weighs 194 lb   _____

4. A child who weighs 72.4 lb and is 40.5 in tall   _____

5. A child who measures 26 in and weighs 36 lb   _____

ANSWERS   1. 1.01 m²   2. 1.94 m²   3. 2.08 m²   4. 0.97 m²   5. 0.55 m²

Dosage Calculation Based on BSA

Once you know the BSA, dosage calculation is simple multiplication.

EXAMPLE 1   Dosage recommended is **5 mg per m²**. The child has a BSA of **1.1 m²**.

1.1 (m²) × 5 mg = **5.5 mg**

EXAMPLE 2   The recommended child's dosage is 25–50 mg per m². The child has a BSA of **0.76 m²**.

Lower dosage   0.76 (m²) × 25 mg = 19 mg

Upper dosage   0.76 (m²) × 50 mg = 38 mg

The dosage range is **19–38 mg**.

PROBLEM

Determine the child's dosage. Express your answers to the nearest whole number.

1. The recommended child's dosage is 5–10 mg/m². The BSA is 0.43 m².   _____

2. A child with a BSA of 0.81 m² is to receive a drug with a recommended dosage of 40 mg/m².   _____

3. Calculate the dosage of a drug with a recommended child's dosage of 20 mg/m² for a child with a BSA of 0.50 m².   _____

4. An adult is to receive a drug with a recommended dosage of 20–40 units per m². The BSA is 1.93 m².   _____

5. The adult recommended dosage is 3–5 mg per m². Calculate dosage for 2.08 m².   _____

ANSWERS   1. 2–4 mg   2. 32 mg   3. 10 mg   4. 39–77 units   5. 6–10 mg

Assessing Orders Based on BSA

In most situations in which you will have to check a dosage against m² recommendations you will refer to drug package inserts, medication protocols, or the *PDR* to determine what the dosage should be.

EXAMPLE 1   Refer to the vinblastine information insert in Figure 13-1 and calculate the first dose for an adult whose BSA is 1.66 m². Calculations are to the nearest whole number.

Recommended first dose = 3.7 mg/m²

1.66 (m²) × 3.7 mg = 6.14 = **6 mg**

EXAMPLE 2   A child with a BSA of 0.96 m² is to receive her fourth dose of vinblastine.

Recommended fourth dose = 6.25 mg/m²

0.96 (m²) × 6.25 mg = **6 mg**

CETUS ONCOLOGY

STERILE VINBLASTINE SULFATE, USP

DOSAGE AND ADMINISTRATION
Caution: It is extremely important that the needle be properly positioned in the vein before this product is injected.

If leakage into surrounding tissue should occur during intravenous administration of vinblastine sulfate, it may cause considerable irritation. The injection should be discontinued immediately, and any remaining portion of the dose should then be introduced into another vein. Local injection of hyaluronidase and the application of moderate heat to the area of leakage help disperse the drug and are thought to minimize discomfort and the possibility of cellulitis.

There are variations in the depth of the leukopenic response which follows therapy with vinblastine sulfate. For this reason, it is recommended that the drug be given no more frequently than *once every 7 days.* It is wise to initiate therapy for adults by administering a single intravenous dose of 3.7 mg/M² of body surface area (bsa); the initial dose for children should be 2.5 mg/M². Thereafter, white-blood-cell counts should be made to determine the patient's sensitivity to vinblastine sulfate. A reduction of 50% in the dose of vinblastine is recommended for patients having a direct serum bilirubin value above 3 mg/100 mL. Since metabolism and excretion are primarily hepatic, no modification is recommended for patients with impaired renal function.

A simplified and conservative incremental approach to dosage *at weekly intervals* may be outlined as follows:

	Adults	Children
First dose	3.7 mg/M² bsa	2.5 mg/M² bsa
Second dose	5.5 mg/M² bsa	3.75 mg/M² bsa
Third dose	7.4 mg/M² bsa	5 mg/M² bsa
Forth dose	9.25 mg/M² bsa	6.25 mg/M² bsa
Fifth dose	11.1 mg/M² bsa	7.5 mg/M² bsa

The above-mentioned increases may be used until a maximum dose (not exceeding 18.5 mg/M² bsa for adults and 12.5 mg/M² bsa for children) is reached. The dose should not be increased after that dose which reduces the white-cell count to approximately 3000 cells/mm³. In some adults, 3.7 mg/M² bsa may produce this leukopenia; other adults may require more than 11.1mg/M² bsa; and, very rarely, as much as 18.5 mg/M² bsa may be necessary. For most adult patients, however, the weekly dosage will prove to be 5.5 to 7.4 mg/M² bsa.

Figure 13-1

PROBLEM

Calculate the dosages of vinblastine from the information available in Figure 13-1. Calculate dosages to the nearest whole number.

1. Calculate the dosage for an adult's third dose. The patient's BSA is 1.91 m². _____

2. Calculate the first child's dosage for a patient with a BSA of 1.2 m². _____

3. Calculate the fifth adult dosage. The BSA is 1.53 m². _____

4. Calculate the second child's dosage for a BSA of 1.01 m². _____

5. Calculate the second adult dose for a BSA of 2.12 m². _____

ANSWERS   1. 14 mg   2. 3 mg   3. 17 mg   4. 4 mg   5. 12 mg

BiCNU®
(carmustine for injection)

DOSAGE AND ADMINISTRATION
The recommended dose of BiCNU as a single agent in previously untreated patients is 150 to 200 mg/m² intravenously every 6 weeks. This may be given as a single dose or divided into daily injections such as 75 to 100 mg/m² on 2 successive days. When BiCNU is used in combination with other myelosuppressive drugs or in patients in whom bone marrow reserve is depleted, the doses should be adjusted accordingly.

Figure 13-2

PROBLEM

Refer to Figure 13-2 for BiCNU® and locate the following information. Express all dosages to the nearest whole number.

1. What is the dosage per m² if the drug is to be given in a single dose?   _____

2. If the BSA IS 1.91 m², what IS the daily dosage range?   _____

3. If the order is for a single dosage of 325 mg, is there any need to question it?   _____

4. If the dosage ordered is 450 mg, is there any need to question it?   _____

ANSWERS   1. 150–200 mg/m²   2. 287–382 mg   3. No   4. Yes; it is too high

Summary

This concludes the chapter on dosage calculation based on BSA. The important points to remember from this chapter are:

BSA is calculated from body weight and height.

BSA is more important than weight alone in calculating some drug dosages because many physiologic processes are more closely related to body surface area than they are to weight.

BSA is calculated in square meters (m²) using a formula.

The formulas for calculation of BSA are:

$$\sqrt{\frac{\text{wt (kg)} \times \text{ht (cm)}}{3600}} \quad and \quad \sqrt{\frac{\text{wt (lb)} \times \text{ht (in)}}{3131}}$$

Once the BSA has been obtained, it can be used to calculate specific drug dosages and assess the accuracy of orders.

Summary Self-Test

Use the formula method to calculate BSA. Express the BSA to the nearest hundredth.

1. A child weighing 58 lb whose height is 36 in _____
2. An adult weighing 74 kg and measuring 160 cm _____
3. A child who is 14.2 kg and measures 64 cm _____
4. An adult weighing 69 kg whose height is 170 cm _____
5. An adolescent who is 55 in and 103 lb _____
6. A child who is 112 cm and weighs 25.3 kg _____
7. An adult who weighs 55 kg and measures 157.5 cm _____
8. An adult who weighs 65.4 kg and is 132 cm in height _____
9. A child whose height is 58 in and whose weight is 26.5 lb _____
10. A child whose height and weight are 60 cm and 13.6 kg, respectively _____

Read the drug insert information provided on pages 188–191 and answer the questions pertaining to each. Calculate dosages to the nearest whole number.

11. Read the information on children's dosage for cyproheptadine HCl in Figure 13-3 and calculate the daily dosage for a 5-year-old child whose BSA is 0.78 m². _____

12. If a dosage of 4 mg is ordered for this 5-year-old, would you question it? _____

13. What is the the daily dosage in mg for a 4-year-old child whose BSA is 0.29 m²? _____

14. What is the daily dosage in mg for a 4-year-old child with a BSA of 0.51 m²? _____

Antibiotic

DOSAGE AND ADMINISTRATION

DOSAGE SHOULD BE INDIVIDUALIZED ACCORDING TO THE NEEDS AND THE RESPONSE OF THE PATIENT.

Each tablet contains 4 mg of antibiotic.

Pediatric Patients

Age 2 to 6 years

The total daily dosage for pediatric patients may be calculated on the basis of body weight or body area using approximately 0.25 mg/kg/day or 8 mg per square meter of body surface (8 mg/m²).

The usual dose is 2 mg ($^{1}/_{2}$ tablet) two or three times a day, adjusted as necessary to the size and response of the patient. The dose is not to exceed 12 mg a day.

Age 7 to 14 years

The usual dose is 4 mg (1 tablet) two or three times a day, adjusted as necessary to the size and response of the patient. The dose is not to exceed 16 mg a day.

Adults

The total daily dose for adults should not exceed 0.5 mg/kg/day.

The therapeutic range is 4 to 20 mg a day, with the majority of patients requiring 12 to 16 mg a day. An occasional patient may require as much as 32 mg a day for adequate relief. It is suggested that dosage be initiated with 4 mg (1 tablet) three times a day and adjusted according to the size and response of the patient.

Figure 13-3

MUTAMYCIN® ℞
[*mū''-tĕ-mī'-sĭn*]
(mitomycin for injection) USP

DOSAGE AND ADMINISTRATION
Mutamycin should be given intravenously only, using care to avoid extravasation of the compound. If extravasation occurs, cellulitis, ulceration, and slough may result.

Each vial contains either mitomycin 5 mg and mannitol 10 mg, mitomycin 20 mg and mannitol 40 mg, or mitomycin 40 mg and mannitol 80 mg. To administer, add Sterile Water for Injection, 10 mL, 40 mL or 80 mL, respectively. Shake to dissolve. If product does not dissolve immediately, allow to stand at room temperature until solution is obtained.

After full hematological recovery (see guide to dosage adjustment) from any previous chemotherapy, the following dosage schedule may be used at 6- to 8-week intervals:

20 mg/m² intravenously as a single dose via a functioning intravenous catheter.

Because of cumulative myelosuppression, patients should be fully reevaluated after each course of Mutamycin, and the dose reduced if the patient has experienced any toxicities. Doses greater than 20 mg/m² have not been shown to be more effective, and are more toxic than lower doses.

The following schedule is suggested as a guide to dosage adjustment:

Figure 13-4

PARAPLATIN® ℞
[*păr-a-plătin*]
(carboplatin for injection)

DOSAGE AND ADMINISTRATION
NOTE: Aluminum reacts with carboplatin causing precipitate formation and loss of potency, therefore, needles or intravenous sets containing aluminum parts that may come in contact with the drug must not be used for the preparation or administration of PARAPLATIN.

PARAPLATIN, as a single agent, has been shown to be effective in patients with recurrent ovarian carcinoma at a dosage of 360 mg/m² IV on day 1 every 4 weeks. In general, however, single intermittent courses of PARAPLATIN should not be repeated until the neutrophil count is at least 2,000 and the platelet count is at least 100,000.

The dose adjustments shown in the table below are modified from a controlled trial in previously treated patients with ovarian carcinoma. Blood counts were done weekly, and the recommendations are based on the lowest posttreatment platelet or neutrophil value.

Figure 13-5

13

15. Calculate the IV dosage of the antineoplastic drug Mutamycin® (Figure 13-4) for an adult with a BSA of 1.46 m². _____

16. An adult with a BSA of 2.12 m² is to receive Mutamycin® IV. Calculate the dosage. _____

17. What dosage of Paraplatin® (Figure 13-5) will be ordered for a woman with ovarian carcinoma whose BSA is 1.61 m²? _____

18. Paraplatin® is ordered for a woman who weighs 130 lb and is 62 in tall. What will her dosage be? _____

19. A dosage of 637 mg of Paraplatin® IV is ordered for a woman who is 161 cm tall and weighs 70 kg. Assess this dosage. _____

BLENOXANE® ℞
[blĕ-nŏk 'sān]
(sterile bleomycin sulfate, USP)
vial, 15 units NSN 6505-01-060-4278(m)

DOSAGE

Because of the possibility of an anaphylactoid reaction, lymphoma patients should be treated with two units or less for the first two doses. If no acute reaction occurs, then the regular dosage schedule may be followed.

The following dose schedule is recommended: Squamous cell carcinoma, lymphosarcoma, reticulum cell sarcoma, testicular carcinoma—0.25 to 0.50 units/kg (10 to 20 units/m^2) given intravenously, intramuscularly, or subcutaneously weekly or twice weekly.

Hodgkin's Disease—0.25 to 0.50 units/kg (10 to 20 units/m^2) given intravenously, intramuscularly, or subcutaneously weekly or twice weekly. After a 50% response, a maintenance dose of one unit daily or five units weekly intravenously or intramuscularly should be given.

Pulmonary toxicity of Blenoxane appears to be dose related with a striking increase when the total dose is over 400 units. Total doses over 400 units should be given with great caution.

Figure 13-6

PLATINOL® ℞
[plă 'tĭ-nŏl "]
(cisplatin for injection, USP)

DOSAGE AND ADMINISTRATION

Note: Needles or intravenous sets containing aluminum parts that may come in contact with PLATINOL® (cisplatin for injection, USP) should not be used for preparation or administration. Aluminum reacts with PLATINOL, causing precipitate formation and a loss of potency.

Metastatic Testicular Tumors—The usual PLATINOL dose for the treatment of testicular cancer in combination with other approved chemotherapeutic agents is 20 mg/m^2 IV daily for 5 days.

Metastatic Ovarian Tumors—The usual PLATINOL dose for the treatment of metastatic ovarian tumors in combination with Cytoxan or other approved chemotherapeutic agents is 75–100 mg/m^2 IV once every 4 weeks, (Day 1).[1,2]

The dose of Cytoxan when used in combination with PLATINOL is 600 mg/m^2 IV once every 4 weeks, (Day 1).[1,2]

For directions for the administration of Cytoxan refer to the Cytoxan package insert.

In combination therapy, PLATINOL and Cytoxan are administered sequentially.

As a single agent, PLATINOL should be administered at a dose of 100 mg/m^2 IV once every 4 weeks.

Figure 13-7

20. Calculate the BSA for an adult with Hodgkin's disease who weighs 60 kg and is 142 cm tall. _____

   What is the IV dosage range of Blenoxane® (Figure 13-6) for this adult? _____

   If the order is for 20 units must you question it? _____

21. What will the dosage range of Blenoxane® be for an adult weighing 91 kg and measuring 190 cm? _____

22. What dosage of Platinol® (Figure 13-7) is required for a woman with a BSA of 1.29 m^2? _____

23. An adult with metastatic testicular carcinoma is to receive Platinol®. He weighs 173 lb and is 65 in tall. Calculate his BSA. _____

   What is his dosage? _____

R

(Acyclovir Sodium)
FOR INTRAVENOUS INFUSION ONLY

DOSAGE AND ADMINISTRATION
CAUTION— RAPID OR BOLUS INTRAVENOUS AND IN-
TRAMUSCULAR OR SUBCUTANEOUS INJECTION MUST
BE AVOIDED. Therapy should be initiated as early as possible following onset of signs and symptoms. For diagnosis—
see INDICATIONS.
Dosage:
HERPES SIMPLEX INFECTIONS
*MUCOSAL AND CUTANEOUS HERPES SIMPLEX (HSV-1
and HSV-2) INFECTIONS IN IMMUNOCOMPROMISED
PATIENTS* —5 mg/kg infused at a constant rate over 1
hour, every 8 hours (15 mg/kg/day) for 7 days in adult patients with normal renal function. In children under 12
years of age, more accurate dosing can be attained by infusing 250 mg/m² at a constant rate over 1 hour, every 8 hours
(750 mg/m²/day) for 7 days.

*SEVERE INITIAL CLINICAL EPISODES OF HERPES
GENITALIS* —The same dose given above—administered
for 5 days.
HERPES SIMPLEX ENCEPHALITIS —10 mg/kg infused
at a constant rate over at least 1 hour, every 8 hours for 10
days. In children between 6 months and 12 years of age, more
accurate dosing is achieved by infusing 500 mg/m², at a constant rate over at least one hour, every 8 hours for 10 days.
VARICELLA ZOSTER INFECTIONS
ZOSTER IN IMMUNOCOMPROMISED PATIENTS —10
mg/kg infused at a constant rate over 1 hour, every 8 hours
for 7 days in adult patients with normal renal function. In
children under 12 years of age, equivalent plasma concentrations are attained by infusing 500 mg/m² at a constant rate
over at least 1 hour, every 8 hours for 7 days. Obese patients
should be dosed at 10 mg/kg (Ideal Body Weight). A maximum dose equivalent to 500 mg/m² every 8 hours should not
be exceeded for any patient.

Figure 13-8

24. Acylclovir sodium (Figure 13-8) is to be given to a child with herpes simplex encephalitis who weighs 34 lb and is 24 in tall. What is the child's BSA?   _____

    What is the dosage for this child?   _____

25. An immunocompromised 10-year-old child with a herpes simplex infection is to be medicated with acyclovir sodium. Her weight is 72 lb and height 40 in. What is her BSA?   _____

    Calculate her per dose dosage.   _____

26. Another immunosuppressed child is to receive acyclovir sodium for a varicella zoster infection. His weight is 43 lb and height 28 in. What is his BSA?   _____

27. What is his dosage?   _____

ANSWERS

1. 0.82 m²	8. 1.55 m²	15. 29 mg	21. 22–44 units
2. 1.81 m²	9. 0.70 m²	16. 42 mg	22. 97–129 mg
3. 0.50 m²	10. 0.48 m²	17. 580 mg	23. 1.90 m²; 38 mg
4. 1.81 m²	11. 6 mg per day	18. 576 mg	24. 0.51 m²; 255 mg
5. 1.35 m²	12. Yes; too low	19. Accurate	25. 0.96 m²; 240 mg
6. 0.89 m²	13. 2 mg per day	20. 1.54 m²;	26. 0.62 m²
7. 1.55 m²	14. 4 mg	15–31 units; No	27. 310 mg

SECTION SIX

Intravenous Calculations

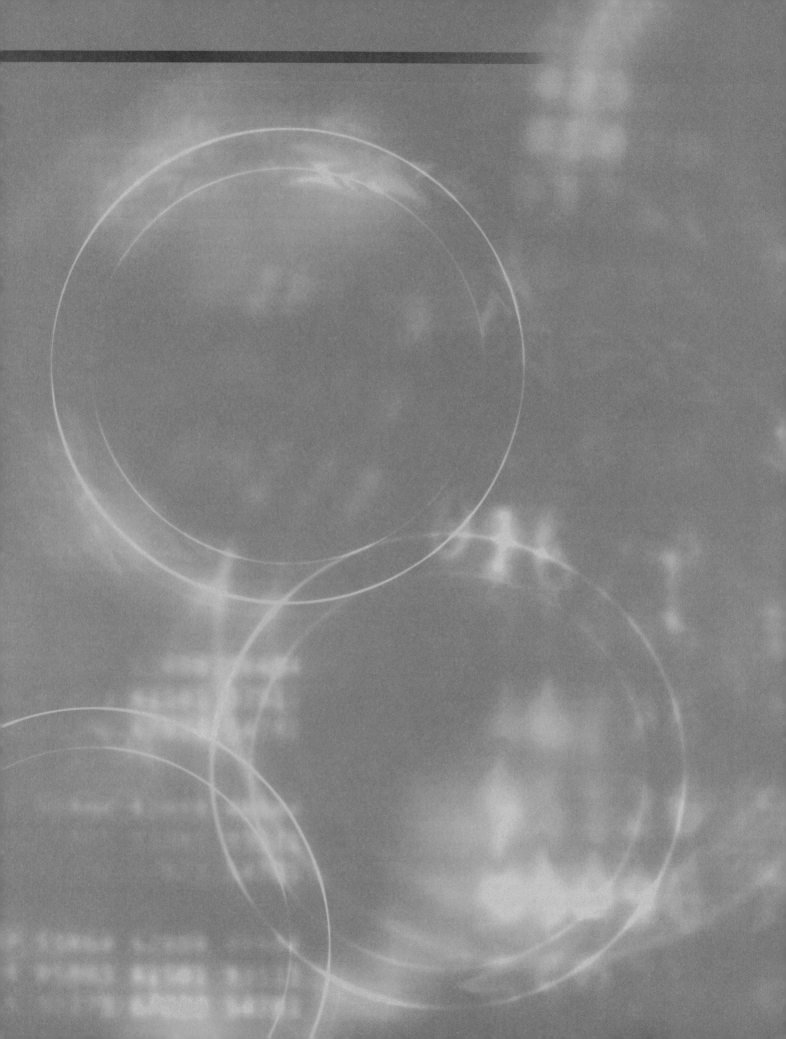

Introduction to IV Therapy

14

The calculations associated with IVs will be easier to understand if you have some general understanding of IV therapy. IV fluid and medication administration is one of the most challenging of all nursing responsibilities. It is estimated that there are currently over 200 different IV fluids being manufactured, and at least as many additives are used with IV fluids, including medications, electrolytes, and nutrients. In addition, there are hundreds of different types of IV administration sets and components, and dozens of different models of electronic infusion devices (EIDs) are used to infuse and monitor IV fluids. This would appear to make the entire subject of IV therapy overwhelming, but it is not. This chapter presents the essentials in understandable segments and gives an excellent base of instruction on which to build. Let's begin by looking at a basic sterile IV setup, which is referred to as a primary line.

Primary Line

Refer to Figure 14-1, which shows a typical primary IV line connecting an IV fluid bag or bottle to the needle or cannula in a vein. The first step is to connect the IV tubing to the IV solution bag using sterile technique.

Close all roller clamps on the tubing before connecting it to the solution bag. This prevents air from entering the tubing.

When connected, the bag is hung on the IV stand. The **drip chamber**, A, is then squeezed to **half fill** it with fluid. This level is very important because **IV flow rates are set and monitored by counting the drops falling in this chamber**. If the chamber is too full the drops cannot be counted. On the other hand, if the outlet at the bottom of the chamber is not completely covered, air can enter the tubing during infusions and, subsequently, the vein and circulatory system. So the half-full fluid level is extremely important.

The correct fluid level for IV drip chambers is half full, to allow drops to be counted and to prevent air from entering the tubing.

OBJECTIVES

The learner will:
1. differentiate between primary and secondary, and peripheral and central IV lines
2. explain the function of drip chambers, roller and slide clamps, and on-line and indwelling injection ports
3. differentiate between volumetric pumps, syringe pumps, and PCAs
4. identify the abbreviations used for IV fluid orders

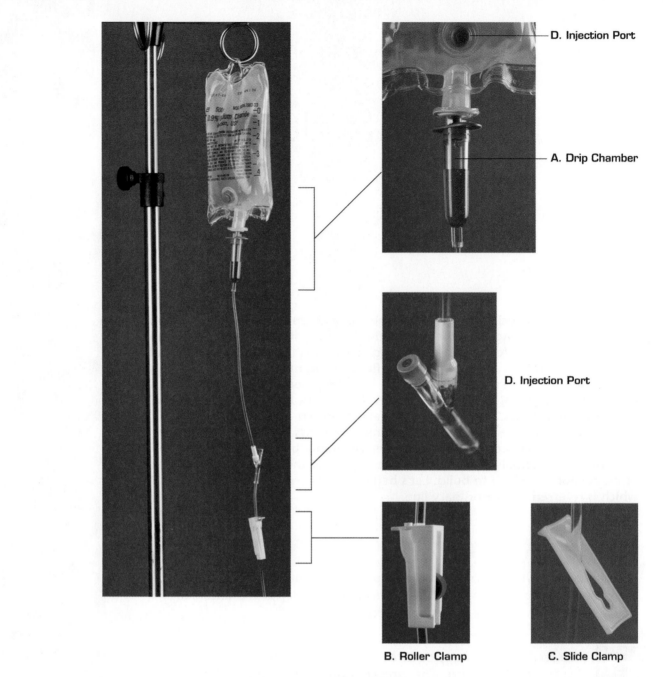

D. Injection Port

A. Drip Chamber

D. Injection Port

B. Roller Clamp

C. Slide Clamp

Figure 14-1

Next notice B, the **roller clamp**. This is opened to fill the line with fluid, and is adjusted after the IV is started, to count the drops falling in the drip chamber and set the flow rate. It provides an extremely accurate control rate. A second type of clamp, C, called a **slide clamp**, is present on tubings. The slide clamp can be used to temporarily stop an IV without disturbing the rate set on the roller clamp.

Next notice D, the **injection port**. Ports are located in several locations on the tubing, typically near the cannula end, drip chamber, and middle of the line, and they are also present on most IV solution bags. Ports allow injection of medication directly into the line or bag, as well as the attachment of secondary IV lines containing compatible IV fluids or medications to the primary line.

Intravenous fluids run by gravity flow. This necessitates that the IV solution bag be hung **above heart level** to exert sufficient pressure to infuse. Three feet is considered an average height for adults.

 The higher an IV bag is hung, the greater the pressure, and the faster the IV will infuse.

This pressure differential also means that if the flow rate is adjusted while an adult is lying in bed, it will slow down if she/he sits or stands and, in fact, it changes slightly with each repositioning. For this reason **monitoring IV flow rate is ongoing**, officially done every hour, but routinely checked after each major position change.

There are two additional terms relating to primary lines that you must know. If an arm or hand (or, less commonly, leg) vein is used for an infusion, it is referred to as a **peripheral line**. This is to distinguish it from a **central line**, which uses a special catheter whose tip is located centrally in a deep chest vein. Central lines may access the chest vein directly through the chest wall, via a neck vein, or through a peripheral vein in the arm or leg.

Secondary Line

Secondary lines attach to the primary line at an injection port. They are used primarily to infuse medications, frequently on an intermittent basis, for example, every 6–8 hours. They may also be used to infuse other compatible IV fluids. Secondary lines are commonly referred to as **IV piggybacks**. They are abbreviated **IVPB**. Refer to Figure 14-2, which illustrates a primary and secondary line setup.

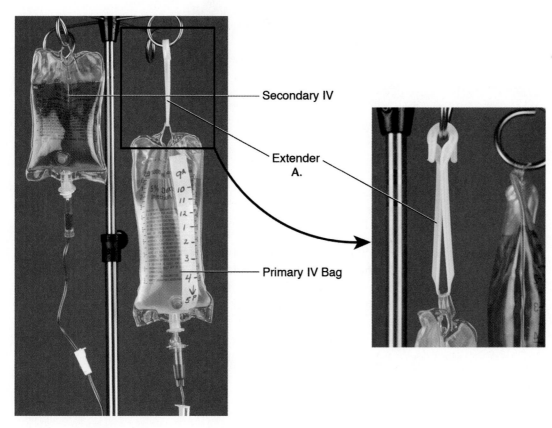

Figure 14-2

The IVPB is connected to a port located below the drip chamber on the primary line. Notice that **the IVPB bag is hung higher than the primary bag**. This gives it greater pressure and causes it to **infuse first**. Each IVPB set includes a plastic or metal **extender**, which is used to lower the primary solution bag to obtain this pressure differential (see Figure 14-2A). The flow rate for the IVPB is set by a separate roller clamp located on the secondary line. When the IVPB bag has emptied the primary line will automatically resume its flow. Secondary medication bags are usually much smaller than primary bags. Fifty, 100, 150, 200, and 250 mL bags are frequently used.

Another type of secondary medication setup is provided by Abbot Laboratories, **ADD-Vantage® system** (Figure 14-3). In this system a specially designed IV fluid bag that contains a **medication vial port** is used. The medication vial containing the ordered drug and dosage is inserted into the port, and the drug (frequently in powdered form) is mixed using IV fluid as the diluent, as illustrated in Figure 14-4. The vial contents are then displaced back into the solution bag and thoroughly mixed in the total solution before infusion. The vial remains in the solution bag port throughout the infusion, making it possible to cross-check the vial label for drug and dosage at any time.

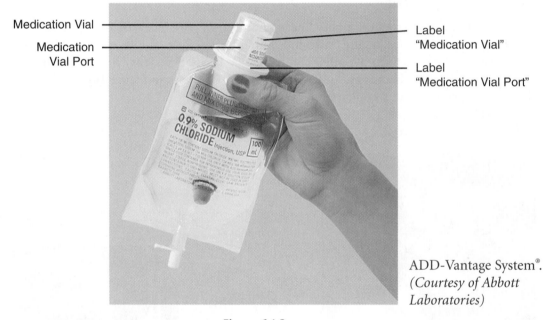

ADD-Vantage System®. *(Courtesy of Abbott Laboratories)*

Figure 14-3

If a drug is not available in either a prepackaged or ADD-Vantage® format, it is often prepared and labeled by the hospital pharmacy. And, finally, an IV medication may be prepared, added to the appropriate IV fluid, thoroughly mixed, labeled and initialed, and administered by the nurse who initiates the infusion.

ADD-Vantage® System **A.** The ADD-Vantage® medication vial is opened first. **B.** The medication vial port on the IV bag is opened. **C.** The vial top is inserted into the IV bag port and twisted to lock tightly in place. **D.** The vial stopper is removed inside the IV bag, and the medication and solution are thoroughly mixed before infusion. *(Courtesy of Abbott Laboratories)*

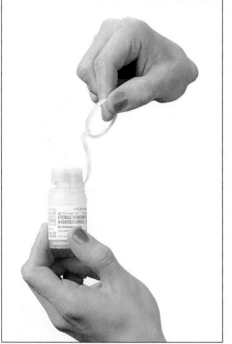

A.

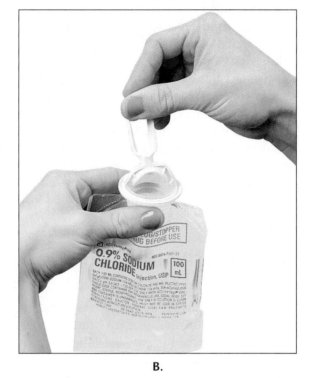

B.

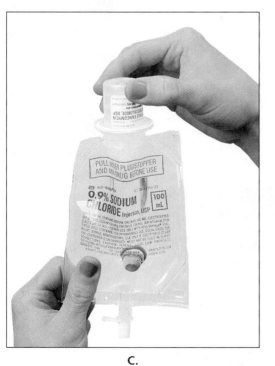

C.

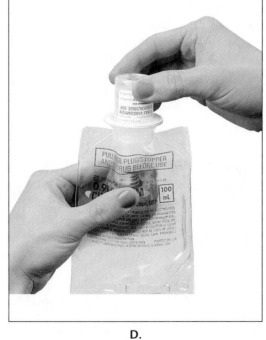

D.

Figure 14-4

Volume-Controlled Burettes

For greater accuracy in measuring **small-volume** IV medications and fluids, a **calibrated burette chamber** such as the one in Figure 14-5 is frequently used. The total capacity of burettes varies from 100 to 150 mL, calibrated in 1 mL increments. Many burettes are calibrated to deliver very small drops (microdrops), which also contributes to their accuracy. Burettes are most often referred to by their trade names, for example, Buretrols®, Solusets®, or Volutrols®. Burette chambers are often connected to a primary line and used as a secondary line, but they can also be primary lines that attach directly to an indwelling cannula. When medication is ordered, it is injected into the burette through its injection port. The exact amount of IV fluid is then added as a diluent. After thorough mixing, the flow rate is set using a separate clamp on the burette line. When IV fluids and/or medications require **exact** measurement, electronic infusion devices such as volumetric pumps are used instead of burettes.

Indwelling Infusion Ports/ Intermittent Locks

When a continuous IV is not necessary, but intermittent IV medication administration is, an **infusion port adapter** (Figure 14-6) can be attached to an indwelling cannula in a vein. Infusion ports are frequently referred to as **heplocks** or **saline locks (or ports)**. This terminology evolved because the ports must be irrigated with 1–2 mL of sterile saline or a heparin lock flush solution (100 units/mL) every 6–8 hours to prevent clotting and blockage. To infuse medication, the port top is cleansed, and the medication line is attached. When the infusion is complete, the line is disconnected until the next dosage is due. Ports are also used for **direct injection of medication using a syringe**, which is called an **IV push**, or **bolus**.

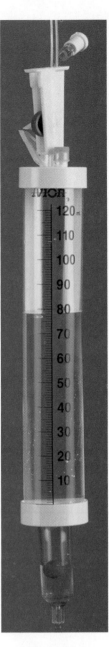

Figure 14-5

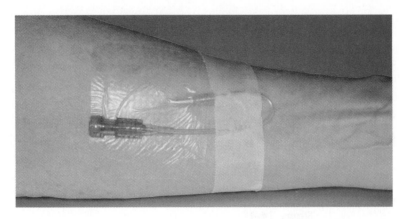

Figure 14-6

Answer the questions about IV administration sets as briefly as possible.

1. What is the correct fluid level for an IV drip chamber? _____

2. Which clamp is used to regulate IV flow rate? _____

3. When might a slide clamp be used? _____

4. What is a peripheral line? _____

5. What is a central line? _____

6. What is the common abbreviation for an intravenous piggyback? _____

7. Is an IV piggyback a primary or secondary line? _____

8. What must the height of a primary solution bag be when a secondary bag is infusing? _____

9. When is a saline lock used? _____

14

ANSWERS 1. Middle of chamber 2. Roller clamp 3. Stop the IV temporarily without disturbing the rate set on the roller clamp 4. Arm or leg vein 5. IV catheter inserted into a large chest vein 6. IVPB 7. Secondary 8. Lower than secondary bag 9. Intermittent infusions when a continuous IV is not necessary

Volumetric Pumps

IV medications are increasingly being administered via two widely used electronic infusion devices: volumetric pumps and syringe pumps. Refer now to Figure 14-7 of the Alaris® SE Single/Dual Channel Pump. Notice that the IV tubing and flow chamber have been inserted

Alaris® SE Single/Dual Channel Pump.
(Courtesy of Cardinal Health)

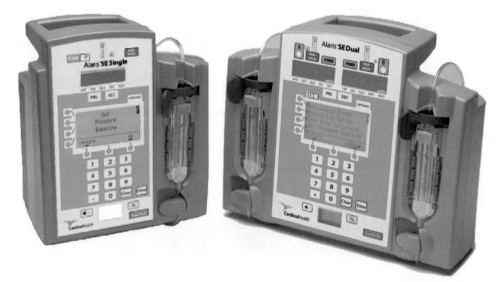

Figure 14-7

into the channel on the right. The unit contains a pumping mechanism that maintains the desired flow rate.

Most of the simpler pumps physically resemble the Alaris® SE Single/Dual Channel Pump, but the functions of different models vary widely. Some models continue to pump fluids even if an IV infiltrates, whereas others have a built-in pressure sensor that will sound an alarm if a resultant increased infusion resistance pressure occurs. Some models sound an alarm when the solution has completely infused; other models do not.

Because of the wide variation in pump models and their functions, caution is mandatory when they are used. It is estimated that as many as 50% of IV medication errors result from errors in pump programming.

Hospital or clinic in-service education is required for the use of all infusion devices.

Infusion devices are now widely used in many households for IV medication administration, and the **precautions in use apply less to the difficulty of the skill than in becoming familiar with the particular infusion model being used.** A single hospital or clinic could realistically have a dozen different models in use, and it is an ongoing nursing responsibility to learn how to use each particular model being used.

Double-checking of programming is mandatory when using infusion devices.

Because errors in infusion device programming are a factor in IV medication errors, it is mandatory that all programming be double-checked. A new generation of sophisticated "smart" pumps that have a built-in library of usual drug dosages, and are capable of detecting programming errors are making their appearance. The B. Braun Outlook™ illustrated in Figure 14-8 is one example. Another dose-specific pump is the Alaris® System shown in Figure 14-9, a lightweight, modular device that integrates infusion, monitoring, and clinical best-practice guidelines.

The B. Braun Outlook™. *(Courtesy of B. Braun Medical Inc.)*

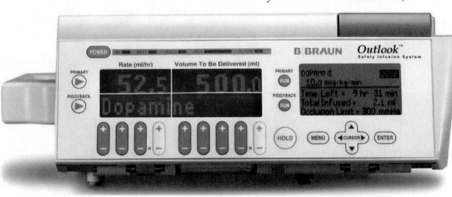

Figure 14-8

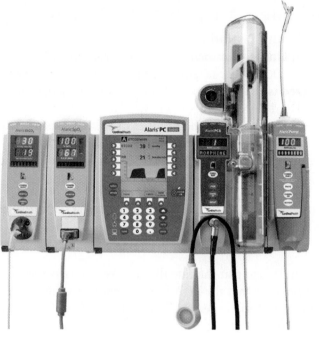

Alaris® System. *(Courtesy of Cardinal Health)*

Figure 14-9

Syringe Pumps

Syringe pumps, as their name implies, are devices that use a syringe to administer medications or fluids such as the B. Braun Perfusor™ Basic Syringe Pump (Figure 14-10). Syringe pumps are particularly valuable when **drugs that cannot be mixed with other solutions or medications** must be administered at a controlled rate over a short period of time, for example, 5, 10, or 20 minutes. The drug is measured in the syringe, which is inserted into the device, and the medication is infused at the rate set.

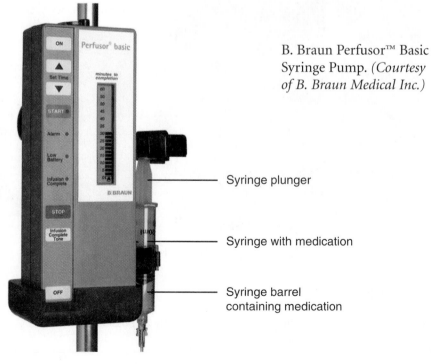

B. Braun Perfusor™ Basic Syringe Pump. *(Courtesy of B. Braun Medical Inc.)*

Syringe plunger

Syringe with medication

Syringe barrel containing medication

Figure 14-10

Patient-Controlled Analgesia (PCA) Devices

PCA devices allow **self-administration of medication to control pain.** A prefilled syringe or medication bag containing pain medication is inserted into a PCA device such as the Abbott Lifecare® PCA 4100 Infuser (Figure 14-11), and the **dosage and frequency of administration ordered is set.** The control button, A, is pressed as medication is needed, and it is administered and recorded by the PCA.

The device also keeps a record of the number of times use is **attempted**, and thus provides a record of the effectiveness of the dosage prescribed. If pain is not being relieved, new orders must be obtained and the PCA reset to administer the new dosage.

All electronic devices must be monitored to ensure they are functioning properly.

Is the IV or medication infusing at the rate that was set? Is activation of the PCA relieving the pain? If not, is it possible that the PCA itself is malfunctioning? Electronic devices have been in use for many years and are relatively trouble free, but if the desired goal is not being obtained, in the absence of other obvious reasons, **the possibility of malfunction must always be considered.**

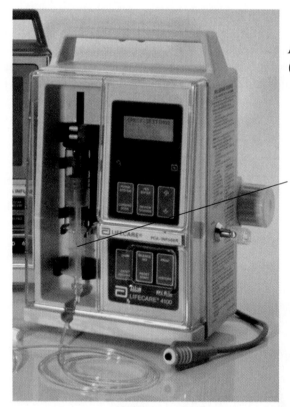

Abbott Lifecare® PCA 4100 Infuser. *(Courtesy of Abbott Laboratories)*

Syringe with medication

A. Control button

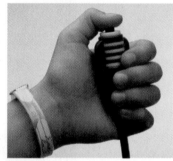

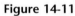

Figure 14-11

PROBLEM

Answer the questions about infusion devices as briefly as possible.

1. What is the function of a volumetric pump? _____

2. List two major precautions in their use. _____

3. When might a syringe pump be used? _____

4. What is a PCA? _____

Introduction to IV Fluids

IV fluids are prepared in plastic solution bags or glass bottles in volumes ranging from 50 mL (bags only) to 1000 mL. The 500 and 1000 mL sizes are the most commonly used. IV bags and bottles are labeled with the **complete name** of the fluid they contain, and the fine print under the solution name identifies the exact amount of each component of the fluid. Some examples of frequently used fluids are: 5% Dextrose in Water and 5% Dextrose in Normal Saline. IV **orders and charting**, however, are most often done **using symbols**.

In IV fluid symbols D always identifies dextrose; W always identifies water; S identifies saline; NS identifies normal saline; and numbers identify percentage (%) strengths.

IV solution symbols may be written in different ways; for example, 5% dextrose in water may be written D5W, 5%D/W, D5%W, or other combinations. But the **symbols and percentage have the identical meaning**. Normal saline solutions are frequently written with the .9 or % sign included, for example, D5 .9NS, or D5 0.9%S. IV fluids with different percentages of saline are also available: 0.45%, often written as 1/2 (0.45% is half of 0.9%), and 0.225%, sometimes written as 1/4 (¼ of 0.9) are examples. Some typical orders might be abbreviated D5 1/2S, or D5 1/4NS.

    Another commonly used solution is **Ringer's lactate**, a balanced electrolyte solution, which is also called lactated Ringer's solution. As you would now expect, this solution is abbreviated **RL** or **LR**, and, possibly, RLS. Electrolytes may also be added to the basic fluids (DW and DS) just discussed. One electrolyte so commonly added that it must be mentioned is potassium chloride, which is abbreviated KCl, and measured in milliequivalents (mEq).

PROBLEM

List as briefly as possible the components and percentage strengths of the IV solutions.

1. D10 NS _____

2. D5 NS _____

3. D2.5 1/2S _____

4. D5 1/4S _____

5. D20W _____

6. D5NS _____

7. D5NS 20 mEq KCl _____

8. D5RL _____

Percentages in IV Fluids

You will recall that **percent means grams of drug per 100 mL of fluid**. This means that a 5% dextrose solution will have 5 g of dextrose in each 100 mL. A 500 mL bag of a 5% solution will contain 5 g × 5, or 25 g of dextrose, whereas 500 mL of a 10% solution contains 10 g × 5, or 50 g of dextrose. The fine print on IV labels always lists the name and amount of all ingredients.

The point being made here is that percentages make IV fluids significantly different from each other. As with drugs, reading labels and making sure the IVs administered are what are actually ordered are critically important.

Parenteral Nutrition

One of the options available for providing nutrition for patients who cannot eat is to administer a nutrient solution via a central vein. This is referred to as parenteral nutrition. The solutions infused are generally high caloric and contain varying percentages of glucose, amino acids, and/or fat emulsions. A number of symbols and descriptions are used for parenteral nutrients. Some of the more common are TPN (total parenteral nutrition), PPN (partial parenteral nutrition), and hyperalimentation (nutrition in excess of maintenance needs). There is a noticeable difference in fluids that contain lipids (fat, intralipids) in that they are opaque-white in appearance, not unlike nonfat milk. These fluids are normally infused slowly, but not usually in excess of 24 hours, because they can spoil and support bacterial growth. All precautions applicable to IVs in general apply equally to parenteral nutrients, with even more meticulous care necessary for the IV site to prevent infection. Flow rate and infusion time calculations covered in subsequent chapters are also applicable for parenteral nutrition solutions.

Summary

This concludes your introduction to IV therapy. The important points to remember from this chapter are:

- Sterile technique is used to set up all IV solutions, tubings, and devices.

- The correct fluid level for an IV drip chamber is half full.

- Injection ports on an IV line are used to connect secondary lines and to infuse medications.

- A peripheral line refers to an IV infusing in a hand, arm, or leg vein.

- A central line refers to an IV infusing into a deep chest vein.

- IVs flow by gravity pressure, and the higher the solution bag, the faster the IV will infuse.

- The average height for an adult IV solution bag is 3 feet above heart level.

- Secondary solution bags must hang higher than the primary bag to infuse first.

- Volume-controlled burettes are used for very exact measurements of IV medications and fluids.

- Intermittent infusion locks or ports are used to infuse IV medications or fluids on an intermittent basis when a continuous IV is not necessary.

- Volumetric pumps are electronic devices that force fluids into a vein under pressure and control infusion rates.

Syringe pumps are used to infuse medications that cannot be mixed with other fluids or medications.

Patient-controlled analgesia (PCA) devices allow self-administration of pain medication.

In IV fluid symbols, D identifies Dextrose, W identifies Water, S identifies Saline, NS identifies Normal Saline, RL and LR identify lactated Ringer's solution, and numbers identify percentage (%) strengths.

Summary Self-Test

You are to assist with some IV procedures. Answer the situational questions concerning IV procedures.

1. An adult is admitted and an IV of 1000 mL D5RL is started. These initials identify what type of solution? _____

   This is referred to as what type of line? _____

2. All roller clamps on the IV tubing are closed before connection to the solution bag. Why? _____

3. The IV is started in the back of the left hand. This makes it what type of line? _____

4. You are asked to check the fluid level in the drip chamber, and you observe that it is correct, which is _____

5. You are then asked to adjust the flow rate. You will use what type of clamp to do this? _____

6. A decision was made to use an electronic infusion control device to administer this IV. The device used is a _____

7. An IV antibiotic is ordered. This is sent from the pharmacy already prepared in a small-volume IV solution bag. The setup used to infuse this medication is referred to as an IV _____

8. This is abbreviated how? _____

9. In order for the antibiotic to infuse first, how must it be hung in relation to the original solution bag? _____

10. Some days later the IV is to be discontinued, but IV antibiotics are to be continued. What is the site used for this intermittent administration called? _____

11. A PCA was used for one day. What do these initials mean? _____

    What symptoms is this device designed to control? _____

Answer the questions as briefly as possible.

12. A small-volume IV medication is to be diluted in 20 mL and infused. This can be most accu-

    rately measured using a _____ _____ .

13. These devices are calibrated in _____ increments.

14. When an IV medication is injected directly into the vein via a port, it is called

    an IV _____ or _____ .

15. Ports may be irrigated with _____ mL of _____ to

    prevent blockage every _____ hr.

16. In IV fluid symbols, D5NS identifies what IV fluid? _____

17. How can an IV be temporarily stopped without changing the flow rate set?

_____

ANSWERS		
1. 5% Dextrose in Ringer's lactate; primary	**7.** Piggyback	**13.** 1 mL
2. To prevent air from entering the tubing	**8.** IVPB	**14.** Push or bolus
	9. Higher	**15.** 1–2; Normal Saline; 6–8
3. Peripheral	**10.** Intermittent infusion port; saline or heparin lock	**16.** 5% Dextrose in Normal Saline
4. Half full	**11.** Patient-controlled analgesia; pain	**17.** By using the slide clamp
5. Roller	**12.** Calibrated burette	
6. Volumetric pump		

IV Flow Rate Calculation

There are two ways to calculate IV flow rates, and this chapter presents both: DA, and the division factor method.

Intravenous fluids are most often ordered on the basis of **mL/hr** to be administered, for example 125 mL/hr. With the widespread use of electronic infusion devices such as volumetric pumps that can be **set to deliver a mL/hr rate**, simply setting the rate ordered and making sure the device is working properly is all that is required for many infusions.

The most common flow rate calculation, which is necessary **when an infusion device is not being used**, involves **converting an IV order to the gtt/min rate necessary to infuse it**. This calculation may be required for **large-volume orders** written designating a **mL/hr** rate, for example, **1000 mL to infuse at 125 mL/hr** or for infusions of **mL per multiple hours**, for example, **3000 mL/24 hr**.

OBJECTIVES

The learner will:
1. identify the calibrations in gtt/mL on IV administration sets
2. calculate flow rates using dimensional analysis
4. calculate flow rates by the division factor method

IV Tubing Calibration

The size of IV drops is regulated by the IV administration set being used, which is **calibrated in number of gtt/mL**. Not all sets (and thus their drop size) are the same. Each hospital uses at least two sizes of infusion sets: the **standard macrodrip set, calibrated at 10, 15, or 20 gtt/mL**, which is used for routine adult IV administrations; and a **mini or microdrip set, calibrated at 60 gtt/mL**, which is used when more exact measurements are needed, for example, in critical care and pediatric infusions.

 IV administration sets are calibrated in gtt/mL.

The **gtt/mL calibration of each administration set is clearly printed on each package**, and the first step in calculating flow rates is to identify the gtt/mL calibration of the set to be used for infusion.

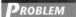

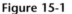

PROBLEM

Refer to the IV administration packages in Figures 15-1 and 15-2 and identify the calibration in gtt/mL of each.

1. _____

2. _____

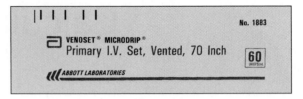

Figure 15-1

Figure 15-2

ANSWERS 1. 60 gtt/mL 2. 15 gtt/mL

Calculation of gtt/min Rates

When an infusion device is not being used, DA can be used to calculate gtt/min manual flow rates. The DA equation is set up exactly the same way as in previous chapters.

EXAMPLE 1

The order is to infuse a solution of D5W at **125 mL/hr** using a macrodrip set calibrated at **10 gtt/mL**. Calculate the flow rate in **gtt/min**.

You will notice an immediate difference in setting up this DA calculation, because **two values are being calculated: gtt and min**. Let's look at how this is done. You are calculating gtt/min. Write this to the left of the equation, followed by an equal sign.

$$\frac{gtt}{min} =$$

Next, begin ratio entries as if you were calculating only the gtt numerator. Locate the complete ratio containing gtt, which is the 10 gtt/mL set calibration. Enter this as the first ratio with 10 gtt as the numerator to match the gtt numerator being calculated; 1 mL becomes the denominator.

$$\frac{gtt}{min} = \frac{10 \ gtt}{1 \ mL}$$

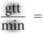

The mL denominator must be matched in the next numerator. Look again at the problem. This is provided by the125 mL/hr flow rate ordered. Enter this ratio with 125 mL as the numerator to match the previous mL denominator; 1 hr becomes the new denominator.

$$\frac{\text{gtt}}{\text{min}} = \frac{10 \text{ gtt}}{1 \text{ mL}} \times \frac{125 \text{ mL}}{1 \text{ hr}}$$

The denominator to be matched now is hr, but there is no hr in the problem data. This indicates the need for a **conversion ratio** between hr and min. Enter this now with 1 hr as the numerator; 60 min becomes the denominator, and it automatically completes the equation.

$$\frac{\text{gtt}}{\text{min}} = \frac{10 \text{ gtt}}{1 \text{ mL}} \times \frac{125 \text{ mL}}{1 \text{ hr}} \times \frac{1 \text{ hr}}{60 \text{ min}}$$

Cancel the alternative denominator/numerator mL/mL and hr/hr units of measure. This leaves only the gtt/min numerator/denominator units being calculated remaining in the equation. Notice how easily the DA equation sets itself up from the data available. Now do the math, which for drop rates can often be completed manually. Answers are rounded to the nearest whole drop.

$$\frac{\text{gtt}}{\text{min}} = \frac{10 \text{ gtt}}{1 \text{ mL}} \times \frac{125 \text{ mL}}{1 \text{ hr}} \times \frac{1 \text{ hr}}{60 \text{ min}} = 20.8 = \textbf{21 gtt/min}$$

A rate of 21 gtt/min is required to infuse an IV at 125 mL/hr using a 10 gtt/mL cali-brated IV set.

 Flow rates are routinely rounded to the nearest whole number.

Let's now look at a **shortcut** that can be used in calculations with **any mL/hr** rate ordered. The **conversion ratio can be eliminated** by immediately substituting 60 min for the 1 hr entry. This will be done in the remaining calculations. Also notice once again that the math of many flow rate calculations can be done by simple reduction instead of using a calculator.

EXAMPLE 2

A **20 gtt/mL** set is to be used to infuse an IV solution at a rate of **90 mL/hr**. Calculate the **gtt/min** flow rate.

Enter the gtt/min to be calculated to the left of the equation followed by an equal sign.

$$\frac{\text{gtt}}{\text{min}}$$

Locate the ratio containing gtt. This is provided by the 20 gtt/mL IV set calibration. Enter it with 20 gtt as the numerator to match the gtt numerator being calculated; 1 mL becomes the denominator.

$$\frac{\text{gtt}}{\text{min}} = \frac{20 \text{ gtt}}{1 \text{ mL}}$$

The mL denominator must be matched in the next numerator entered. This is provided by the 90 mL/hr rate. Enter this now with 90 mL as the numerator; **enter 60 min for the 1 hr conversion to complete the equation.**

$$\frac{\text{gtt}}{\text{min}} = \frac{20 \text{ gtt}}{1 \text{ mL}} \times \frac{90 \text{ mL}}{60 \text{ min}}$$

Cancel the alternate mL/mL units of measure, leaving only the gtt/min being calculated remaining in the equation. Do the math, noticing that simple reduction of the numbers in this equation can solve this flow rate calculation.

$$\frac{\text{gtt}}{\text{min}} = \frac{\overset{1}{\cancel{20}} \text{ gtt}}{1 \text{ } \cancel{\text{mL}}} \times \frac{\overset{30}{\cancel{90}} \cancel{\text{mL}}}{\underset{1}{\underset{3}{\cancel{60}}} \text{ min}} = \textbf{30 gtt/min}$$

A 30 gtt/min flow rate will be required to obtain an infusion rate of 90 mL/hr using a set calibrated at 20 gtt/mL.

<hr>

EXAMPLE 3

Calculate the **gtt/min** flow rate to administer an IV at **100 mL/hr** using a set calibrated at **15 gtt/mL.**

Enter the gtt/min being calculated first to the left of the equation, followed by an equal sign.

$$\frac{\text{gtt}}{\text{min}} =$$

The gtt numerator being calculated must be matched by a gtt numerator entry in the first ratio entered. This is provided by the 15 gtt/mL set calibration. Enter 15 gtt as the numerator; 1 mL becomes the denominator.

$$\frac{\text{gtt}}{\text{min}} = \frac{15 \text{ gtt}}{1 \text{ mL}}$$

The mL denominator must now be matched in the next numerator. This is provided by the 100 mL of the 100 mL/hr rate ordered. Enter 100 mL as the next numerator, and substitute 60 min for the hr rate to complete to equation.

$$\frac{\text{gtt}}{\text{min}} = \frac{15 \text{ gtt}}{1 \text{ mL}} \times \frac{100 \text{ mL}}{60 \text{ min}}$$

Cancel the alternate denominator/numerator mL/mL entries to be sure you entered the ratios correctly. Only the gtt/min being calculated remains in the equation. Do the math, using simple reduction to obtain the answer.

$$\frac{\text{gtt}}{\text{min}} = \frac{\overset{1}{\cancel{15}} \text{ gtt}}{1 \text{ } \cancel{\text{mL}}} \times \frac{\overset{25}{\cancel{100}} \cancel{\text{mL}}}{\underset{1}{\underset{4}{\cancel{60}}} \text{ min}} = \textbf{25 gtt/min}$$

The gtt/min rate required for a 100 mL/hr infusion using a 15 gtt/mL set is 25 gtt/min.

Calculate the gtt/min manual flow rate for the IV infusions. If possible, use simple reduction to obtain the answers.

1. Administer 110 mL/hr using a set calibrated at 20 gtt/mL. _____

2. A 20 mL/hr rate is ordered using a microdrip set calibrated at 60 gtt/mL. _____

3. A 20 gtt/mL set is used to infuse an IV at 100 mL/hr. _____

4. A rate of 80 mL/hr is ordered using a 10 gtt/mL calibrated set. _____

5. A set calibrated at 15 gtt/mL is used for an infusion of 90 mL/hr. _____

ANSWERS 1. 37 gtt/min 2. 20 gtt/min 3. 33 gtt/min 4. 13 gtt/min 5. 23 gtt/min

15

Small Volume gtt/min Calculations

Many small volume IVs are administered by manually set rates, frequently using a volume-controlled burette. An example would be a volume of 100 mL to infuse in 40 min. The calculation for these rates is much simpler, because the rate is usually ordered per min, and no hr to min time conversion is needed.

EXAMPLE 1

Calculate the **gtt/min** flow rate for **100 mL** to be infused in **40 min** using a set calibrated at **15 gtt/mL**.

Enter the gtt/min being calculated to the left of the equation followed by an equal sign.

$$\frac{gtt}{min} =$$

The gtt numerator being calculated must be matched in the first numerator entered. This is provided by the 15 gtt of the calibration set. Enter 15 gtt as the first or starting numerator; 1 mL becomes the denominator.

$$\frac{gtt}{min} = \frac{15\ gtt}{1\ mL}$$

The mL denominator must be matched in the next numerator. This is provided by the 100 mL of the 100 mL in 40 min infusion rate ordered. Enter this ratio now with 100 mL as the numerator; 40 min becomes the new denominator and completes the equation.

$$\frac{gtt}{min} = \frac{15\ gtt}{1\ mL} \times \frac{100\ mL}{40\ min}$$

Cancel the alternate denominator/numerator mL/mL entries to check for accurate ratio entry, then do the math.

$$\frac{gtt}{min} = \frac{15\ gtt}{1\ \cancel{mL}} \times \frac{\overset{5}{\cancel{100\ mL}}}{\underset{2}{\cancel{40}\ min}} = 37.5 = \textbf{38 gtt/min}$$

To infuse 100 mL in 40 min using a 15 gtt/mL calibrated set, the rate must be manually adjusted to 38 gtt/min.

EXAMPLE 2

An IV with a **15 mL** volume is to infuse in **30 min** using a **microdrip** set calibrated at **60 gtt/mL**. Calculate the manual gtt/min flow rate.

Enter the gtt/min to be calculated to the left of the equation followed by an equal sign.

$$\frac{gtt}{min} =$$

The gtt numerator being calculated must be matched by the numerator of the first ratio entered. This is provided by the 60 gtt/mL set calibration. Enter this ratio with 60 gtt as the numerator; 1 mL becomes the denominator.

$$\frac{gtt}{min} = \frac{60\ gtt}{1\ mL}$$

The mL denominator must be matched in the following numerator. The ratio containing mL is the 15 mL volume in 30 min infusion rate. Enter 15 mL as the numerator; 30 min becomes the final denominator to complete the equation.

$$\frac{gtt}{min} = \frac{60\ gtt}{1\ \cancel{mL}} \times \frac{15\ \cancel{mL}}{30\ min}$$

Cancel the alternate denominator/numerator mL/mL entries to check for correct ratio entry, then do the math.

$$\frac{gtt}{min} = \frac{\overset{2}{\cancel{60}}\ gtt}{1\ \cancel{mL}} \times \frac{15\ \cancel{mL}}{\underset{1}{\cancel{30}}\ min} = \textbf{30 gtt/min}$$

To infuse 15 mL in 30 min using a 60 gtt/mL microdrip set, the drip rate must be adjusted to deliver 30 gtt/min.

EXAMPLE 3

Calculate the gtt/min manual flow rate for a volume of **50 mL** to infuse in **20 min** using a **20 gtt/mL** infusion set.

Enter the gtt/min being calculated to the left of the equation followed by an equal sign.

$$\frac{gtt}{min} =$$

The gtt numerator being calculated must be matched in the numerator of the first ratio enter. This is provided by 20 gtt/mL calibration of the infusion set. Enter this ratio now with 20 gtt as the numerator; 1 mL becomes the denominator.

$$\frac{gtt}{min} = \frac{20\ gtt}{1\ mL}$$

The mL denominator must now be matched in the following numerator. The 50 mL volume to be infused in 20 min provides the next ratio. Enter it now with 50 mL as the numerator; 20 min becomes the denominator and completes the equation.

$$\frac{gtt}{min} = \frac{20\ gtt}{1\ mL} \times \frac{50\ mL}{20\ min}$$

Cancel the alternate denominator/numerator mL/mL entries to check for correct ratio entry, and do the math.

$$\frac{gtt}{min} = \frac{\overset{1}{\cancel{20}}\,gtt}{1\,\cancel{mL}} \times \frac{50\,\cancel{mL}}{\underset{1}{\cancel{20}}\,min} = \textbf{50 gtt/min}$$

To infuse 50 mL in 20 min using a set calibrated at 20 gtt/mL, the manual rate must be set at 50 gtt/min.

PROBLEM

Calculate the flow rates necessary to infuse the IVs in the time specified. If possible, use simple reduction to calculate the flow rates.

1. A volume of 75 mL in 50 min using a 10 gtt/mL set _____

2. An 80 mL volume in 50 min using a 15 gtt/mL set _____

3. A set calibrated at 20 gtt/mL to infuse 40 mL in 20 min _____

4. A 10 gtt/mL set to infuse 20 mL in 20 min _____

5. A 30 mL volume to infuse in 40 min using a 60 gtt/mL set _____

ANSWERS   **1.** 15 gtt/min   **2.** 24 gtt/min   **3.** 40 gtt/min   **4.** 10 gtt/min   **5.** 45 gtt/min

Division Factor Method of Calculation

In a clinical setting where **all the macrodrip IV sets have the same calibration**, either 10, 15, or 20 gtt/mL, an alternate **division factor method** can be used to calculate flow rates. However, **this method can only be used if the rate is expressed in mL/hr (mL/60 min)**. Let's start by looking at how the division factor is obtained.

EXAMPLE

Calculate the **gtt/min** rate to administer an IV at **125 mL/hr** using a set calibrated at **10 gtt/mL**.

$$\frac{gtt}{min} = \frac{\overset{1}{\cancel{10}}\,(gtt)}{1\,(mL)} \times \frac{125\,(mL)}{\underset{6}{\cancel{60}}\,(min)} = 20.8 = \textbf{21 gtt/mL}$$

Because the time is restricted to 60 min the set calibration, 10, can be divided into 60 min to obtain a constant number, 6. This number is the **division factor**, and for all 10 gtt/mL calibrated sets the division factor is 6.

 The division factor can be obtained for any IV set by dividing 60 by the calibration of the set.

PROBLEM

Determine the division factor for the IV sets.

1. 20 gtt/mL   _____

2. 15 gtt/mL   _____

3. 60 gtt/mL   _____

4. 10 gtt/mL   _____

ANSWERS 1. 3   2. 4   3. 1   4. 6

15

Once the division factor is known, the gtt/min rate can be calculated in one step, by dividing the mL/hr rate by the division factor. Look once again at both the DA and division factor examples.

$$\frac{\text{gtt}}{\text{min}} = \frac{\overset{1}{\cancel{10}}\,(\text{gtt})}{1\,(\text{mL})} \times \frac{125\,(\text{mL})}{\underset{6}{\cancel{60}}\,(\text{min})} = 20.8 = \textbf{21 gtt/mL}$$

or 125 (mL/hr) ÷ 6 = 20.8 = **21 gtt/min**

The 125 mL/hr flow rate divided by the division factor 6 gives the same 21 gtt/min rate.

 The gtt/min flow rate can be calculated for mL/hr IV orders in one step by dividing the mL/hr to be infused by the division factor of the administration set.

EXAMPLE 1

Infuse an IV at **100 mL/hr** using a set calibrated at **10 gtt/mL**.

Determine the division factor: 60 ÷ 10 = **6**

Calculate the flow rate: 100 mL ÷ 6 = 16.6 = **17 gtt/min**

EXAMPLE 2

Infuse an IV at **125 mL/hr** using a set calibrated at **15 gtt/mL**.

60 ÷ 15 = **4**   125 mL ÷ 4 = 31.2 = **31 gtt/min**

EXAMPLE 3

A set calibrated at **20 gtt/mL** is used to infuse **90 mL per hr.**

60 ÷ 20 = **3**   90 mL ÷ 3 = **30 gtt/min**

The division factor is of enormous assistance in clinical practice because hospitals and clinics generally use only one size macrodrip set. This means that the same division factor can be used for all mL/hr IV flow rate calculations.

PROBLEM

Calculate the flow rates in gtt/min for the infusions using the division factor method.

1. A rate of 110 mL/hr via a set calibrated at 20 gtt/mL. _____

2. A set is calibrated at 15 gtt/mL. Infuse at 130 mL/hr. _____

3. Infuse 150 mL/hr using a 10 gtt/mL set. _____

4. A set calibrated at 20 gtt/mL is used to infuse 45 mL/hr. _____

5. Infusion is ordered at 75 mL/hr with a set calibrated at 15 gtt/mL. _____

ANSWERS 1. 37 gtt/min 2. 33 gtt/min 3. 25 gtt/min 4. 15 gtt/min 5. 19 gtt/min

All of the preceding examples and problems using the division factor method were for **macrodrip** sets. Let's now look at what happens when a **microdrip** set calibrated at **60 gtt/mL** is used.

EXAMPLE

Infuse at **50 mL/hr** using a **60 gtt/mL** microdrip.

$$60 \div 60 = 1 \qquad 50\,mL \div 1 = \mathbf{50\,gtt/min}$$

Because the set calibration is 60, and the division factor is based on a 60-min (1 hr) time, the division factor is 1. So, **for microdrip sets the gtt/min flow rate will be identical to the mL/hr ordered.**

 When a 60 gtt/mL microdrip set is used, the flow rate in gtt/min is identical to the volume in mL/hr to be infused.

PROBLEM

What is the drip rate in gtt/min for the infusions if a microdrip is used?

1. 120 mL/hr _____

2. 90 mL/hr _____

3. 100 mL/hr _____

4. 75 mL/hr _____

5. 80 mL/hr _____

ANSWERS 1. 120 gtt/min 2. 90 gtt/min 3. 100 gtt/min 4. 75 gtt/min 5. 80 gtt/min

The division factor method can be used to calculate the flow rate of **any volume that can be expressed in mL/hr.** Larger volumes can be divided and smaller volumes can be multiplied and expressed in mL/hr. This does require an extra step, and if you find it confusing you may elect not to use it.

EXAMPLE 1 2400 mL/24 hr = 2400 ÷ 24 = **100 mL/hr**

EXAMPLE 2 1800 mL/8 hr = 1800 ÷ 8 = **225 mL/hr**

EXAMPLE 3   10 mL/30 min = 10 × 2 (2 × 30 min) = **20 mL/hr**

EXAMPLE 4   15 mL/20 min = 15 × 3 (3 × 20 min) = **45 mL/hr**

Regulating Flow Rate

Manual flow rates are regulated by **counting the number of drops falling in the drip chamber.** The standard procedure for doing this is to hold a watch next to the drip chamber and actually **count the number of drops falling.** The roller clamp is adjusted during the count until the required rate has been set. A 15-sec count is most commonly used because it's easier to focus on the count for a shorter period of time. This means that the ordered gtt/min (60 sec) rate must be divided by 4 to obtain the 15-second drip count (60 sec ÷ 4 = 15 sec).

EXAMPLE 1

An IV is to run at a rate of **60 gtt/min.** What will the 15-sec count be?

60 gtt/min ÷ 4 = **15 gtt**

Adjust the rate to 15 gtt/15 sec.

EXAMPLE 2

A **70 gtt/min** IV rate is ordered. What will the 15-sec count be?

70 gtt/min ÷ 4 = 17.5 = **18 gtt**

Adjust the rate to 18 gtt/15 sec.

EXAMPLE 3

Adjust an IV to a rate of **50 gtt/min** using a 15-sec count.

50 gtt/min ÷ 4 = **13 gtt**

Adjust the rate to 13 gtt/15 sec.

PROBLEM

Answer the questions about 15-second drip rates.

1. The 15-second count of an IV flow rate is 7 gtt. A 29 gtt/min rate is required. Is this rate correct?   _____

2. You are to regulate a newly started IV to deliver 67 gtt/min. Using a 15-second count, how would you set the flow rate?   _____

3. An IV is to run at 48 gtt/min. What must the 15-second drip rate be?   _____

4. How many gtt will you count in 15 seconds if the rate is 55 gtt/min?   _____

5. An IV is to run at 84 gtt/min. What will the 15-second rate be?   _____

ANSWERS   1. Yes   2. 17 gtt/15 sec   3. 12 gtt/15 sec   4. 14 gtt/15 sec   5. 21 gtt/15 sec

Individual hospitals, and states or provinces, may require a 30- or 60-sec (1 min) count. When a 60-sec count is required, particular care must be taken not to let your attention wander during the count, which can easily happen in this longer time frame. A 60-sec count will require a full minute count, whereas a 30-sec count will require the gtt/min rate to be divided by 2 (60 sec ÷ 2 = 30 sec).

EXAMPLE 1

An IV is to be infused at 56 gtt/min. What is the 30-sec rate?

56 gtt/min ÷ 2 = 28 gtt

Adjust the rate to 28 gtt/30 sec.

EXAMPLE 2

A rate of 72 gtt/min has been ordered. What will the 30-sec count be?

72 gtt/min ÷ 2 = 36 gtt

Adjust the rate to 36 gtt/30 sec.

PROBLEM

Calculate the 30-sec count for the IVs.

1. An IV is to be run at a rate of 48 gtt/min. Calculate a 30-sec count. _____

2. An IV is ordered to infuse at 52 gtt/min. _____

ANSWERS   1. 24 gtt/30 sec   2. 26 gtt/30 sec

Summary

This concludes the chapter on IV flow rate calculation and monitoring. The important points to remember from this chapter are:

IVs are ordered as mL/hr or mL/min to be administered.

Manual flow rates are counted in gtt/min.

IV tubings are calibrated in gtt/mL.

Macrodrip IV sets will have a calibration of 10, 15, or 20 gtt/mL.

Mini or microdrip sets have a calibration of 60 gtt/mL.

The division factor method can be used to calculate flow rates only if the volume to be administered is specified in mL/hr (60 min).

The division factor is obtained by dividing 60 by the gtt/mL set calibration.

Flow rate by the division factor method is determined by dividing the mL/hr to be administered by the division factor.

Because micro/minidrip sets have a calibration of 60 gtt/mL, their division factor is 1, and the flow rate in gtt/min is the same as the mL/hr ordered.

15

Summary Self-Test

Answer the questions as briefly as possible.

1. Determine the division factor for the following IV sets.

   a) 60 gtt/mL _____

   b) 15 gtt/mL _____

   c) 20 gtt/mL _____

   d) 10 gtt/mL _____

2. How is the flow rate determined in the division factor method? _____

3. The division factor method can only be used if the volume to be administered is expressed in _____

4. An IV is to infuse at 50 gtt/min. How will you set it using a 15-sec count? _____

5. You are to adjust an IV at a rate of 60 gtt/min. What will the 15-sec count be? _____

Calculate the flow rate in gtt/min for the IV solutions and medications. Don't let the types of solutions confuse you. Concentrate on locating the information you need for your calculations.

6. D5W 2000 mL has been ordered to run 16 hr. Set calibration is 10 gtt/mL. _____

7. The order is for 500 mL of normal saline in 8 hr. The set is calibrated at 15 gtt/mL. _____

8. Administer 150 mL of sodium chloride 0.45% over 3 hr. A microdrip is used. _____

9. 1500 mL D5W with 40 mEq KCl/L has been ordered to run over 12 hr. Set calibration is 20 gtt/mL. _____

10. An IV medication of 30 mL is to be administered over 30 min using a 15 gtt/mL set. _____

11. Administer 100 mL of 0.9% NaCl in 1 hr using a 15 gtt/mL set. _____

12. Infuse 500 mL of intralipids IV in 6 hr. Set calibration is 10 gtt/mL. _____

13. An IV of 1000 mL D5 1/4 NaCl with 20 mEq KCl is ordered to run at 25 mL/hr using a microdrip set. _____

14. Ringer's lactate 800 mL has been ordered to run in 5 hr. Set calibration is 10 gtt/mL. _____

15. Administer 1500 mL of D5 lactated Ringer's solution over 8 hr using a set calibrated at 20 gtt/mL. _____

16. The order is for D5 1/2 NaCl 750 mL to run in 6 hr. Set calibration is 15 gtt/mL. _____

17. The order is to infuse 50 mL of a piggyback antibiotic over 1 hr. The set calibration is a microdrip. _____

18. An IV of 500 mL D5W is to infuse over 6 hr. You will be using a set calibration of 10 gtt/mL. _____

19. Infuse 120 mL gentamicin via IVPB over 1 hr. Set calibration is 10 gtt/mL. _____

20. Administer 12 mL of an IV medication in 22 min using a microdrip set. _____

21. A client is to receive 3000 mL of D5W in 20 hr. Set is calibrated at 20 gtt/mL. _____

22. Infuse 1 liter of D5W in 5 hr using a set calibration of 15 gtt/mL. _____

23. A hyperalimentation solution of 1180 mL is to infuse in 12 hr using a set calibration of 20 gtt/mL. _____

24. Two 500 mL units of whole blood are ordered. Both units are to be completed in 5 hr. The set calibration is 20 gtt/mL. _____

25. Infuse 15 mL of IV medication in the next 14 min using a 20 gtt/mL set. _____

26. An IV of 1000 mL 0.9% NaCl is to be infused in 10 hr using a 20 gtt/mL calibration. _____

27. A minidrip is used to administer 12 mL in 17 min. _____

28. Infuse 2750 mL in 20 hr using a 10 gtt/mL set. _____

29. D5W 1800 mL is to infuse in the next 15 hr with a 15 gtt/mL set. _____

30. Infuse 600 mL of intralipids IV in 6 hr with a 10 gtt/mL set. _____

31. Administer 22 mL of an IV antibiotic solution in 18 min using a minidrip set. _____

32. 1800 mL of D5W with 30 mEq of KCl per liter have been ordered to infuse in 10 hr. Set calibration is 20 gtt/mL. _____

33. Infuse 8 mL in 9 min using a minidrip. _____

34. An IV of 4000 mL D5W IV is to be infused in the next 20 hr. A 20 gtt/mL set is used. _____

35. Infuse 150 mL D5W in 90 minutes on a 15 gtt/mL set. _____

ANSWERS

1. a) 1 b) 4 c) 3	8. 50 gtt/min	18. 14 gtt/min	28. 23 gtt/min
d) 6	9. 42 gtt/min	19. 20 gtt/min	29. 30 gtt/min
2. mL/hr ÷ division	10. 15 gtt/min	20. 33 gtt/min	30. 17 gtt/min
factor	11. 25 gtt/min	21. 50 gtt/min	31. 73 gtt/min
3. mL/hr	12. 14 gtt/min	22. 50 gtt/min	32. 60 gtt/min
(mL/60 min)	13. 25 gtt/min	23. 33 gtt/min	33. 53 gtt/min
4. 13 gtt/15 sec	14. 27 gtt/min	24. 67 gtt/min	34. 67 gtt/min
5. 15 gtt/15 sec	15. 63 gtt/min	25. 21 gtt/min	35. 25 gtt/min
6. 21 gtt/min	16. 31 gtt/min	26. 33 gtt/min	
7. 16 gtt/min	17. 50 gtt/min	27. 42 gtt/min	

Calculating IV Infusion and Completion Times

The three main reasons for calculating IV infusion times are: (1) to know when a particular solution bag will be completed so that any additional solutions ordered can be prepared in advance and ready to hang; (2) to discontinue an IV when it has completed; and (3) to label an IV bag with the start, progress, and completion times so that the infusion can be monitored and adjusted as necessary to keep it on schedule. Knowing the infusion time is also important because laboratory studies are sometimes made before, during, or after specified amounts of IV solutions have infused. The infusion time may be calculated in hours and/or minutes, depending on the amount and type of solution and individual need.

Calculating from Volume and Hourly Rate Ordered

Most IV orders are written specifying the total volume to be infused and the hourly rate of administration, for example, 2000 mL at 100 mL per hr. The largest IV solution bag is 1000 mL, so this 2000 mL volume (or any volume) may require a combination of several 1000 mL, 500 mL, or 250 mL bags.

Because most large-volume IVs take several hours to infuse, the unit of time being calculated is most often hours (hr). An easy one-step calculation is used to obtain the infusion time. To use it you will divide the **total volume to be infused** by the **mL/hr rate** of infusion.

 IV infusion time is calculated by dividing the total volume to be infused by the mL/hr flow rate.

EXAMPLE 1

Calculate the infusion time for an IV of **500 mL** D5W ordered to infuse at **50 mL/hr.**

$$\text{Infusion Time} = \text{total volume} \div \text{mL/hr rate}$$

$$= 500 \text{ mL} \div 50 \text{ mL/hr} = \textbf{10 hr}$$

The infusion time for an IV of 500 mL infusing at 50 mL/hr is 10 hr.

EXAMPLE 2

The order is to infuse **1000 mL** of D5NS at **75 mL/hr.** Calculate the infusion time.

$$1000 \text{ mL} \div 75 \text{ mL/hr} = \textbf{13.33 hr}$$

In this example, the 13 represents hr, whereas the **.33 represents the fraction of an additional hr.**

 Fractional hr are converted to min by multiplying 60 min by the fraction obtained.

Calculate the min by multiplying 60 min by the fractional hr.

$$60 \text{ min} \times .33 = 19.8 = \textbf{20 min}$$

The total infusion time is 13 hr 20 min.

EXAMPLE 3

An IV of **1000 mL** D5W is infusing at **90 mL/hr.** How long will it take to complete?

$$1000 \text{ mL} \div 90 \text{ mL/hr} = \textbf{11.11 hr}$$

Remember that .11 represents the fraction of an additional hr. Convert this to minutes by multiplying 60 min by .11.

$$60 \text{ min} \times .11 = 6.6 = \textbf{7 min}$$

The total infusion time is 11 hr 7 min.

EXAMPLE 4

Calculate the infusion time for an IV of **750 mL** RL ordered at a rate of **80 mL/hr.**

$$750 \text{ mL} \div 80 \text{ mL/hr} = \textbf{9.38 hr}$$

$$60 \text{ min} \times .38 = 22.8 = \textbf{23 min}$$

The infusion time is 9 hr 23 min.

EXAMPLE 5

A rate of **75 mL/hr** is ordered for a total volume of **500 mL** D5W. Calculate the infusion time.

$$500 \text{ mL} \div 75 \text{ mL/hr} = \textbf{6.67 hr}$$

$$60 \text{ min} \times .67 = 40.2 = \textbf{40 min}$$

The infusion time is 6 hr 40 min.

PROBLEM

Calculate infusion times for the IVs.

1. An IV of 900 mL RL ordered to infuse at 80 mL/hr   _____

2. A volume of 250 mL to be infused at 30 mL/hr   _____

3. An infusion of 180 mL of NS to run at a rate of 25 mL/hr   _____

4. A volume of 1000 mL D5W ordered at a rate of 60 mL/hr   _____

5. An IV of 150 mL ordered to infuse at 80 mL/hr   _____

> **ANSWERS** **1.** 11 hr 15 min **2.** 8 hr 20 min **3.** 7 hr 12 min **4.** 16 hr 40 min **5.** 1 hr 53 min
> Note: Answers may vary due to rounding or calculator setting, so variations of 1–2 min may be considered correct.

Calculating Infusion Time from gtt/min Rate and Set Calibration

In some instances, the only information you may have to calculate the infusion time is the gtt/min rate at which the IV is infusing, the set calibration, and the total volume to be infused. DA is used for the calculation.

EXAMPLE 1

Calculate the infusion time for an IV of **1000 mL** of D5W running at **25 gtt/min** on a set calibrated at **10 gtt/mL**.

Write the hr being calculated first to the left of the equation, followed by an equal sign.

$$hr =$$

There is no hr in the data, so a 1 hr = 60 min conversion must be entered as the first (starting) ratio. Enter this now with 1 hr as the numerator to match the hr being calculated; 60 min becomes the denominator.

$$hr = \frac{1\ hr}{60\ min}$$

The min denominator must be matched in the next numerator. This is provided by the 25 gtt/min flow rate. Enter this ratio now with 1 min as the numerator; 25 gtt becomes the denominator.

$$hr = \frac{1\ hr}{60\ min} \times \frac{1\ min}{25\ gtt}$$

The gtt denominator must be matched in the next numerator. This is provided by the 10 gtt/mL set calibration; enter 10 gtt as the numerator and 1 mL as the denominator.

$$hr = \frac{1\ hr}{60\ min} \times \frac{1\ min}{25\ gtt} \times \frac{10\ gtt}{1\ mL}$$

The denominator to be matched next is mL, and this is provided by the 1000 mL volume being infused. Enter 1000 mL now as the final numerator to complete the equation. •

$$hr = \frac{1\ hr}{60\ min} \times \frac{1\ min}{25\ gtt} \times \frac{10\ gtt}{1\ mL} \times \frac{1000\ mL}{}$$

Cancel the alternate denominator/numerator min/min, gtt/gtt, and mL/mL entries to check for correct ratio entry. Then do the math.

$$hr = \frac{1 \text{ hr}}{60 \text{ min}} \times \frac{1 \text{ min}}{25 \text{ gtt}} \times \frac{10 \text{ gtt}}{1 \text{ mL}} \times \frac{1000 \text{ mL}}{} = \textbf{6.67 hr}$$

This infusion will complete in 6.67 hr. However, one last step is necessary. **The fractional hr of the answer must be converted to min.** This is done by **multiplying 60 min by the .67 fraction obtained.**

$$60 \text{ min} \times .67 = 40.2 = \textbf{40 min}$$

The infusion time for a 1000 mL volume being administered at a rate of 25 gtt/min using a set calibrated at 10 gtt/mL is 6 hr 40 min.

EXAMPLE 2

A volume of **750 mL** D5RL is running at **12 gtt/min** on a set calibrated at **10 gtt/mL**. Calculate the infusion time.

Write the hr being calculated first to the left of the equation, followed by an equal sign.

$$hr =$$

Enter the 1 hr = 60 min conversion as the first ratio, with 1 hr as the numerator; 60 min becomes the denominator.

$$hr = \frac{1 \text{ hr}}{60 \text{ min}}$$

The denominator to be matched is hr. This is provided by the 12 gtt/min infusion rate ratio. Enter this with 1 min as the numerator; 12 gtt becomes the denominator.

$$hr = \frac{1 \text{ hr}}{60 \text{ min}} \times \frac{1 \text{ min}}{12 \text{ gtt}}$$

The gtt denominator must now be matched in the next numerator. This is provided by the 10 gtt/mL set calibration; enter 10 gtt now as the numerator and 1 mL the denominator.

$$hr = \frac{1 \text{ hr}}{60 \text{ min}} \times \frac{1 \text{ min}}{12 \text{ gtt}} \times \frac{10 \text{ gtt}}{1 \text{ mL}}$$

The mL denominator must now be matched. This is provided by the 750 mL volume to be infused. Enter 750 mL as the final matching numerator to complete the equation.

$$hr = \frac{1 \text{ hr}}{60 \text{ min}} \times \frac{1 \text{ min}}{12 \text{ gtt}} \times \frac{10 \text{ gtt}}{1 \text{ mL}} \times \frac{750 \text{ mL}}{}$$

Cancel the alternate denominator/numerator min/min, gtt/gtt, and mL/mL entries to check for correct ratio entry. Then do the math.

$$hr = \frac{1 \text{ hr}}{60 \text{ min}} \times \frac{1 \text{ min}}{12 \text{ gtt}} \times \frac{10 \text{ gtt}}{1 \text{ mL}} \times \frac{750 \text{ mL}}{} = \textbf{10.42 hr}$$

Convert the fractional hr to min by multiplying 60 min by the .42 fraction obtained.

$$60 \text{ min} \times .42 = 25.2 = \textbf{25 min}$$

The infusion time for a 750 mL volume being administered at a rate of 12 gtt/min using a set calibrated at 10 gtt/mL is 10 hr 25 min.

EXAMPLE 3

Determine the infusion time for **100 mL** D5NS infusing at a rate of **40 gtt/min** using a **microdrip set**.

Write the hr being calculated first to the left of the equation, followed by an equal sign.

$$hr =$$

Enter the 1 hr = 60 min conversion as the first ratio with 1 hr as the numerator to match the hr being calculated; 60 min becomes the denominator.

$$hr = \frac{1 \text{ hr}}{60 \text{ min}}$$

Match the new min denominator in the next numerator with the 1 min of the 40 gtt/min rate of infusion; 40 gtt becomes the new denominator.

$$hr = \frac{1 \text{ hr}}{60 \text{ min}} \times \frac{1 \text{ min}}{40 \text{ gtt}}$$

The gtt denominator must now be matched in the next numerator. This is provided by the 60 gtt/mL microdrip set calibration. Enter 60 gtt now as the numerator and 1 mL as the denominator.

$$hr = \frac{1 \text{ hr}}{60 \text{ min}} \times \frac{1 \text{ min}}{40 \text{ gtt}} \times \frac{60 \text{ gtt}}{1 \text{ mL}}$$

The denominator to be matched next is mL, and this is provided by the 100 mL volume to be infused. Enter 100 mL now as the final numerator to complete the equation.

$$hr = \frac{1 \text{ hr}}{60 \text{ min}} \times \frac{1 \text{ min}}{40 \text{ gtt}} \times \frac{60 \text{ gtt}}{1 \text{ mL}} \times \frac{100 \text{ mL}}{}$$

Cancel the alternate denominator/numerator min/min, gtt/gtt, and mL/mL entries to check for correct ratio entry. Do the math.

$$hr = \frac{1 \text{ hr}}{60 \text{ min}} \times \frac{1 \text{ min}}{40 \text{ gtt}} \times \frac{60 \text{ gtt}}{1 \text{ mL}} \times \frac{100 \text{ mL}}{} = \textbf{2.5 hr}$$

Convert the fractional hr to min by multiplying 60 min by the .5 fraction.

$$60 \text{ min} \times .5 = \textbf{30 min}$$

The infusion time for a 100 mL volume being administered at a rate of 40 gtt/min using a set calibrated at 60 gtt/mL is 2 hr 30 min.

EXAMPLE 4

Calculate the infusion time for a volume of **150 mL** D5RL is running at **20 gtt/min** on a set calibrated at **15 gtt/mL**.

Write the hr being calculated first to the left of the equation, followed by an equal sign.

$$hr =$$

Enter the 1 hr = 60 min conversion as the first ratio with 1 hr as the numerator to match the hr being calculated; 60 min becomes the denominator.

$$hr = \frac{1 \text{ hr}}{60 \text{ min}}$$

The min denominator must be matched in the next numerator. This is provided by the 20 gtt/min infusion rate ratio. Enter this with 1 min as the numerator; 20 gtt becomes the denominator.

$$hr = \frac{1 \text{ hr}}{60 \text{ min}} \times \frac{1 \text{ min}}{20 \text{ gtt}}$$

The gtt denominator must now be matched in the next numerator. The needed ratio is provided by the 15 gtt/mL set calibration. Enter 15 gtt now as the numerator and 1 mL as the denominator.

$$hr = \frac{1 \text{ hr}}{60 \text{ min}} \times \frac{1 \text{ min}}{20 \text{ gtt}} \times \frac{15 \text{ gtt}}{1 \text{ mL}}$$

The denominator to be matched next is mL, and this is provided by the 150 mL volume to be infused. Enter 150 mL now as the final numerator to complete the equation.

$$hr = \frac{1 \text{ hr}}{60 \text{ min}} \times \frac{1 \text{ min}}{20 \text{ gtt}} \times \frac{15 \text{ gtt}}{1 \text{ mL}} \times \frac{150 \text{ mL}}{}$$

Cancel the alternate denominator/numerator min/min, gtt/gtt, and mL/mL entries to check for correct ratio entry. Do the math.

$$hr = \frac{1 \text{ hr}}{60 \text{ min}} \times \frac{1 \text{ min}}{20 \text{ gtt}} \times \frac{15 \text{ gtt}}{1 \text{ mL}} \times \frac{150 \text{ mL}}{} = \textbf{1.88 hr}$$

Convert the fractional hr to min by multiplying 60 min by the .88 fraction.

$$60 \text{ min} \times .92 = 52.8 = \textbf{53 min}$$

The infusion time for a 150 mL volume being administered at a rate of 20 gtt/min using a set calibrated at 15 gtt/mL is 1 hr 53 min.

PROBLEM

Determine the infusion times for the following infusions.

1. An IV of 1 L D5W to infuse at a flow rate of 33 gtt/min using a set calibrated at 15 gtt/mL _____

2. An IV of 250 mL D5RL infusing on a 10 gtt/mL set at a rate of 25 gtt/min _____

3. A volume of 300 mL to infuse at 20 gtt/min using a 10 gtt/mL set _____

4. A volume of 900 mL running at a rate of 60 gtt/min using a 20 gtt/mL calibrated set _____

5. A volume of 1500 mL infusing on a 15 gtt/mL calibrated set and running at a rate of 45 gtt/min _____

ANSWERS 1. 7 hr 35 min 2. 1 hr 40 min 3. 2 hr 30 min 4. 5 hr 5. 8 hr 20 min

Calculating Small-Volume Infusion Times of Less Than 1 hr

Many small-volume infusions will complete in less than 1 hr. Because the infusion time being calculated is **min**, the calculation will be one ratio shorter, and simple math will provide most answers.

EXAMPLE 1

An IV medication with a volume of **40 mL** is ordered to infuse at **45 gtt/min**. A **microdrip** set is being used.

Enter the min being calculated first followed by an equal sign.

$$\text{min} =$$

The numerator must be matched with a min entry. This is provided by the 45 gtt/min flow rate. Enter this now with 1 min as the numerator; 45 gtt becomes the denominator.

$$\text{min} = \frac{1 \text{ min}}{45 \text{ gtt}}$$

The denominator to be matched is gtt. This is provided by the 60 gtt/mL administration set ratio. Enter this now with 60 gtt as the numerator; 1 mL becomes the denominator.

$$\text{min} = \frac{1 \text{ min}}{45 \text{ gtt}} \times \frac{60 \text{ gtt}}{1 \text{ mL}}$$

The mL denominator is matched in the next numerator by the 40 mL volume to be infused to complete the equation.

$$\text{min} = \frac{1 \text{ min}}{45 \text{ gtt}} \times \frac{60 \text{ gtt}}{1 \text{ mL}} \times \frac{40 \text{ mL}}{}$$

Cancel the alternate denominator/numerator gtt/gtt and mL/mL entries to check for correct ratio entry. Do the math.

$$\text{min} = \frac{1 \text{ min}}{45 \text{ gtt}} \times \frac{60 \text{ gtt}}{1 \text{ mL}} \times \frac{40 \text{ mL}}{} = 53.3 = \textbf{53 min}$$

A 40 mL volume infusing on a microdrip set at a rate of 45 gtt/min will complete in 53 min.

EXAMPLE 2

An IV volume of **60 mL** is ordered to infuse at **50 gtt/min**. A **10 gtt/mL** set is being used.

Enter the min being calculated first followed by an equal sign.

$$\text{min} =$$

The min numerator must be matched with a min entry. This is provided by the 50 gtt/min flow rate. Enter this with 1 min as the numerator; 50 gtt becomes the denominator.

$$\text{min} = \frac{1 \text{ min}}{50 \text{ gtt}}$$

The gtt denominator must be matched in the next numerator. This is provided by the 10 gtt/mL administration set. Enter this with 10 gtt as the numerator; 1 mL becomes the denominator.

$$\text{min} = \frac{1 \text{ min}}{50 \text{ gtt}} \times \frac{10 \text{ gtt}}{1 \text{ mL}}$$

The mL denominator is matched in the final numerator with the 60 mL volume to be infused and completes the equation.

$$\text{min} = \frac{1 \text{ min}}{50 \text{ gtt}} \times \frac{10 \text{ gtt}}{1 \text{ mL}} \times \frac{60 \text{ mL}}{}$$

Cancel the alternate denominator/numerator gtt/gtt and mL/mL entries to check for correct ratio entry. Do the math.

$$\text{min} = \frac{1 \text{ min}}{50 \text{ gtt}} \times \frac{10 \text{ gtt}}{1 \text{ mL}} \times \frac{60 \text{ mL}}{} = \textbf{12 min}$$

A 60 mL volume infusing on a 10 gtt/mL set at a rate of 50 gtt/min will complete in 12 min.

EXAMPLE 3

An IV volume of **20 mL** is ordered to infuse at **20 gtt/min**. A **15 gtt/mL** set is being used.

Enter the min being calculated first followed by an equal sign.

$$\text{min} =$$

The min being calculated must be matched with a min numerator entry. This is provided by the 20 gtt/min flow rate. Enter this with 1 min as the numerator, 20 gtt becomes the denominator.

$$\text{min} = \frac{1 \text{ min}}{20 \text{ gtt}}$$

Match the gtt denominator in the next numerator by entering the 15 gtt of the 15 gtt/mL administration set calibration; 1 mL becomes the denominator.

$$\text{min} = \frac{1 \text{ min}}{20 \text{ gtt}} \times \frac{15 \text{ gtt}}{1 \text{ mL}}$$

The mL denominator must be matched in the next numerator. This is provided by the 20 mL volume to be infused. Enter it now to complete the equation.

$$\text{min} = \frac{1 \text{ min}}{20 \text{ gtt}} \times \frac{15 \text{ gtt}}{1 \text{ mL}} \times \frac{20 \text{ mL}}{}$$

Cancel the alternate denominator/numerator gtt/gtt and mL/mL entries to check for correct ratio entry. Do the math.

$$\text{min} = \frac{1 \text{ min}}{20 \text{ gtt}} \times \frac{15 \text{ gtt}}{1 \text{ mL}} \times \frac{20 \text{ mL}}{} = \textbf{15 min}$$

A 20 mL volume infusing on a 15 gtt/mL set at a rate of 20 gtt/min will complete in 15 min.

Calculate the infusion times for the following IVs.

1. A volume of 25 mL to infuse at 30 gtt/min using a 60 gtt/mL set _____

2. A 35 mL volume to run at 25 gtt/min using a 15 gtt/mL set _____

3. A rate of 40 gtt/min ordered for a 70 mL volume using a 20 gtt/mL set _____

4. A volume of 55 mL to infuse on a 10 gtt/mL calibrated set at
45 gtt/min _____

5. A 10 mL volume to infuse at 40 gtt/min on a microdrip set _____

16

ANSWERS 1. 50 min   2. 21 min   3. 35 min   4. 12 min   5. 15 min

Determining Infusion Completion Time

The reason for calculating infusion times is to know when an IV solution or medication will be completely infused. To obtain the **completion time** for an IV, you must now **add the infusion time** you calculated **to the start time**. This is not complicated; it just requires the same care you have been using for the other calculations in this text. The safest way to calculate the completion time is to **add the minutes first**. With them out of the way, only the hours are left to add. This approach is much less confusing. It's also safer to **write the times down** as you calculate them. So, do that in the following examples and problems. Only the first example will show calculation for the 24-hour military time (0–2400 hr), because these calculations are simple additions.

EXAMPLE 1

An IV started at **1450** has an infusion time of **3 hr 40 min**. What is the completion time?

Add the minutes first.

50 min (current time in min) + 40 min (infusion time) = **90 min**

Use 60 min of the 90 min total to change the 14 hr current time to 15 hr; add the additional 30 min for a total of **1530**.

Now add the hours.

1530 + 3 hr = **1830**

Completion time = **1830**

EXAMPLE 2

An IV medication will infuse in **20 minutes**. It is now **6:14 p.m.** When will it be complete?

Add the minutes.

6:14 p.m. + **20 min** = **6:34 p.m.**

Completion time = **6:34 p.m.**

Minutes alone are easy to add, even if the answer crosses the a.m./p.m. time change.

EXAMPLE 3

An IV is calculated to infuse in **2 hr 33 min**. It is now **4:43 p.m.** When will it complete?

Add the minutes first.

> 4:43 p.m. + **33 min** = **5:16 p.m.**

Now that the minutes are out of the way you only have to add 2 hours; much safer.

Add the hours.

> 5:16 p.m. + **2 hr** = **7:16 p.m.**

The infusion will complete at 7:16 p.m.

EXAMPLE 4

An IV infusion time is **13 hr 20 min**. What is its completion time if it was started at **10:45 a.m.**?

Add the minutes first.

> 10:45 a.m. + **20 min** = **11:05 a.m.**

You must now **add** the **13 hours** to the **11:05 a.m.** you just calculated.

Add the hours.

> 11:05 a.m. + **13 hr** = **12:05 a.m.**

The completion time will be 12:05 a.m.

EXAMPLE 5

A IV with an infusion time of **10 hr 7 min** is started at **9:42 a.m.** When will it complete?

Add the minutes.

> 9:42 a.m. + **7 min** = **9:49 a.m.**

Add the hours.

> 9:49 a.m. + **10 hr** = **7:49 p.m.**

The completion time will be 7:49 p.m.

EXAMPLE 6

An IV with an infusion time of **12 hr 30 min** is started at **2:10 a.m.** When will it complete?

Add the minutes.

> 2:10 a.m. + **30 min** = **2:40 a.m.**

Add the hours.

> 2:40 a.m. + **12 hr** = **2:40 p.m.**

The completion time will be 2:40 p.m.

Calculate the completion times for the infusions.

1. An IV started at 0440 that has an infusion time of 9 hr 42 min. Use military time.   _____

2. An IV medication started at 7:30 a.m. that has an infusion time of 45 min.   _____

3. An IV with an infusion time of 7 hr 7 min that was restarted at 10:42 a.m.   _____

4. An IV with a restart time of 9:07 p.m. that has an infusion time of 6 hr 27 min.   _____

5. An IV with an infusion time of 3 hr 30 min that was started at 11:49 p.m.   _____

> **ANSWERS** **1.** 1422 **2.** 8:15 a.m. **3.** 5:49 p.m. **4.** 3:34 a.m. **5.** 3:19 a.m. **Note:** Consider answers that vary by 1–2 min correct.

Labeling Solution Bags with Infusion and Completion Times

IV bags/bottles are calibrated so that the amount of fluid remaining can be checked at any time. In the majority of hospitals it is routine to label bags when they are hung with start, progress, and finish times to provide a visual reference of the status of the infusion. Commercially prepared labels are available for this purpose; however, you can prepare one using any opaque tape available.

Refer to Figure 16-2 on page 234, where you can see close-up calibrations on a 1000 mL bag. Notice that each 50 mL is calibrated, but that only the 100 mL calibrations are numbered: 1, 2, 3 (for 100, 200, 300), etc. Notice also that the calibrations on the IV bag are not all the same width: they are somewhat wider at the bottom, because gravity and the pressure of the solution force more fluid to the bottom of the bag.

The tape on the IV solution bag in Figure 16-1 is for an 8-hour infusion, from 9 a.m. to 5 p.m. The 9A represents the start time of 9 a.m., and the 5P at the bottom represents the completion time of 5 p.m. An 8-hr infusion time for 1000 mL means that 125 mL are to be infused per hour (1000 mL ÷ 8 hr = 125 mL/hr). Each 125 mL is labeled on the calibrated scale along with the hour the IV should be at this level. This tape allows for constant monitoring of the IV by all staff. No matter what your responsibility is you must be aware of IV drip rates and develop the habit of reading IV labeling, particularly if you have been giving personal care that involves movement or repositioning.

Let's look at an example of how you could label an IV that is just being started. You may use a commercial time tape provided by your instructor, or copy the calibrations from one of the photos in this text to make up your own scale on scratch paper.

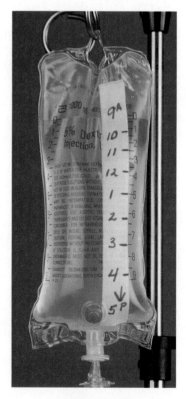

Figure 16-1

(Courtesy of Abbott Laboratories)

EXAMPLE 1

An IV of **1000 mL** has been ordered to run at **150 mL/hr**. It was started at **1:40 p.m.** Tape the bag with start, progress, and completion times.

Add the tape to the bag/bottle so that it is near but does not cover the calibrations. Enter the start time as 1:40 p.m. at the 1000 mL level. Next, mark each 150 mL from top to bottom with the successive hours the IV will run.

1000 mL − 150 mL = 850 mL		Label 850 mL for 2:40 p.m.
850 mL − 150 mL = 700 mL		Label 700 mL for 3:40 p.m.
700 mL − 150 mL = 550 mL		Label 550 mL for 4:40 p.m.
550 mL − 150 mL = 400 mL		Label 400 mL for 5:40 p.m.
400 mL − 150 mL = 250 mL		Label 250 mL for 6:40 p.m.
250 mL − 150 mL = 100 mL		Label 100 mL for 7:40 p.m.

Calculate the infusion time for the remaining 100 mL.

$$100 \text{ mL} \div 150 \text{ mL/hr} = 0.666 = \textbf{0.67 hr}$$

$$60 \text{ min} \times 0.67 = 40.2 = \textbf{40 min}$$

$$7:40 \text{ p.m.} + \textbf{40 min} = \textbf{8:20 p.m.}$$

The completion time is 8:20 p.m.

EXAMPLE 2

An infiltrated IV with **625 mL** remaining is restarted at **5:30 p.m.** to run at **150 mL/hr**. Relabel the bag with the new start, progress, and completion times.

Label the 625 mL level with the 5:30 p.m. restart time.

625 mL − 150 mL = 475 mL		Label 475 mL for 6:30 p.m.
475 mL − 150 mL = 325 mL		Label 325 mL for 7:30 p.m.
325 mL − 150 mL = 175 mL		Label 175 mL for 8:30 p.m.
175 mL − 150 mL = 25 mL		Label 25 mL for 9:30 p.m.

Calculate the infusion time for the remaining 25 mL.

$$25 \text{ mL} \div 150 \text{ mL/hr} = 0.166 = \textbf{0.17 hr}$$

$$60 \text{ min} \times 0.17 = 10.2 = \textbf{10 min}$$

$$9:30 \text{ p.m.} + \textbf{10 min} = \textbf{9:40 p.m.}$$

The completion time is 9:40 p.m.

EXAMPLE 3

An infiltrated IV with **340 mL** remaining is restarted at **4:15 a.m.** to run at **70 mL/hr**. Relabel the bag with the new start, progress, and completion times.

Label the 340 mL level with the 4:15 a.m. restart time.

340 mL − 70 mL = 270 mL		Label 270 mL for 5:15 a.m.
270 mL − 70 mL = 200 mL		Label 200 mL for 6:15 a.m.
200 mL − 70 mL = 130 mL		Label 130 mL for 7:15 a.m.
130 mL − 70 mL = 60 mL		Label 60 mL for 8:15 a.m.

Calculate the infusion time for the remaining 60 mL.

$$60 \text{ mL} \div 70 \text{ mL/hr} = 0.857 = \textbf{0.86 hr}$$

$$60 \text{ min} \times 0.86 = 51.6 = \textbf{52 min}$$

$$8{:}15 \text{ a.m.} + \textbf{52 min} = \textbf{9:17 a.m.}$$

The completion time is 9:17 a.m.

PROBLEM

Calculate the infusion and completion times for the IVs pictured. Label the IV bags provided with start, progress, and completion times. Have your instructor check your labeling.

1. The IV in Figure 16-2 of 1000 mL was started at 0710 to run at 75 mL/hr.

   Infusion time _____ Completion time _____

2. The 1000 mL IV in Figure 16-3 has an ordered rate of 125 mL/hr. It was started at 6:30 p.m.

   Infusion time _____ Completion time _____

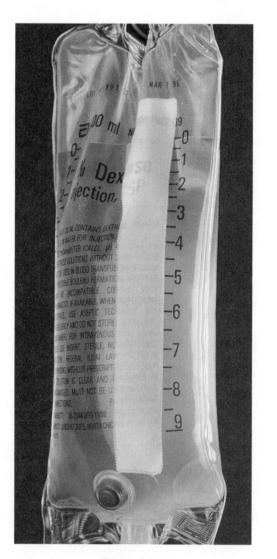

Figure 16-2

(Courtesy of Abbott Laboratories)

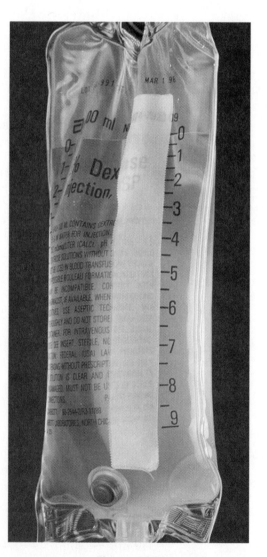

Figure 16-3

(Courtesy of Abbott Laboratories)

3. The IV in Figure 16-4 of 1000 mL has an ordered rate of 80 mL/hr.
It was started at 5:40 a.m.

Infusion time _____   Completion time _____

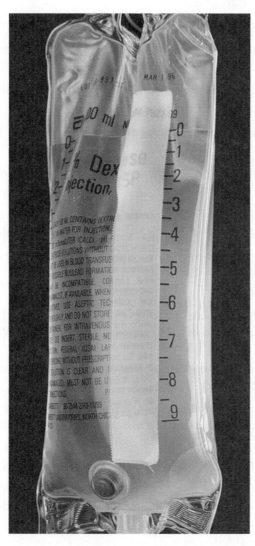

Figure 16-4

(Courtesy of Abbott Laboratories)

ANSWERS **1.** 13 hr 20 min; 2030 **2.** 8 hr; 2:30 a.m. **3.** 12 hr 30 min; 6.10 p.m. **Note:** Consider answers
that vary by 1–2 min correct.

Summary

This concludes the chapter on calculation of infusion and completion times and labeling of IV bags with start, progress, and completion times. The important points to remember from this chapter are:

- The infusion time is the time necessary for an IV bag to infuse completely.

- The infusion time is calculated by dividing the total volume to infuse by the mL/hr rate ordered.

- Infusion times also may be calculated using the volume of the bag being hung, the mL/hr or gtt/min rate ordered, and set calibration.

- The completion time is calculated by adding the infusion time to the start time.

- When adding the infusion time to the start time it is safer to add the minutes first, then the hours.

- When the total minutes are 60 or more, an additional hour is added, and 60 minutes are subtracted from the total minutes calculated.

- Calculating infusion and completion times provides an opportunity to plan ahead and have the next solution ordered ready to hang, or to discontinue the IV when it is completed.

- It is routine in many hospitals to label IV solutions with start, finish, and progress times to provide a visual record of the infusion status.

Summary Self-Test

Calculate the infusion and completion times for the following IVs. Don't let the solution abbreviations confuse you; concentrate on locating the information you need for your calculations.

1. The order is for 50 mL D5W to infuse at 50 gtt/min using a microdrip. The infusion was started at 10:10 a.m.

    Infusion time _____ Completion time _____

2. An infusion of 1150 mL of hyperalimentation is ordered to run at 80 mL/hr. It was started at 8:02 a.m.

    Infusion time _____ Completion time _____

3. A total of 280 mL of D10W remain in an IV bag. The flow rate is 70 mL/hr. It is now 11:03 a.m.

    Infusion time _____ Completion time _____

4. The order is to infuse 500 mL of whole blood at 90 mL/hr. The transfusion was started at 2:40 p.m.

    Infusion time _____ Completion time _____

5. An infiltrated IV with 850 mL of D5W remaining is restarted at 10 a.m. at a rate of 150 mL/hr.

    Infusion time _____ Completion time _____

6. At 4:04 a.m. an IV of 500 mL of intralipids is started at a rate of 50 mL/hr.

    Infusion time _____ Completion time _____

7. An IV medication with a volume of 50 mL is started at 1:45 p.m. to infuse at 30 gtt/min using a set calibrated at 15 gtt/mL.

    Infusion time _____ Completion time _____

8. An IV of 520 mL of RL is restarted at 0420 at a rate of 125 mL/hr.

   Infusion time _____   Completion time _____

9. It is 12.00 p.m. and an IV of 900 mL D10NS is infusing at a rate of 100 mL/hr.

   Infusion time _____   Completion time _____

10. An IV of 150 mL is started at 7:10 a.m. to infuse at 33 gtt/min with a set calibrated at 10 gtt/mL.

    Infusion time _____   Completion time _____

11. An infusion of 250 mL of normal saline is started at 11:20 a.m. to infuse at a rate of 20 mL/hr.

    Infusion time _____   Completion time _____

12. The flow rate ordered for 1 L of D5W is 80 mL/hr. It was started at 8:07 p.m.

    Infusion time _____   Completion time _____

13. One unit of packed cells with a 250 mL volume is started at 3:40 p.m. to be infused at 30 gtt/min using a 20 gtt/mL set.

    Infusion time _____   Completion time _____

14. An IV volume of 100 mL is started at 4:00 p.m. to infuse at 42 gtt/min using a microdrip.

    Infusion time _____   Completion time _____

15. At 11:00 p.m. 200 mL of D5W remain in an IV. The rate is 20 gtt/min and set calibration is 10 gtt/mL.

    Infusion time _____   Completion time _____

16. An infusion of 350 mL of RL is restarted to run at 50 gtt/min using a 10 gtt/mL set. It is now 9:47 a.m.

    Infusion time _____   Completion time _____

17. An IV volume of 25 mL is started at 8:17 a.m. using a microdrip to run at 25 gtt/min.

    Infusion time _____   Completion time _____

18. An IV of 425 mL of D5 1/4NaCl is restarted at 0814 to infuse at 15 gtt/min using a 10 gtt/mL set.

    Infusion time _____   Completion time _____

19. At 10:30 p.m. there are 180 mL left in an IV of D5 0.45%NaCl that is infusing at 25 mL/hr.

    Infusion time _____   Completion time _____

20. At 2 p.m. 500 mL of D5NS is started to run at a rate of 20 gtt/min using a 20 gtt/mL set.

    Infusion time _____   Completion time _____

21. An infusion of 250 mL of NS is started at 3:04 a.m. to run at 50 gtt/min using a 15 gtt/mL set.

    Infusion time _____   Completion time _____

22. With 525 mL of D10W remaining a rate change to 35 gtt/min is ordered. It is 2:10 a.m. and a 10 gtt/mL set is being used.

    Infusion time _____   Completion time _____

23. A liter of D5 1/4NaCl is started at 8:42 a.m. at a rate of 22 gtt/min using a set calibrated at 20 gtt/mL.

    Infusion time _____   Completion time _____

24. An infusion of 1000 mL of sodium chloride 0.9% is to run at 200 mL/hr. It is started at 6:40 p.m.

Infusion time _____ Completion time _____

25. An IV of 100 mL is started at 7:50 a.m. to run at 33 gtt/min using a 10 gtt/mL set.

Infusion time _____ Completion time _____

26. A volume of 500 mL of RL is started at 4:04 p.m. at a rate of 50 gtt/min using a microdrip.

Infusion time _____ Completion time _____

27. An IV of 950 mL NS is restarted at 2:10 a.m. at 25 gtt/min using a 15 gtt/mL set.

Infusion time _____ Completion time _____

28. An IV of 30 mL is started at 0915 at a rate of 10 gtt/min using a 10 gtt/mL set.

Infusion time _____ Completion time _____

29. A volume of 90 mL was started at 6:15 a.m. to be infused at 30 gtt/min using a 20 gtt/mL set.

Infusion time _____ Completion time _____

30. A set calibrated at 15 gtt/mL is used at 4:20 p.m. to infuse a volume of 100 mL. The rate ordered is 45 gtt/min.

Infusion time _____ Completion time _____

31. A 20 gtt/mL set is used for a restart of 750 mL of D5W at 3:03 p.m. at a rate of 32 gtt/min.

Infusion time _____ Completion time _____

ANSWERS

1. 60 min; 11:10 a.m.	**12.** 12 hr 30 min; 8:37 a.m.	**22.** 2 hr 30 min; 4:40 a.m.
2. 14 hr 23 min; 10:25 p.m.	**13.** 2 hr 47 min; 6:27 p.m.	**23.** 15 hr 9 min; 11:51 p.m.
3. 4 hr; 3:03 p.m.	**14.** 143 min or 2 hr 23 min;	**24.** 5 hr; 11:40 p.m.
4. 5 hr 34 min; 8:14 p.m.	6:23 p.m.	**25.** 30 min; 8:20 a.m.
5. 5 hr 40 min; 3:40 p.m.	**15.** 1 hr 40 min; 12:40 a.m.	**26.** 10 hr; 2:04 a.m.
6. 10 hr; 2:04 p.m.	**16.** 1 hr 10 min; 10:57 a.m.	**27.** 9 hr 30 min; 11:40 a.m.
7. 25 min; 2:10 p.m.	**17.** 60 min; 9:17 a.m.	**28.** 30 min; 0945
8. 4 hr 10 min; 0830	**18.** 4 hr 43 min; 1257	**29.** 60 min; 7:15 a.m.
9. 9 hr; 9 p.m.	**19.** 7 hr 12 min; 5:42 a.m.	**30.** 33 min; 4:53 p.m.
10. 45 min; 7:55 a.m.	**20.** 8 hr 20 min; 10:20 p.m.	**31.** 7 hr 48 min; 10:51 p.m.
11. 12 hr 30 min; 11:50 p.m.	**21.** 1 hr 15 min; 4:19 a.m.	

Note: Answers may vary slightly due to rounding.

Label the solution bags for the times and rates indicated. Have your instructor check your labeling.

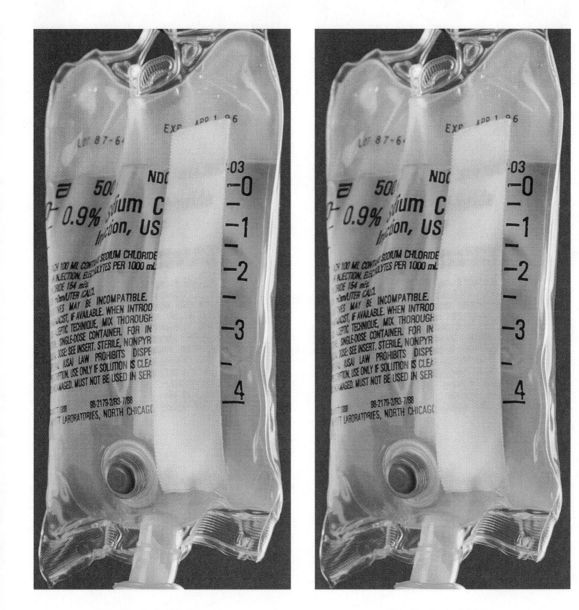

32. Started: 10:47 a.m.
Rate: 80 mL/hr

33. Started: 1315
Rate: 100 mL/hr

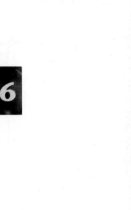

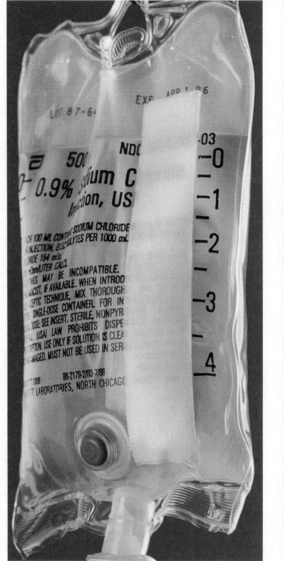

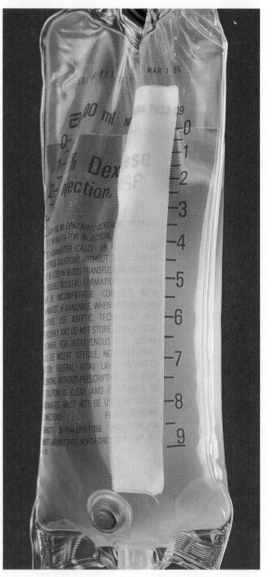

34. Started: 2:10 p.m.
Rate: 90 mL/hr

35. Started: 0440
Rate: 75 mL/hr

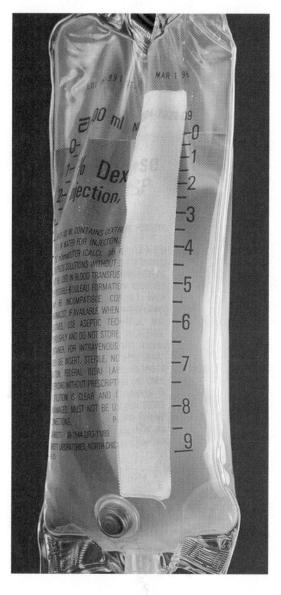

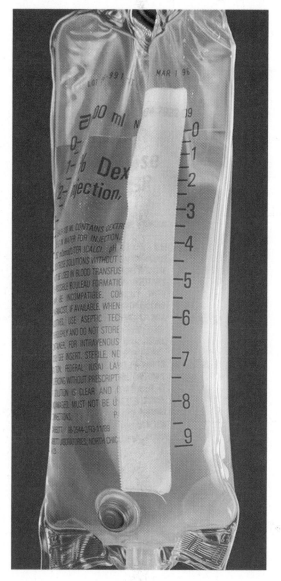

36. Started: 0730
Rate: 50 mL/hr

37. Started: 6:20 p.m.
Rate: 25 mL/hr

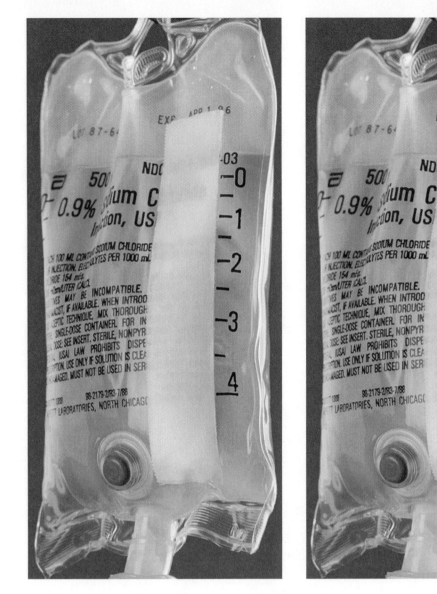

38. Started: 3:03 a.m.
Rate: 50 mL/hr

39. Started: 0744
Rate: 125 mL/hr

16

40. Started: 2140
Rate: 100 mL/hr

17

IV Medication and Titration Calculations

Many IV drugs are used in critical and life-threatening situations to alter or maintain vital physiologic functions, for example, heart rate, cardiac output, blood pressure, respiration, and renal function. In general, these drugs have a very rapid action and short duration. They may be administered by IV push or bolus, but also may be diluted in 250–500 mL of IV solution, most commonly D5W.

Intravenous medications may be ordered by dosage (mcg/mg/units per min/hr), or based on body weight (mcg/mg/units per kg per min/hr). They may also be ordered to infuse within a specific dosage range, for example, 1–3 mcg/min, to elicit a measurable physiologic response; an example would be to maintain a systolic BP above 100 mm Hg. This **rate adjustment is called titration**, and dosage increments are made within the ordered range until the desired response has been established. Most IV drugs require close and continuous monitoring. An electronic infusion device (EID), either volumetric pump or syringe pump, is used for their administration. **All calculations are for an EID or microdrip, and the mL/hr and gtt/min rates are interchangeable.**

The calculations in this chapter include: (1) converting ordered dosages to the flow rates necessary to administer them, and (2) using flow rates to calculate the dosage infusing at any given moment. A client's weight is often a critical factor in IV dosages, and its use in calculations will also be covered. A variety of EIDs display average or usual dosage and flow rate equivalents, but you must know how to do these calculations yourself, because you are likely to encounter situations in which you will have to do so. IV drugs that alter a basic physiologic function generally have narrow margins of safety, and accuracy is imperative in their calculation. Double-checking of math is both mandatory and routine. As a general rule, dosages are calculated to the nearest tenth. Flow rates may be rounded to the nearest mL, or, if the EID can be set to tenths, to the nearest tenth mL.

Calculating mL/hr Rate from Dosage Ordered

One of the most common IV calculations is to determine the mL/hr flow rate for a specific drug dosage ordered. So let's start by looking at some examples of these.

EXAMPLE 1

A cardiac medication with a strength of **125 mg/100 mL** D5W is to infuse at a rate of **20 mg/hr.** Calculate the **mL/hr** flow rate.

$$\frac{mL}{hr} = \frac{100 \text{ mL}}{125 \text{ mg}} \times \frac{20 \text{ mg}}{1 \text{ hr}}$$

$$= \frac{100 \text{ mL}}{125 \text{ mg}} \times \frac{20 \text{ mg}}{1 \text{ hr}}$$

$$= \textbf{16 mL/hr}$$

To infuse 20 mg/hr set the flow rate at 16 mL/hr.

EXAMPLE 2

A maintenance dose of a BP elevating medication with a strength of **2 mcg/min** has been ordered using an **8 mg in 250 mL** D5W solution. Calculate the **mL/hr** flow rate.

This equation will need a 60 min = 1 hr, and a 1 mg = 1000 mcg conversion

$$\frac{mL}{hr} = \frac{250 \text{ mL}}{8 \text{ mg}} \times \frac{1 \text{ mg}}{1000 \text{ mcg}} \times \frac{2 \text{ mcg}}{1 \text{ min}} \times \frac{60 \text{ min}}{1 \text{ hr}}$$

$$= \frac{250 \text{ mL}}{8 \text{ mg}} \times \frac{1 \text{ mg}}{1000 \text{ mcg}} \times \frac{2 \text{ mcg}}{1 \text{ min}} \times \frac{60 \text{ min}}{1 \text{ hr}}$$

$$= 3.75 = \textbf{4 mL/hr}$$

To infuse 2 mcg/min set the flow rate at 4 mL/hr.

EXAMPLE 3

A medication with a strength of **50 mg in 250 mL** D5W is used to infuse a dosage of **200 mcg/min.** Calculate the flow rate in **mL/hr.**

This equation will need a 60 min = 1 hr, and 1 mg = 1000 mcg conversion.

$$\frac{mL}{hr} = \frac{250 \text{ mL}}{50 \text{ mg}} \times \frac{1 \text{ mg}}{1000 \text{ mcg}} \times \frac{200 \text{ mcg}}{1 \text{ min}} \times \frac{60 \text{ min}}{1 \text{ hr}}$$

$$= \frac{250 \text{ mL}}{50 \text{ mg}} \times \frac{1 \text{ mg}}{1000 \text{ mcg}} \times \frac{200 \text{ mcg}}{1 \text{ min}} \times \frac{60 \text{ min}}{1 \text{ hr}}$$

$$= \textbf{60 mL/hr}$$

To infuse 200 mcg/min set the flow rate at 60 mL/hr.

EXAMPLE 4

Medication has been ordered for a cardiac patient at the rate of **3 mcg/min** using a **1 mg/250 mL** D5W solution. Calculate the **mL/hr** flow rate for a pump infusion.

$$\frac{mL}{hr} = \frac{250\ mL}{1\ mg} \times \frac{1\ mg}{1000\ mcg} \times \frac{3\ mcg}{1\ min} \times \frac{60\ min}{1\ hr}$$

$$= \frac{250\ mL}{1\ mg} \times \frac{1\ mg}{1000\ mcg} \times \frac{3\ mcg}{1\ min} \times \frac{60\ min}{1\ hr}$$

$$= \textbf{45 mL/hr}$$

To infuse 3 mcg/min set the pump at 45 mL/hr.

EXAMPLE 5

A **500 mL** D5W solution with **2 g** of medication is to be infused at a rate of **1 mg/min** via volumetric pump. Calculate the **mL/hr** flow rate.

$$\frac{mL}{hr} = \frac{500\ mL}{2\ g} \times \frac{1\ g}{1000\ mg} \times \frac{1\ mg}{1\ min} \times \frac{60\ min}{1\ hr}$$

$$= \frac{500\ mL}{2\ g} \times \frac{1\ g}{1000\ mg} \times \frac{1\ mg}{1\ min} \times \frac{60\ min}{1\ hr}$$

$$= \textbf{15 mL/hr}$$

Set the pump at 15 mL/hr to infuse 1 mg/min.

PROBLEM

Calculate the mL/hr flow rates to administer the following IV dosages. Round answers to the nearest whole mL.

1. A 20 mg/hr dosage is ordered using a 100 mg/100 mL solution.　　　＿＿＿＿＿＿

2. A medication is ordered at the rate of 3 mcg/min. The solution strength is 8 mg in 250 mL D5W.　　　＿＿＿＿＿＿

3. A solution of 2 g medication in 500 mL D5W is used to administer a dosage of 2 mg/min.　　　＿＿＿＿＿＿

4. A 2 mcg/min infusion is ordered. The solution strength is 1 mg/250 mL.　　　＿＿＿＿＿＿

5. An initial dose of a cardiac drug is ordered at 25 mg/hr. The solution strength is 125 mg/100 mL.　　　＿＿＿＿＿＿

ANSWERS　1. 20 mL/hr　2. 6 mL/hr　3. 30 mL/hr　4. 30 mL/hr　5. 20 mL/hr

Calculating mL/hr Rate from Dosage per kg Ordered

Many IV medication infusions are calculated based on body weight, for example 95.9 mcg/kg/hr. **Body weight to the nearest tenth kg** is used for these calculations. There are two ways the mL/hr flow rate can be calculated. The methods may result in answers whose tenths vary slightly, but they are considered equivalent. The first method requires two steps. The dosage for the body weight is calculated to the nearest tenth first, then used to determine the flow rate. The examples below illustrate **two-step mL/hr flow rate calculation**.

Two-Step mL/hr Flow Rate Calculation

EXAMPLE 1

Medication is ordered at the rate of **3 mcg/kg/min** for an adult weighing **95.9 kg**. The solution strength is **400 mg** in **250 mL** D5W. Calculate flow rate to the nearest tenth mL.

Calculate the dosage.

$$3 \text{ mcg/kg/min} \times 95.9 \text{ kg} = \textbf{287.7 mcg/min}$$

Calculate the flow rate.

$$\frac{mL}{hr} = \frac{250 \text{ mL}}{400 \text{ mg}} \times \frac{1 \text{ mg}}{1000 \text{ mcg}} \times \frac{287.7 \text{ mcg}}{1 \text{ min}} \times \frac{60 \text{ min}}{1 \text{ hr}}$$

$$= \frac{250 \text{ mL}}{400 \text{ mg}} \times \frac{1 \text{ mg}}{1000 \text{ mcg}} \times \frac{287.7 \text{ mcg}}{1 \text{ min}} \times \frac{60 \text{ min}}{1 \text{ hr}}$$

$$= 10.79 = \textbf{10.8 mL/hr}$$

To infuse 3 mcg/kg/min set the flow rate at 10.8 mL/hr.

EXAMPLE 2

A dosage of **2.5 g in 250 mL** D5W has been ordered at a rate of **100 mcg/kg/min** for an adult weighing **104.6 kg**. Calculate the flow rate to the nearest tenth mL.

Calculate the dosage.

$$100 \text{ mcg/kg/min} \times 104.6 \text{ kg} = \textbf{10,460 mcg/min or 10.5 mg/min}$$

Calculate the flow rate.

$$\frac{mL}{hr} = \frac{250 \text{ mL}}{2.5 \text{ g}} \times \frac{1 \text{ g}}{1000 \text{ mcg}} \times \frac{10.5 \text{ mg}}{1 \text{ min}} \times \frac{60 \text{ min}}{1 \text{ hr}}$$

$$= \frac{250 \text{ mL}}{2.5 \text{ g}} \times \frac{1 \text{ g}}{1000 \text{ mcg}} \times \frac{10.5 \text{ mg}}{1 \text{ min}} \times \frac{60 \text{ min}}{1 \text{ hr}}$$

$$= 63 = \textbf{63 mL/hr}$$

To infuse 100 mcg/kg/min set the flow rate at 63 mL/hr.

EXAMPLE 3

A medication has been ordered at **4 mcg/kg/min** from a solution of **50 mg in 250 mL** D5W. The body weight is **107.3 kg**. Calculate flow rate to the nearest tenth mL.

Calculate the dosage.

$$4 \text{ mcg/kg/min} \times 107.3 \text{ kg} = \textbf{429.2 mcg/min}$$

Calculate the flow rate.

$$\frac{\text{mL}}{\text{hr}} = \frac{250 \text{ mL}}{50 \text{ mg}} \times \frac{1 \text{ mg}}{1000 \text{ mcg}} \times \frac{429.2 \text{ mcg}}{1 \text{ min}} \times \frac{60 \text{ min}}{1 \text{ hr}}$$

$$= \frac{250 \text{ mL}}{50 \cancel{\text{ mg}}} \times \frac{1 \cancel{\text{ mg}}}{1000 \cancel{\text{ mcg}}} \times \frac{429.2 \cancel{\text{ mcg}}}{1 \cancel{\text{ min}}} \times \frac{60 \cancel{\text{ min}}}{1 \text{ hr}}$$

$$= 128.76 = \textbf{128.8 mL/hr}$$

To infuse 4 mcg/kg/min set the flow rate at 128.8 mL/hr.

EXAMPLE 4

A **5 mcg/kg/min** dosage has been ordered using a **500 mg/250 mL** D5W strength solution. The adult weighs **99.4 kg**. Calculate the flow rate to the nearest tenth mL.

Calculate the dosage.

$$5 \text{ mcg/kg/min} \times 99.4 \text{ kg} = \textbf{497 mcg/min}$$

Calculate the flow rate.

$$\frac{\text{mL}}{\text{hr}} = \frac{250 \text{ mL}}{500 \text{ mg}} \times \frac{1 \text{ mg}}{1000 \text{ mcg}} \times \frac{497 \text{ mcg}}{1 \text{ min}} \times \frac{60 \text{ min}}{1 \text{ hr}}$$

$$= \frac{250 \text{ mL}}{500 \cancel{\text{ mg}}} \times \frac{1 \cancel{\text{ mg}}}{1000 \cancel{\text{ mcg}}} \times \frac{497 \cancel{\text{ mcg}}}{1 \cancel{\text{ min}}} \times \frac{60 \cancel{\text{ min}}}{1 \text{ hr}}$$

$$= 14.91 = \textbf{14.9 mL/hr}$$

To infuse 5 mcg/kg/min set the flow rate at 14.9 mL/hr.

EXAMPLE 5

A **100 mcg/kg/min** dosage has been ordered using a **5 g/500 mL** D5W solution. The body weight is **77.6 kg**. Calculate the flow rate to the nearest tenth mL.

Calculate the dosage.

$$100 \text{ mcg/kg/min} \times 77.6 \text{ kg} = \textbf{7760 mcg} \text{ or } 7.76 = \textbf{7.8 mg/min}$$

Calculate the flow rate.

$$\frac{\text{mL}}{\text{hr}} = \frac{500 \text{ mL}}{5 \text{ g}} \times \frac{1 \text{ g}}{1000 \text{ mg}} \times \frac{7.8 \text{ mg}}{1 \text{ min}} \times \frac{60 \text{ min}}{1 \text{ hr}}$$

$$= \frac{500 \text{ mL}}{5 \cancel{\text{ g}}} \times \frac{1 \cancel{\text{ g}}}{1000 \cancel{\text{ mg}}} \times \frac{7.8 \cancel{\text{ mg}}}{1 \cancel{\text{ min}}} \times \frac{60 \cancel{\text{ min}}}{1 \text{ hr}}$$

$$= 46.8 = \textbf{46.8 mL/hr}$$

To infuse 100 mcg/min set the flow rate at 46.8 mL/hr.

Use the two-step method to calculate the flow rates necessary to infuse the dosages based on body weight. Express all flow rates to the nearest tenth mL.

1. A 3 mcg/kg/min dosage has been ordered for an adult weighing 87.4 kg. The solution being used has a strength of 50 mg in 250 mL D5W. _____ _____

2. IV medication has been ordered to infuse at 4 mcg/kg/min using a 400 mg/250 mL D5W solution. The body weight is 92.4 kg. _____ _____

3. A 2.5 mcg/kg/min dosage has been ordered. The solution strength is 0.5 g/250 mL D5W. The body weight is 80.7 kg. _____ _____

4. A rate of 150 mcg/kg/min has been ordered for a 92.1 kg body weight. The solution strength is 2.5 g in 250 mL D5W. _____ _____

5. A 5 mcg/kg/min infusion has been ordered for a body weight of 80.3 kg. The solution to be used has 1 g in 500 mL D5W. _____ _____

17

ANSWERS 1. 262.2 mcg/min; 78.7 mL/hr   2. 369.6 mcg/min; 13.9 mL/hr   3. 201.8 mcg/min; 6.1 mL/hr   4. 13,815 mcg or 13.8 mg/min; 82.8 mL/hr   5. 401.5 mcg/min; 12 mL/hr

One-Step DA Equation Calculation

The second method is to use one-step DA equation flow rate calculation DA for the entire calculation. This method requires very careful entry of ratios, and equally careful cancellation of measurement units to verify accuracy in ratio entry. Let's look at the entire process step by step. Express flow rates to the nearest tenth mL.

EXAMPLE 1

Medication is ordered at the rate of **3 mcg/kg/min** for an adult weighing **95.9 kg**. The solution strength is **400 mg** in **250 mL** D5W. Calculate flow rate to the nearest tenth mL.

The first two ratios entered are the same as in the two-step method.

$$\frac{mL}{hr} = \frac{250 \text{ mL}}{400 \text{ mg}} \times \frac{1 \text{ mg}}{1000 \text{ mcg}}$$

The denominator to be matched next is mcg. This is provided by the 3 mcg/kg/min dosage. Enter this with 3 mcg as the numerator; two measures, kg and min, become the new denominator.

$$\frac{mL}{hr} = \frac{250 \text{ mL}}{400 \text{ mg}} \times \frac{1 \text{ mg}}{1000 \text{ mcg}} \times \frac{3 \text{ mcg}}{kg/min}$$

Both kg and min must be matched in the next numerators. Either can be entered first, but min is the best choice, because a conversion ratio is needed to change min to the hr being calculated. Enter the 60 min = 1 hour conversion, with 60 min as the numerator, to match the previous min denominator.

$$\frac{mL}{hr} = \frac{250 \text{ mL}}{400 \text{ mg}} \times \frac{1 \text{ mg}}{1000 \text{ mcg}} \times \frac{3 \text{ mcg}}{kg/min} \times \frac{60 \text{ min}}{1 \text{ hr}}$$

Only one measure remains to be entered, the 95.9 kg body weight. Enter this as the final numerator, to match the remaining kg denominator. This completes the equation.

$$\frac{mL}{hr} = \frac{250\ mL}{400\ mg} \times \frac{1\ mg}{1000\ mcg} \times \frac{3\ mcg}{kg/min} \times \frac{60\ min}{1\ hr} \times \frac{95.9\ kg}{}$$

Cancel the alternate denominator/numerator measures. Only mL and hr remain in the equation. Do the math. Some of the quantities cancel easily, but a calculator will be of use here.

$$\frac{mL}{hr} = \frac{250\ mL}{400\ \cancel{mg}} \times \frac{1\ \cancel{mg}}{1000\ \cancel{mcg}} \times \frac{3\ \cancel{mcg}}{\cancel{kg/min}} \times \frac{60\ \cancel{min}}{1\ hr} \times \frac{95.9\ \cancel{kg}}{}$$

$$= 10.79 = \mathbf{10.8\ mL/hr}$$

The 10.8 mL/hr answer is identical to the 10.8 mL/hr answer obtained in the two-step calculation previously demonstrated.

EXAMPLE 2

A dosage of **2.5 g in 250 mL** D5W has been ordered at a rate of **100 mcg/kg/min** for an adult weighing **104.6 kg**. Calculates flow rate to the nearest tenth mL.

Enter the mL/hr being calculated. The first mL numerator is provided by the 250 mL containing 2.5 g medication. Enter it now.

$$\frac{mL}{hr} = \frac{250\ mL}{2.5\ g}$$

The dosage ordered is in mcg, so g-to-mg and mg-to-mcg conversion ratios are needed. Enter these now.

$$\frac{mL}{hr} = \frac{250\ mL}{2.5\ g} \times \frac{1\ g}{1000\ mg} \times \frac{1\ mg}{1000\ mcg}$$

Enter the 100 mcg/kg/min dosage next, with mcg as the numerator to match the previous mcg denominator.

$$\frac{mL}{hr} = \frac{250\ mL}{2.5\ g} \times \frac{1\ g}{1000\ mg} \times \frac{1\ mg}{1000\ mcg} \times \frac{100\ mcg}{kg/min}$$

Enter the min/hr conversion ratio.

$$\frac{mL}{hr} = \frac{250\ mL}{2.5\ g} \times \frac{1\ g}{1000\ mg} \times \frac{1\ mg}{1000\ mcg} \times \frac{100\ mcg}{kg/min} \times \frac{60\ min}{1\ hr}$$

Enter the 104.6 kg body weight to complete the equation.

$$\frac{mL}{hr} = \frac{250\ mL}{2.5\ g} \times \frac{1\ g}{1000\ mg} \times \frac{1\ mg}{1000\ mcg} \times \frac{100\ mcg}{kg/min} \times \frac{60\ min}{1\ hr} \times \frac{104.6\ kg}{}$$

Cancel the alternate denominator/numerator entries to double-check the accuracy of ratio entry. Do the math.

$$\frac{mL}{hr} = \frac{250\ mL}{2.5\ \cancel{g}} \times \frac{1\ \cancel{g}}{1000\ \cancel{mg}} \times \frac{1\ \cancel{mg}}{1000\ \cancel{mcg}} \times \frac{100\ \cancel{mcg}}{\cancel{kg/min}} \times \frac{60\ \cancel{min}}{1\ hr} \times \frac{104.6\ \cancel{kg}}{}$$

$$= 62.76 = \mathbf{62.8\ mL/hr}$$

The 62.8 mL/hr answer is identical to the 62.8 mL/hr answer obtained in the two-step calculation.

17

EXAMPLE 3

A medication has been ordered at 4 mcg/kg/min from a solution of **50 mg** in **250 mL** D5W. The body weight is **107.3 kg**. Express the flow rate to the nearest tenth.

$$\frac{mL}{hr} = \frac{250\ mL}{50\ mg}$$

$$\frac{mL}{hr} = \frac{250\ mL}{50\ mg} \times \frac{1\ mg}{1000\ mcg}$$

$$\frac{mL}{hr} = \frac{250\ mL}{50\ mg} \times \frac{1\ mg}{1000\ mcg} \times \frac{4\ mcg}{kg/min}$$

$$\frac{mL}{hr} = \frac{250\ mL}{50\ mg} \times \frac{1\ mg}{1000\ mcg} \times \frac{4\ mcg}{kg/min} \times \frac{60\ min}{1\ hr}$$

$$\frac{mL}{hr} = \frac{250\ mL}{50\ mg} \times \frac{1\ mg}{1000\ mcg} \times \frac{4\ mcg}{kg/min} \times \frac{60\ min}{1\ hr} \times \frac{107.3\ kg}{}$$

$$= 128.76 = \textbf{128.8 mL/hr}$$

The 128.8 mL/hr answer is identical to the 12.8 mL/hr rate calculated in the two-step method.

EXAMPLE 4

A **5 mcg/kg/min** dosage has been ordered using a **500 mg/250 mL** D5W strength solution. An adult weighs **99.4 kg**. Calculate the flow rate to the nearest tenth mL.

$$\frac{mL}{hr} = \frac{250\ mL}{500\ mg}$$

$$\frac{mL}{hr} = \frac{250\ mL}{500\ mg} \times \frac{1\ mg}{1000\ mcg}$$

$$\frac{mL}{hr} = \frac{250\ mL}{500\ mg} \times \frac{1\ mg}{1000\ mcg} \times \frac{5\ mcg}{kg/min}$$

$$\frac{mL}{hr} = \frac{250\ mL}{500\ mg} \times \frac{1\ mg}{1000\ mcg} \times \frac{5\ mcg}{kg/min} \times \frac{60\ min}{1\ hr}$$

$$\frac{mL}{hr} = \frac{250\ mL}{500\ mg} \times \frac{1\ mg}{1000\ mcg} \times \frac{5\ mcg}{kg/min} \times \frac{60\ min}{1\ hr} \times \frac{99.4\ kg}{}$$

$$= \textbf{14.9 mL/hr}$$

The 14.9 mL/hr rate is identical to the 14.9 mL/hr rate calculated in the two-step method.

EXAMPLE 5

A **100 mcg/kg/min** dosage has been ordered using a **5 g/500 mL** D5W solution. The body weight is **77.6 kg**. Calculate the flow rate to the nearest tenth mL.

$$\frac{mL}{hr} = \frac{500 \text{ mL}}{5 \text{ g}}$$

$$\frac{mL}{hr} = \frac{500 \text{ mL}}{5 \text{ g}} \times \frac{1 \text{ g}}{1000 \text{ mg}}$$

$$\frac{mL}{hr} = \frac{500 \text{ mL}}{5 \text{ g}} \times \frac{1 \text{ g}}{1000 \text{ mg}} \times \frac{1 \text{ mg}}{1000 \text{ mcg}}$$

$$\frac{mL}{hr} = \frac{500 \text{ mL}}{5 \text{ g}} \times \frac{1 \text{ g}}{1000 \text{ mg}} \times \frac{1 \text{ mg}}{1000 \text{ mcg}} \times \frac{100 \text{ mcg}}{kg/min}$$

$$\frac{mL}{hr} = \frac{500 \text{ mL}}{5 \text{ g}} \times \frac{1 \text{ g}}{1000 \text{ mg}} \times \frac{1 \text{ mg}}{1000 \text{ mcg}} \times \frac{100 \text{ mcg}}{kg/min} \times \frac{60 \text{ min}}{1 \text{ hr}}$$

$$\frac{mL}{hr} = \frac{500 \text{ mL}}{5 \text{ g}} \times \frac{1 \text{ g}}{1000 \text{ mg}} \times \frac{1 \text{ mg}}{1000 \text{ mcg}} \times \frac{100 \text{ mcg}}{kg/min} \times \frac{60 \text{ min}}{1 \text{ hr}} \times \frac{77.6 \text{ kg}}{}$$

$$= 46.56 = \textbf{46.6 mL/hr}$$

The 46.6 mL/hr answer is equivalent to the 4.8 mL/hr answer obtained in the two-step method.

PROBLEM

Use the one-step method to calculate the flow rates necessary to infuse the dosages based on body weight. Express all flow rates to the nearest tenth mL.

1. A 3.5 mcg/kg/min dosage has been ordered for an adult weighing 90.3 kg. The solution being used has a strength of 40 mg in 150 mL D5W. _____

2. IV medication has been ordered to infuse at 3 mcg/kg/min using a 250 mg/250 mL D5W solution. The body weight is 87.3 kg. _____

3. A 4 mcg/kg/min dosage has been ordered. The solution strength is 600 mg/250 mL D5W. The weight is 90.3 kg. _____

4. A rate of 200 mcg/kg/min has been ordered for a 83.3 kg weight. The solution strength is 3.5 g in 250 mL D5W. _____

5. A 4.5 mcg/kg/min infusion has been ordered for an 79.9 kg body weight. The solution to be used has 1.5 g in 200 mL D5W. _____

ANSWERS   1. 71.1 mL/hr   2. 15.7 mL/hr   3. 9 mL/hr   4. 71.4 mL/hr   5. 2.9 mL/hr

Calculating Dosage Infusing from Flow Rate

It is possible to calculate the dosage being administered at any moment from the **flow rate infusing**, and the **solution concentration**.

EXAMPLE 1

An IV of **500 mL** D5W containing **800 mg** of medication is infusing at a rate of **25 mL/hr**. Calculate the dosage infusing, in **mg/hr** and **mcg/min**.

$$\frac{mg}{hr} = \frac{800 \; mg}{500 \; mL} \times \frac{25 \; mL}{1 \; hr}$$

$$= \frac{800 \; mg}{500 \; mL} \times \frac{25 \; mL}{1 \; hr}$$

$$= \textbf{40 mg/hr}$$

mg/min $= 40 \; mg \div 60 \; min = 0.67 \; mg = \textbf{670 mcg/min}$

EXAMPLE 2

A post-op cardiac medication is infusing at **30 gtt/min**. The solution strength is **100 mg** in **500 mL** D5W. Calculate the **mcg/min** and **mg/hr** infusing.

$$\frac{mcg}{min} = \frac{1000 \; mcg}{1 \; mg} \times \frac{100 \; mg}{500 \; mL} \times \frac{1 \; mL}{60 \; gtt} \times \frac{30 \; gtt}{1 \; min}$$

$$= \frac{1000 \; mcg}{1 \; mg} \times \frac{100 \; mg}{500 \; mL} \times \frac{1 \; mL}{60 \; gtt} \times \frac{30 \; gtt}{1 \; min}$$

$$= \textbf{100 mcg/min}$$

mg/hr $= 100 \; mcg \times 60 \; min = 6000 \; mcg = \textbf{6 mg/hr}$

EXAMPLE 3

A continuous infusion at a flow rate of **15 mL/hr** has been ordered. The solution strength is **2 g** medication in **500 mL** D5W. Calculate the **mg/hr** and **mg/min** being infused. The average dosage of this medication is **1–4 mg/min**. Is the dosage within normal range?

$$\frac{mg}{hr} = \frac{1000 \; mg}{1 \; g} \times \frac{2 \; g}{500 \; mL} \times \frac{15 \; mL}{1 \; hr}$$

$$= \frac{1000 \; mg}{1 \; g} \times \frac{2 \; g}{500 \; mL} \times \frac{15 \; mL}{1 \; hr}$$

$$= \textbf{60 mg/hr}$$

mg/min $= 60 \; mg \div 60 \; min = \textbf{1 mg/min}$

The dosage is within the normal range of 1–4 mg/min.

EXAMPLE 4

A solution of **5 g (5000 mg)** medication in **500 mL** D5W is infusing at **30 mL/hr.** Calculate the **mcg/min** infusing.

$$\frac{\text{mcg}}{\text{min}} = \frac{1000 \text{ mcg}}{1 \text{ mg}} \times \frac{5000 \text{ mg}}{500 \text{ mL}} \times \frac{30 \text{ mL}}{1 \text{ hr}} \times \frac{1 \text{ hr}}{60 \text{ min}}$$

$$= \frac{1000 \text{ mcg}}{1 \text{ mg}} \times \frac{5000 \text{ mg}}{500 \text{ mL}} \times \frac{30 \text{ mL}}{1 \text{ hr}} \times \frac{1 \text{ hr}}{60 \text{ min}}$$

$$= \textbf{5,000 mcg/min}$$

PROBLEM

Calculate the dosages indicated in the problems. Express dosages to the nearest tenth.

1. A continuous medication infusion is ordered. The solution strength is 2 mg in 500 mL D5W, and the rate of infusion is 40 mL/hr. Calculate the mcg/min infusing. _____

   Is the infusion within the normal 1–5 mcg/min range? _____

2. The order is to infuse 500 mg in 250 mL at a rate of 7 mL/hr. Calculate the mg/hr and mcg/min being received. _____

   _____

3. A 2 g in 500 mL D5W solution strength is ordered to run at 30 mL/hr. Calculate the number of mg/min being administered. _____

   The normal dosage range for this drug is between 1–6 mg/min. Is the dosage within these limits? _____

4. The order is for 6 mL/hr of a medication by volumetric pump. The solution strength is 50 mg/250 mL. How many mcg/min are being infused? _____

5. A drug is ordered to control heart rate during surgery. The solution available has a strength of 2.5 g in 250 mL D5W. The order is to infuse at 32 mL/hr. Calculate the mg/hr and mg/min being infused. _____

   _____

ANSWERS 1. 2.7 mcg/min; yes 2. 14 mg/hr; 233.3 mcg/min 3. 2 mg/min; yes 4. 20 mcg/min 5. 320 mg/hr; 5.3 mg/min

Titration of Infusions

Titration refers to the **adjustment of dosage within a specific range to obtain a measurable physiologic response,** for example a blood pressure drug at 2–4 mcg/min to maintain systolic BP >100. The dosage is increased or decreased within the ordered range until the desired response is obtained. The **lowest dosage is set first, and adjusted upwards and downwards as necessary.** The **upper dosage is never exceeded** unless a new order is obtained.

Volumetric pumps are used for administration. Flow rates are calculated in mL/hr for the lowest and highest dosage ordered, and adjusted within this range to elicit the desired physiologic response. Let's look at some examples.

EXAMPLE 1

A **2–4 mcg/min** dosage has been ordered. The solution being titrated has **8 mg** in **250 mL** D5W. Calculate the flow rate of medication for the **2–4 mcg range**. Express answers to the nearest tenth.

Calculate the lower 2 mcg/min flow rate first.

$$\frac{mL}{hr} = \frac{250\ mL}{8\ mg} \times \frac{1\ mg}{1000\ mcg} \times \frac{2\ mcg}{1\ min} \times \frac{60\ min}{1\ hr}$$

$$= \frac{250\ mL}{8\ mg} \times \frac{1\ mg}{1000\ mcg} \times \frac{2\ mcg}{1\ min} \times \frac{60\ min}{1\ hr}$$

$$= 3.75 = \textbf{3.8 mL/hr}$$

Next calculate the upper 4 mcg/min flow rate.

$$\frac{mL}{hr} = \frac{250\ mL}{8\ mg} \times \frac{1\ mg}{1000\ mcg} \times \frac{4\ mcg}{1\ min} \times \frac{60\ min}{1\ hr}$$

$$= \frac{250\ mL}{8\ mg} \times \frac{1\ mg}{1000\ mcg} \times \frac{4\ mcg}{1\ min} \times \frac{60\ min}{1\ hr}$$

$$= 7.5 = \textbf{7.5 mL/hr}$$

A dosage of 2–4 mcg/min is delivered by a flow rate of 3.8–7.5 mL/hr.

Let's assume that several changes in mL/hr have been made, and that the BP has now stabilized at **5 mL/hr**. Look how simple it is to determine how many **mcg/min** (or per hr) is being administered.

$$\frac{mcg}{min} = \frac{1000\ mcg}{1\ mg} \times \frac{8\ mg}{250\ mL} \times \frac{5\ mL}{1\ hr} \times \frac{1\ hr}{60\ min}$$

$$= \frac{1000\ mcg}{1\ mg} \times \frac{8\ mg}{250\ mL} \times \frac{5\ mL}{1\ hr} \times \frac{1\ hr}{60\ min}$$

$$= 2.67 = \textbf{2.7 mcg/min}$$

At a flow rate of 5 mL/hr 2.7 mcg/min is being administered.

EXAMPLE 2

A medication is to be titrated between **415–830 mcg/min**. The solution concentration is **100 mg** in **40 mL** NS. Calculate the **mL/hr** flow rate range. Express answers to the nearest tenth.

Calculate the flow rate for the lower 415 mcg/min dosage.

$$\frac{mL}{hr} = \frac{40\ mL}{100\ mg} \times \frac{1\ mg}{1000\ mcg} \times \frac{415\ mcg}{1\ min} \times \frac{60\ min}{1\ hr}$$

$$= \frac{40\ mL}{100\ mg} \times \frac{1\ mg}{1000\ mcg} \times \frac{415\ mcg}{1\ min} \times \frac{60\ min}{1\ hr}$$

$$= 9.96 = \textbf{10 mL/hr}$$

Calculate the flow rate for the upper 830 mcg/min dosage.

$$\frac{mL}{hr} = \frac{40\ mL}{100\ mg} \times \frac{1\ mg}{1000\ mcg} \times \frac{830\ mcg}{1\ min} \times \frac{60\ min}{1\ hr}$$

$$= \frac{40\ mL}{100\ mg} \times \frac{1\ mg}{1000\ mcg} \times \frac{415\ mcg}{1\ min} \times \frac{60\ min}{1\ hr}$$

$$= 19.92 = \textbf{19.9 mL/hr}$$

A dosage of 415–830 mcg/min requires a flow rate of 10–19.9 mL/hr.

This rate is adjusted several times, and the IV is now infusing at **14 mL/hr**. How many **mcg/min** are now infusing?

$$\frac{mcg}{min} = \frac{1000\ mcg}{1\ mg} \times \frac{100\ mg}{40\ mL} \times \frac{14\ mL}{1\ hr} \times \frac{1\ hr}{60\ min}$$

$$= \frac{1000\ mcg}{1\ mg} \times \frac{100\ mg}{40\ mL} \times \frac{14\ mL}{1\ hr} \times \frac{1\ hr}{60\ min}$$

$$= 583.33 = \textbf{583.3 mcg/min}$$

A 14 mL/hr flow rate will infuse 583.3 mcg/min.

EXAMPLE 3

An adult weighing **103.1 kg** has orders for a drug to be titrated between **0.3–3 mcg/kg/min**. The solution concentration is **50 mg in 250 mL** D5W. Express answers to the nearest tenth.

Calculate the dosage range for this 103.1 kg weight first.

      Lower dosage: 0.3 mcg/kg/min × 103.1 kg = 30.93 = **30.9 mcg/min**

      Upper dosage: 3 mcg/kg/min × 103 .1 kg = **309.3 mcg/min**

The dosage range for this 103.1 kg adult is 30.9–309.3 mcg/min.

Calculate the flow rate for the lower 30.9 mcg/min dosage.

$$\frac{mL}{hr} = \frac{250\ mL}{50\ mg} \times \frac{1\ mg}{1000\ mcg} \times \frac{30.9\ mcg}{1\ min} \times \frac{60\ min}{1\ hr}$$

$$= \frac{250\ mL}{50\ mg} \times \frac{1\ mg}{1000\ mcg} \times \frac{30.9\ mcg}{1\ min} \times \frac{60\ min}{1\ hr}$$

$$= 9.2 = \textbf{9.2 mL/hr}$$

Calculate the flow rate for the upper 309.3 mcg/min dosage.

$$\frac{mL}{hr} = \frac{250\ mL}{50\ mg} \times \frac{1\ mg}{1000\ mcg} \times \frac{309.3\ mcg}{1\ min} \times \frac{60\ min}{1\ hr}$$

$$= \frac{250\ mL}{50\ mg} \times \frac{1\ mg}{1000\ mcg} \times \frac{309.3\ mcg}{1\ min} \times \frac{60\ min}{1\ hr}$$

$$= 92.7 = \textbf{92.7 mL/hr}$$

To deliver 0.3–3 mcg/kg/min the flow rate must be titrated between 9.2–92.7 mL/hr.

If after several titrations the adult stabilizes at a rate of **22 mL/hr**, how many **mcg/min** will be infusing?

$$\frac{mcg}{min} = \frac{1000\ mcg}{1\ mg} \times \frac{50\ mg}{250\ mL} \times \frac{22\ mL}{1\ hr} \times \frac{1\ hr}{60\ min}$$

$$= \frac{1000\ mcg}{1\ mg} \times \frac{50\ mg}{250\ mL} \times \frac{22\ mL}{1\ hr} \times \frac{1\ hr}{60\ min}$$

$$= 73.3\ \textbf{mcg/min}$$

A flow rate of 22 mL/hr will infuse 73.3 mcg/min.

EXAMPLE 4

A drug has been ordered to titrate at **3–6 mcg/kg/min**. The solution strength is **50 mg in 250 mL**. Calculate the flow rate range for a **72.4 kg** adult. Round answers to the nearest whole mL.

Calculate the dosage range for the 72.4 kg weight.

> **Lower dosage:** 3 mcg/kg/min × 72.4 kg = **217.2 mcg/min**
>
> **Upper dosage:** 6 mcg/kg/min × 72.4 kg = **434.4 mcg/min**

Calculate the flow rate for the lower 217.2 mcg/min dosage.

$$\frac{mL}{hr} = \frac{250\ mL}{50\ mg} \times \frac{1\ mg}{1000\ mcg} \times \frac{217.2\ mcg}{1\ min} \times \frac{60\ min}{1\ hr}$$

$$= \frac{250\ mL}{50\ mg} \times \frac{1\ mg}{1000\ mcg} \times \frac{217.2\ mcg}{1\ min} \times \frac{60\ min}{1\ hr}$$

$$= 65.1 = \textbf{65 mL/hr}$$

Calculate the flow rate for the upper 434.4 mcg/min dosage.

$$\frac{mL}{hr} = \frac{250\ mL}{50\ mg} \times \frac{1\ mg}{1000\ mcg} \times \frac{434.4\ mcg}{1\ min} \times \frac{60\ min}{1\ hr}$$

$$= \frac{250\ mL}{50\ mg} \times \frac{1\ mg}{1000\ mcg} \times \frac{434.4\ mcg}{1\ min} \times \frac{60\ min}{1\ hr}$$

$$= 130.3 = \textbf{130 mL/hr}$$

To deliver 3–6 mcg/kg/min to this 72.4 kg adult, the flow rate must be titrated between 65–130 mL/hr.

If after several adjustments upwards the flow rate is stabilized at **75 mL/hr**, what will the **mcg/min** dosage be?

$$\frac{mcg}{min} = \frac{1000\ mcg}{1\ mg} \times \frac{50\ mg}{250\ mL} \times \frac{75\ mL}{1\ hr} \times \frac{1\ hr}{60\ min}$$

$$= \frac{1000\ mcg}{1\ mg} \times \frac{50\ mg}{250\ mL} \times \frac{75\ mL}{1\ hr} \times \frac{1\ hr}{60\ min}$$

$$= \textbf{250 mcg/min}$$

An infusion rate of 75 mL/hr will deliver 250 mcg/min.

PROBLEM

Calculate the dosage range, mL/hr flow rate, and stabilizing dosages as indicated for the titrations. Express fractional dosages to the nearest tenth, and mL/hr flow rates to the nearest whole mL.

1. A 2 g in 500 mL D5W solution is ordered to titrate at 1–2 mg/min. After several titrations the rate is stabilized at 18 mL/hr.

   Flow rate range _____ Stabilizing dosage/min _____

2. A drug is ordered to titrate between 1–3 mcg/min to sustain heart rate. The solution strength is 1 mg per 250 mL D5W. The heart rate is stabilized at 35 mL/hr.

   Flow rate range _____ Stabilizing dosage/min _____

3. A stabilizing dosage of medication is established at a rate of 14 mL/hr. The dosage range being titrated is 5–8 mcg/kg/min. The body weight is 103.7 kg, and the solution strength is 100 mg in 40 mL NS.

   Dosage range mcg/min _____ Flow rate range mL/hr _____

   Stabilizing dosage/min _____

4. A drug is to titrate between 50–100 mcg/kg/min. The body weight is 78.7 kg, and the solution strength is 2500 mg in 250 mL D5W. After several titrations the rate is stabilized at 30 mL/hr.

   Dosage range mcg/min _____ Flow rate range mL/hr _____

   Stabilizing dosage/min _____

5. An adult weighing 73.2 kg has a solution of 500 mg medication in 250 mL D5W ordered to titrate between 3–10 mcg/kg/min. After many adjustments, the rate is stabilized at 27 mL/hr.

   Dosage range mcg/min _____ Flow rate range mL/hr _____

   Stabilizing dosage/min _____

ANSWERS 1. 15–30 mL/hr; 1.2 mg/min 2. 15–45 mL/hr; 2.3 mcg/min 3. 518.5–829.6 mcg/min; 12–20 mL/hr; 583.3 mcg/min 4. 3935–7870 mcg/min; 24–47 mL/hr; 5000 mcg/min 5. 219.6–732 mcg/min; 7–22 mL/hr; 900 mcg/min

Summary

This concludes the chapter on titration of IV medications. The important points to remember about these medications are:

They have a rapid action and short duration.

They have a narrow margin of safety, and continuous monitoring is required in their use.

They are frequently titrated within a specific dosage/flow rate to elicit a measurable physiologic response.

When titrated they are initiated at the lowest dosage ordered, and increased or decreased slowly to obtain the desired response.

They are infused using an EID.

The mL/hr flow rate for EIDs can be calculated to the nearest whole mL, or tenth mL, depending on the EID available.

Calculations for dosage and flow rates must always be double-checked.

Summary Self-Test

Read each question thoroughly, and calculate only the dosages and flow rates indicated. Express dosages to the nearest tenth, and flow rates to the nearest whole mL.

1. A dosage of 6 mcg/kg/min is ordered to infuse IV to sustain the blood pressure of an adult weighing 75.4 kg. The solution available is 500 mg in 250 mL D5W.

   mcg/min dosage _____ mL/hr flow rate _____

2. The order is to infuse a solution of 50 mg in 250 mL D5W at 0.8 mcg/kg/min. Calculate the flow rate in mL/hr for 65.9 kg.

   mcg/min dosage _____ mL/hr flow rate _____

3. An adult has an order for 250 mg in 500 mL D5W to infuse between 0.5 and 0.7 mg/kg/hr. His weight is 82.4 kg. He stabilizes at 75 mL/hr.

   mg/hr dosage range _____ mL/hr flow rate range _____

   stabilizing dosage/hr _____

4. A solution of 400 mg in 250 mL D5W is infusing at 20 gtt/min.

   mcg/min dosage _____

5. A 1–6 mg/min rate is ordered. The solution strength is 2 g/500 mL. Stabilization is obtained at a rate of 80 mL/hr.

   mL/hr flow rate range _____ stabilizing dosage mg/min _____

6. The orders are for an infusion of 2 g in 500 mL D5W at 60 mL/hr. Is this dosage within the normal 1–4 mg/min range?

   mg/min dosage _____ mg/hr dosage _____

   normal range? _____

7. The IV solution available is 25 mg in 50 mL. The order is to infuse at 8 mg/hr.

   mL/hr flow rate _____

8. A solution strength of 100 mg in 40 mL NS is ordered to infuse at 5 mcg/kg/min for a body weight of 77.1 kg.

   mL/hr flow rate _____

9. Medication has been ordered at 4 mcg/min. The solution available is 1 mg in 250 mL D5W.

   gtt/min flow rate _____

10. An adult weighing 80 kg has an order for medication to infuse at 8 mcg/kg/min. The solution strength is 800 mg in 500 mL D5W.

    mcg/min dosage _____ gtt/min flow rate _____

11. A 400 mg dosage is added to 250 mL D5W and infused at 45 gtt/min. Calculate the mcg/min and mg/hr infusing.

    mcg/min dosage _____ mg/hr dosage _____

12. Orders are for a 1 mg/min medication titration. The solution strength is 250 mg in 250 mL D5W.

    gtt/min flow rate _____

13. An adult weighing 77.9 kg is to receive 80 mcg/kg/min of a medication. The solution strength is 2.5 g in 250 mL D5W.

    mcg/min dosage _____ mL/hr flow rate _____

14. A 4 mcg/min dosage has been ordered using an 8 mg in 250 mL D5W solution.

    gtt/min flow rate _____

15. The body weight is 81.7 kg and the order is for an 8–10 mcg/kg/min infusion. The solution strength is 400 mg in 250 mL D5W. The IV is infusing at 25 mL/hr.

     mcg/min dosage range _____ mcg/min infusing _____

     Within ordered range? _____

16. A 6 mcg/kg/min dosage has been ordered for a 90.7 kg body weight. The solution strength is 50 mg in 250 mL D5W.

     mcg/min dosage _____ mL/hr flow rate _____

17. A rate of 5 mcg/kg/min is ordered. The solution available is 400 mg in 250 mL D5W. The body weight is 70.7 kg.

     mcg/min dosage _____ gtt/min flow rate _____

18. A 3 mg/min rate is ordered. The solution strength is 2 g in 500 mL D5W.

     mL/hr flow rate _____

19. A solution of 50 mg/250 mL D5W is infusing at 15 gtt/min.

     mcg/min infusing _____

20. A 2 g in 500 mL D5W solution is to infuse at a rate of 2 mg/min.

     mL/hr flow rate _____

21. An adult whose weight is 102.4 kg is to receive 2 mg/kg/hr of medication. The solution strength is 1 g in 500 mL D5W.

     mg/hr dosage _____ mL/hr flow rate _____

22. A 1 g in 100 mL D5W solution is to infuse at a rate of 15 mcg/kg/min. The body weight is 94.4 kg.

     mcg/min dosage _____ gtt/min flow rate _____

23. An adult is receiving 4 gtt/min of a solution that contains 8 mg in 250 mL D5W. Is this within the normal range of 2–4 mcg/min?

     mcg/min infusing _____ Normal range? _____

24. Medication is ordered to titrate between 5–10 mcg/kg/min. The body weight is 97.1 kg, and the solution strength is 100 mg/40 mL NS. The stabilizing flow rate is 17 mL/hr.

     mcg/min range _____ mL/hr flow rate range _____

     mcg/min stabilizing dosage _____

25. A solution of 500 mg in 250 mL D5W is ordered for a 101.2 kg body weight to titrate between 3–10 mcg/kg/min. The stabilization is reached at 23 mL/hr.

     mcg/min dosage range _____ mL/hr flow rate range _____

     mcg/min stabilizing dosage _____

26. An infusion of 500 mg in 250 mL D5W has a stabilizing rate of 14 mL/hr.

     mcg/min infusing _____

27. A 5–10 mcg/kg/min rate is to be titrated for an adult weighing 79.6 kg. The solution strength is 100 mg in 40 mL NS. Stabilization is achieved at 12 mL/hr.

     mcg/min dosage range _____ mL/hr flow rate range _____

     mcg/min stabilizing dosage _____

28. A 400 mg in 250 mL D5W solution is to be titrated at 2–20 mcg/kg/min. The body weight is 62.3 kg. The BP stabilizes at 32 mL/hr.

     mcg/min dosage range _____ mL/hr flow rate range _____

     mcg/min stabilizing dosage _____

29. Medication has been ordered for an adult weighing 84.9 kg to titrate at 2.5–10 mcg/kg/min. The solution strength is 500 mg in 250 mL D5W. Stabilization is achieved at a rate of 18 mL/hr.

        mcg/min dosage range _____ mL/hr flow rate range _____

        mcg/min stabilizing dosage _____

30. Medication is ordered at a rate of 1–4 mg/min. The solution strength is 2 g in 500 mL D5W.

        mL/hr flow rate range _____

ANSWERS

1. 452.4 mcg/min; 14 mL/hr
2. 52.7 mcg/min; 16 mL/hr
3. 41.2–57.7 mg/hr; 82–115 mL/hr; 37.5 mg/hr
4. 533.3 mcg/min
5. 15–90 mL/hr; 5.3 mg/min
6. 4 mg/min; 240 mg/hr; yes
7. 16 mL/hr
8. 9 mL/hr
9. 60 gtt/min
10. 640 mcg/min; 24 gtt/min
11. 1200 mcg/min; 72 mg/hr
12. 60 gtt/min

13. 6232 mcg/min; 37 mL/hr
14. 8 gtt/min
15. 653.6–817 mcg/min; 666.7 mcg/min; yes
16. 544.2 mcg/min; 163 mL/hr
17. 353.5 mcg/min; 13 gtt/min
18. 45 mL/hr
19. 50 mcg/min
20. 30 mL/hr
21. 204.8 mg/hr; 102 mL/hr
22. 1416 mcg/min; 9 gtt/min
23. 2.1 mcg/min; yes

24. 485.5–971 mcg/min; 12–23 mL/hr; 708.3 mcg/min
25. 303.6–1012 mcg/min; 9–30 mL/hr; 766.7 mcg/min
26. 466.7 mcg/min
27. 398–796 mcg/min; 10–19 mL/hr; 500 mcg/min
28. 124.6–1246 mcg/min; 5–47 mL/hr; 853.3 mcg/min
29. 212.3–849 mcg/min; 6–25 mL/hr; 600 mcg/min
30. 15–60 mL/hr

18

Heparin Intravenous Calculations

OBJECTIVES

The learner will calculate the:

1. amount of heparin to be added to prepare IV solutions
2. mL/hr flow rates for EID administration
3. hourly dosage from mL/hr infusing

Heparin is an anticoagulant drug that inhibits new blood clot formation or the extension of already existing clots. Heparin dosages are expressed in USP units, and are commonly administered intravenously. Dosages may be ordered on the basis of units/hr, or, if a standard concentration of IV solution is used, by mL/hr flow rate. Heparin dosages are ordered on a very individualized basis, and blood tests to monitor coagulation times are essential.

 The usual heparinizing dosage for adults is 20,000–40,000 units every 24 hours.

This means that the average daily dosage will fall within the 20,000 units to 40,000 units parameters. Dosages larger or smaller may be ordered based on coagulation time, but dosages markedly different from the average would need to be questioned.

In this chapter you will be introduced to several of the commercially prepared IV solutions containing heparin, as well as to heparin vial labels, which you will use to calculate the preparation of a variety of IV heparin solution strengths using standard IV solutions. You will also practice calculating heparin flow rates; calculating hourly dosage being administered; and assessing the accuracy of prescribed heparin dosages. The calculations are identical to those you have already practiced in previous chapters except that heparin is measured in units. Heparin is administered IV using a volumetric pump.

Reading Heparin Labels and Preparing IV Solutions

Commercially prepared IV solutions containing heparin are available in several strengths. Refer to the IV bag labeling in Figure 18-1, and notice the blue "Heparin Sodium 1,000 units in 0.9% Sodium Chloride Injection" on this 500 mL bag label, and the additional red dosage labeling "Heparin 1,000 units (2 units/mL)." The red dosages draw particular attention to the fact that these bags contain heparin, to make the bags instantly recognizable. They serve as an important safety factor in solution identification.

If a commercially prepared intravenous heparin dosage strength is not available, you may be required to prepare the solution yourself from **a number of available vial dosage strengths**. Let's stop and look at several vial labels now, so that you can refresh your memory with some typical calculations.

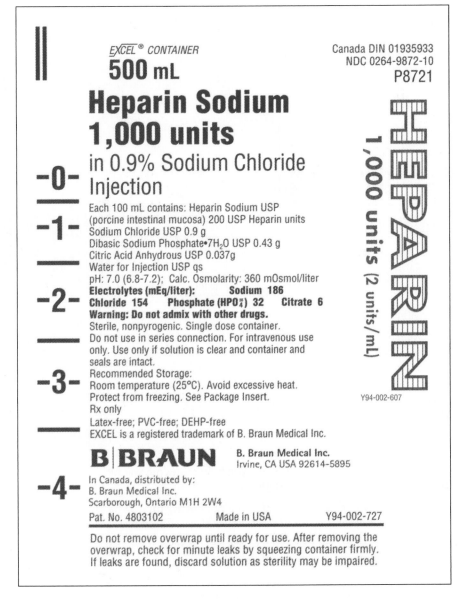

Figure 18-1

(Courtesy of B. Braun Medical Inc., Irvine, CA)

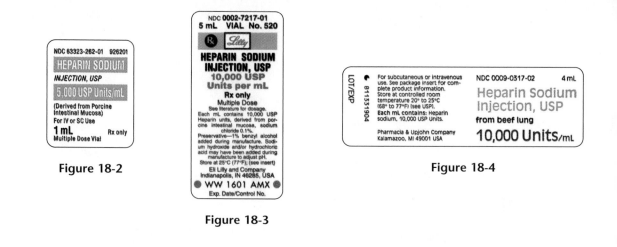

Figure 18-2

Figure 18-3

Figure 18-4

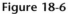

Figure 18-5

Figure 18-6

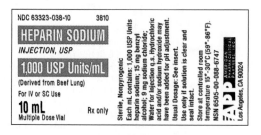

PROBLEM

Read the heparin labels provided and determine how many mL of heparin will be necessary to prepare the solutions indicated.

1. Refer to the label in Figure 18-2 and determine how many mL will be required to add 4,000 units to an IV solution.

_____

2. Refer to the label in Figure 18-3 and determine how many mL will be required to add 30,000 units to an IV solution.

_____

3. Refer to the label in Figure 18-4 and determine how many mL will be required to add 20,000 units to an IV solution.

_____

4. Refer to the label in Figure 18-5 and determine how many mL of heparin will be required to add 25,000 units to an IV solution.

_____

5. Refer to the label in Figure 18-6 and determine how many mL will be required to add 10,000 units to an IV solution.

_____

ANSWERS   1. 0.8 mL   2. 3 mL   3. 2 mL   4. 5 mL   5. 10 mL

Calculating mL/hr Flow Rate from units/hr Ordered

Because heparin is most frequently ordered in units/hr to be administered, for example, 1000 units/hr, and infused using an EID, a common calculation will be the mL/hr flow rate needed for the infusion.

EXAMPLE 1

The order is to infuse heparin **1000 units/hr** from a solution of **20,000 units in 500 mL** D5W. Calculate the **mL/hr** flow rate.

Enter the mL/hr being calculated first. Locate the ratio containing mL, the 20,000 units/500 mL strength, and enter this as the starting ratio with mL as the numerator, to match the mL numerator of the units being calculated; 20,000 units becomes the denominator.

$$\frac{mL}{hr} = \frac{500 \text{ mL}}{20,000 \text{ units}}$$

The starting ratio denominator, units, must be matched in the next numerator. Enter the 1000 units/hr rate ordered with units as the numerator. This completes the equation.

$$\frac{mL}{hr} = \frac{500 \text{ mL}}{20,000 \text{ units}} \times \frac{1000 \text{ units}}{1 \text{ hr}}$$

Cancel alternate denominator/numerator units in the equation to double-check that the ratios have been entered correctly. Only mL and hr should remain. Do the math.

$$\frac{mL}{hr} = \frac{500 \text{ mL}}{20,000 \text{ units}} \times \frac{1000 \text{ units}}{1 \text{ hr}} = \textbf{25 mL/hr}$$

EXAMPLE 2

The order is for heparin **800 units/hr**. The solution available is **40,000 units in 1000 mL** D5W. Calculate the **mL/hr** flow rate.

Enter the mL/hr being calculated. Enter the 1000 mL/40,000 units ratio with mL as the numerator.

$$\frac{mL}{hr} = \frac{1000 \text{ mL}}{40,000 \text{ units}}$$

Enter the next ratio, 800 units/hr, with 800 units as the numerator to match the starting ratio denominator.

$$\frac{mL}{hr} = \frac{1000 \text{ mL}}{40,000 \text{ units}} \times \frac{800 \text{ units}}{1 \text{ hr}}$$

Cancel to double-check for correct ratio entry, and do the math.

$$\frac{mL}{hr} = \frac{1000 \text{ mL}}{40,000 \text{ units}} \times \frac{800 \text{ units}}{1 \text{ hr}} = \textbf{20 mL/hr}$$

EXAMPLE 3

The order is to infuse heparin **1100 units/hr** from a solution strength of **60,000 units in 1 L** D5W. Calculate the **mL/hr** flow rate.

$$\frac{mL}{hr} = \frac{1000 \text{ mL}}{60,000 \text{ units}} \times \frac{1100 \text{ units}}{1 \text{ hr}}$$

$$\frac{mL}{hr} = \frac{1000 \text{ mL}}{60,000 \text{ units}} \times \frac{1100 \text{ units}}{1 \text{ hr}} = 18.33 = \textbf{18 mL/hr}$$

18

PROBLEM

Calculate the mL/hr flow rates for the heparin infusions.

1. The order is to infuse 1000 units heparin per hour from an available solution strength of 25,000 units in 500 mL D5W. _____

2. Heparin has been ordered at 2500 units per hour. The solution strength is 50,000 units in 1000 mL D5W. _____

3. The order is to infuse 1100 units per hour from a 15,000 units in 1 L D5W solution. _____

4. An adult has orders for 50,000 units of heparin in 1000 mL D5W to infuse at a rate of 2000 units per hour. _____

5. Administer 1500 units per hour of heparin from an available strength of 40,000 units in 1 L. _____

ANSWERS 1. 20 mL/hr 2. 50 mL/hr 3. 73 mL/hr 4. 40 mL/hr 5. 38 mL/hr

Calculating units/hr Infusing from mL/hr Infusing

If a heparin order specifies infusion at a predetermined mL/hr flow rate, the physician has already calculated the dosage per hour/day. However, it remains a nursing responsibility to double-check dosages to determine if they are within the normal heparinizing range of 20,000–40,000 units per day. Here's how you would do this. The units/hr infusing is calculated first.

EXAMPLE 1

An IV of **1000 mL** D5W containing **40,000 units** of heparin has been ordered to infuse at **30 mL/hr**. Calculate the **units/hr** infusing and assess the accuracy of this dosage.

Enter the units/hr being calculated first. Locate the ratio containing units, the 40,000 units/1000 mL strength, and enter this as the starting ratio with the 40,000 units as numerator to match the units numerator being calculated.

$$\frac{units}{hr} = \frac{40,000 \text{ units}}{1000 \text{ mL}}$$

The starting ratio mL denominator must now be matched in the next numerator. Look back at the problem, and you'll see the 30 mL/hr rate. This becomes the last ratio entered. Enter it with 30 mL as the numerator; 1 hr becomes the denominator.

$$\frac{units}{hr} = \frac{40,000 \text{ units}}{1000 \text{ mL}} \times \frac{30 \text{ mL}}{1 \text{ hr}}$$

Cancel the alternate denominator mL units of measure to double-check for correct ratio entry, and do the math.

$$\frac{\text{units}}{\text{hr}} = \frac{40,000 \text{ units}}{1000 \text{ mL}} \times \frac{30 \text{ mL}}{1 \text{ hr}} = \textbf{1200 units/hr}$$

At a rate of 30 mL/hr, 1200 units/hr are infusing.

1200 units/hr $\times$ 24 hr = **28,000 units/24 hr. This dosage is within the normal 20,000–40,000 units heparinizing range.**

EXAMPLE 2

The order is to infuse a solution of heparin **20,000 units to 1 L** D5W at **80 mL/hr.** Calculate the **units/hr** infusing and assess the accuracy of the order.

Enter the units/hr being calculated first, then the 20,000 units/1000 mL starting ratio, with units as the numerator to match the units numerator being calculated.

$$\frac{\text{units}}{\text{hr}} = \frac{20,000 \text{ units}}{1000 \text{ mL}}$$

Enter the 80 units/1 hr rate ordered next, with 80 mL as the numerator to match the starting ratio mL denominator to complete the equation.

$$\frac{\text{units}}{\text{hr}} = \frac{20,000 \text{ units}}{1000 \text{ mL}} \times \frac{80 \text{ mL}}{1 \text{ hr}}$$

Cancel the alternate denominator/numerator mL units of measure to double-check for accurate ratio entry, and do the math.

$$\frac{\text{units}}{\text{hr}} = \frac{20,000 \text{ units}}{1000 \text{ mL}} \times \frac{80 \text{ mL}}{1 \text{ hr}} = \textbf{1600 units/hr}$$

1600 units/hr $\times$ 24 hr = **38,400 units/24 hr. The dosage is within the normal 20,000–40,000 units range.**

EXAMPLE 3

An IV of D5W **500 mL** with **10,000 units** heparin is infusing at **30 mL/hr.** Calculate the **units/hr** dosage and determine if this dose is within the normal range.

$$\frac{\text{units}}{\text{hr}} = \frac{10,000 \text{ units}}{500 \text{ mL}} \times \frac{30 \text{ mL}}{1 \text{ hr}}$$

$$= \frac{10,000 \text{ units}}{500 \text{ mL}} \times \frac{30 \text{ mL}}{1 \text{ hr}}$$

$$= \textbf{600 units/hr}$$

600 units/hr $\times$ 24 hr = **14,400 units/day. This is less than the normal 20,000–40,000 units heparinizing dose,** so the order should be reconfirmed.

PROBLEM

Calculate the units/hr heparin dosages, and determine if they are within the normal daily range.

1. The order is to add 30,000 units heparin to 750 mL D5W and infuse at 25 mL/hr.

   units/hr _____ units/day _____ Within normal range? _____

2. A solution of 20,000 units heparin in 500 mL D5W is to be infused at 30 mL/hr.

   units/hr _____ units/day _____ Within normal range? _____

3. One liter of D5NS with heparin 60,000 units is ordered to infuse at 40 mL/hr.

   units/hr _____ units/day _____ Within normal range? _____

4. The order is to add 20,000 units heparin to 1 L D5W and infuse at 30 mL/hr.

   units/hr _____ units/day _____ Within normal range? _____

5. A 25,000 units in 500 mL D5W heparin solution is infusing at 30 mL/hr.

   units/hr _____ units/day _____ Within normal range? _____

ANSWERS 1. 1000 units/hr; 24,000 units/day; yes 2. 1200 units/hr; 28,800 units/day; yes 3. 2400 units/hr; 57,600 units/day; high 4. 600 units/hr; 14,400 units/day; low 5. 1500 units/hr; 36,000 units/day; yes

Summary

This concludes the chapter on heparin administration. The important points to remember are:

Heparin is a potent anticoagulant that is frequently added to IV solutions.

It is measured in USP units.

The normal heparinizing dosage is 20,000–40,000 units/day.

The patient on heparin therapy will have frequent blood tests to check coagulation times.

Heparin may be ordered by mL/hr flow rate, or by units/hr to infuse.

An EID is used for infusion.

Commercially prepared IV solutions are available for several heparin strengths.

Additional strengths may require the preparation of heparin from a variety of available vial strengths.

Summary Self-Test

Calculate the heparin flow rates and hourly dosages as indicated in the questions.

1. An adult is to receive heparin 1000 units/hr. The IV solution available has 25,000 units in 1 L D5W, and a pump will be used. Flow rate _____

2. A solution of 35,000 units heparin in 1 L D51/2S is to infuse via volumetric pump at 1200 units/hr. Flow rate _____

3. The order is for 20,000 units heparin in 500 mL D5W to infuse at 40 mL/hr. Dosage per hr _____

4. Calculate the hourly heparin dosage infusing at 50 mL/hr from a 35,000 units heparin in 1 L D5W solution. Dosage per hour   _____

5. An adult who recently had open heart surgery has an IV of 500 mL D5W with 20,000 units heparin infusing at 20 mL/hr. Dosage per hr   _____

6. An accident victim with a fractured pelvis has orders for 1 L D51/2S with 60,000 units heparin to infuse at 30 mL/hr. Dosage per hour   _____

   Within normal range?   _____

7. The order is for 1000 units heparin per hour. The solution strength is 20,000 units in 500 mL D5NS. Flow rate   _____

8. A newly admitted adult has an order for 1250 units/hr heparin from a solution strength of 15,000 units in 500 mL D5W. A pump is used to monitor the infusion. Flow rate   _____

9. Calculate the hourly dosage infusing with a 25 mL/hr rate from a 1 L D51/4S with 45,000 units heparin solution. Dosage   _____

10. A solution of 10,000 units heparin in 500 mL D5W is ordered to infuse at 1000 units/hr. Flow rate   _____

11. A solution of 500 mL D5NS with 30,000 units heparin is infusing at 25 mL/hr. Dosage per hour   _____

    Within normal limits?   _____

12. An adult with multiple fractures has an order for 2 L D51/2S each to contain 20,000 units heparin to infuse at 50 mL/hr using a microdrip. Dosage per hour   _____

13. An IV of 1000 mL D51/4S with 40,000 units heparin is to infuse at 1200 units/hr via pump. Flow rate   _____

14. The order is to infuse 500 mL D51/4S with 25,000 units heparin at 1500 units/hr. Flow rate   _____

15. A liter of D5W with 40,000 units heparin is infusing at 25 mL/hr. Dosage per hour   _____

16. A 500 mL IV with 25,000 units heparin is infusing at 30 mL/hr. Dosage per hour   _____

17. 500 mL D5W with 30,000 units of heparin is to infuse via pump at 1500 units/hr. Flow rate   _____

18. The order is to infuse 1 L D51/2S with 45,000 units of heparin at 1875 units/hr. Flow rate   _____

ANSWERS

1. 40 mL/hr	**6.** 1800 units/hr;	**10.** 50 mL/hr	**14.** 30 mL/hr
2. 34 mL/hr	high	**11.** 1500 units/hr;	**15.** 1000 units/hr
3. 1600 units/hr	**7.** 25 mL/hr	yes	**16.** 1500 units/hr
4. 1750 units/hr	**8.** 42 mL/hr	**12.** 1000 units/hr	**17.** 25 mL/hr
5. 800 units/hr	**9.** 1125 units/hr	**13.** 30 mL/hr	**18.** 42 mL/hr

SECTION SEVEN
Pediatric Medication Calculations

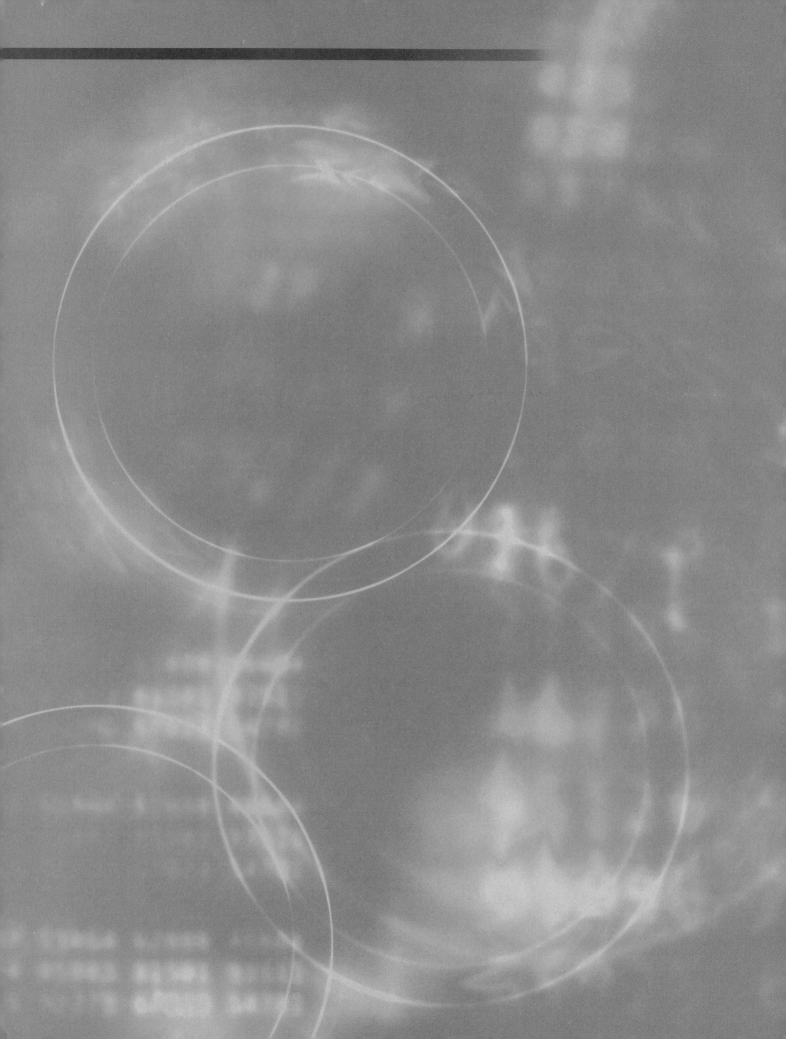

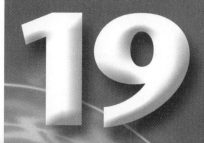

Pediatric Oral and Parenteral Medications

Two differences between adult and pediatric dosages will be immediately apparent: **most oral drugs are prepared as liquids** because infants and small children cannot be expected to swallow tablets easily, if at all, and **dosages are dramatically smaller**. The oral route is used whenever possible, but when a child cannot swallow, or the drug is ineffective given orally, drugs are administered by a parenteral route.

Both the subcutaneous and intramuscular routes may be used depending on the type of drug to be administered. However, the small muscle size of infants and children limits the use of the intramuscular route, as does the nature of the drug being used. For example, most antibiotics are administered intravenously rather than intramuscularly.

Oral Medications

Most oral pediatric drugs are prepared as liquids to facilitate ease in swallowing. If the child is old enough to cooperate, these dosages may be measured in a medication cup. Solutions may also be measured using oral syringes, such as the ones shown in Figure 19-1. Notice that oral syringes have the same metric calibrations as hypodermic syringes, but also include household measures, for example, tsp. Oral syringes have different-sized tips to prevent their being mistakenly used with hypodermic needles. On some oral syringes the tip is positioned off center (termed *eccentric*), to further distinguish them from hypodermic syringes, or they may be amber colored, as in the Figure 19-1 illustration.

If oral syringes are not available, hypodermic syringes (**without the needle**) can also be used for dosage measurement. In addition to accuracy, syringes provide an excellent method of administering oral liquid drugs to infants and small children. Some oral liquids are prepared using a calibrated medication dropper that is an integral part of the medication bottle. These may be calibrated in mL as on the dropper shown in Figure 19-2, or in actual dosage, for example, 25 mg or 50 mg. Animal-shaped measures such as those shown in Figure 19-3 are also helpful in enticing reluctant toddlers to take necessary medications. In each instance the goal is to ensure that the infant or child actually swallows the total dosage.

OBJECTIVES
The learner will:
1. explain how suspensions are measured and administered
2. calculate pediatric oral dosages
3. list the precautions of IM and subcutaneous injection in infants and children
4. calculate pediatric IM and subcutaneous dosages

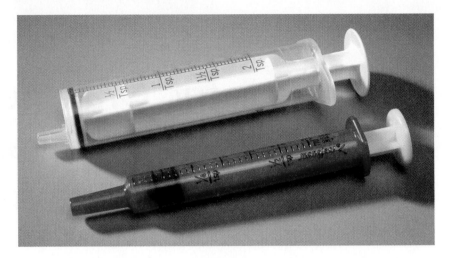

Figure 19-1

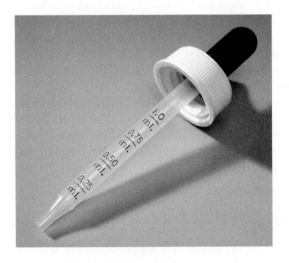

Figure 19-2

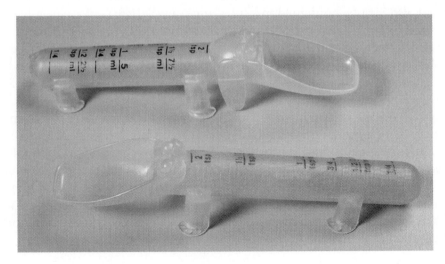

Figure 19-3

Care must be taken with liquid oral drugs to identify those prepared as **suspensions**. A **suspension consists of an insoluble drug in a liquid base** as for example in the Augmentin® suspension in Figure 19-4. The drug in a suspension settles to the bottom of the bottle between uses, and **thorough mixing immediately prior to pouring** is mandatory. Suspensions must also be **administered promptly after measurement** to prevent the drug from settling out again and an incomplete dosage being administered.

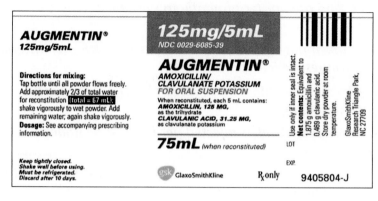

Figure 19-4

Suspensions must be thoroughly mixed before measurement and promptly administered to prevent settling out of their insoluble drugs.

When a tablet or capsule is administered, the child's mouth must be checked to be certain it has actually been swallowed. If swallowing is a problem, some tablets can be crushed and given in a small amount of applesauce, ice cream, or juice if the child has no dietary restrictions to contraindicate this. Keep in mind, however, that **enteric coated and timed release tablets or capsules cannot be crushed** because this would destroy the coating that allows them to function on a delayed action basis.

IM and Subcutaneous Medications

The drugs most often given subcutaneously are insulin and immunizations that specifically require the subcutaneous route. Any site with sufficient subcutaneous tissue may be used, with the upper arm being the site of choice for immunizations. The intramuscular route is used most frequently for preoperative and postoperative medications for sedation and pain, and for immunizations such as DPT (diphtheria, pertussis, tetanus), which must be administered deep IM. The intramuscular site of choice for infants and small children is the vastus lateralis or rectus femoris of the thigh, because the gluteal muscles do not develop until a child has learned to walk. Usually not more than 1 mL is injected per site, and sites are rotated regularly.

Dosage calculation is the same as for adults, except **dosages are usually calculated to the nearest hundredth and measured using a tuberculin (TB) syringe** (refer to Chapter 7 if you need to review the calibrations and use of a TB syringe). There is less margin for error in pediatric dosages, and calculations and measurements must be double-checked carefully.

Summary

This concludes the introduction to pediatric oral and IM and subcutaneous medication administration. The important points to remember from this chapter are:

- *Care must be taken when administering oral drugs to ensure that the child has actually swallowed the dosage.*

- *If liquid medications are prepared as suspensions, mix thoroughly prior to measurement, and administer promptly to prevent settling out of their insoluble drugs.*

- *Care must be taken not to confuse oral syringes, which are unsterile, with hypodermic syringes, which are sterile.*

- *The IM site of choice for infants and small children is the vastus lateralis or rectus femoris of the thigh.*

- *Usually not more than 1 mL is injected per IM or subcutaneous site, and sites are rotated regularly.*

- *Pediatric parenteral dosages are usually calculated to the nearest hundredth and measured using a TB syringe.*

Summary Self-Test

Use the pediatric medication labels provided to measure the oral dosages. Indicate in the second column if the medication is a suspension.

PART I	mL	Suspension
1. Prepare a 125 mg dosage of Augmentin®.	_____	_____
2. Prepare a 125 mg dosage of Amoxil®.	_____	_____

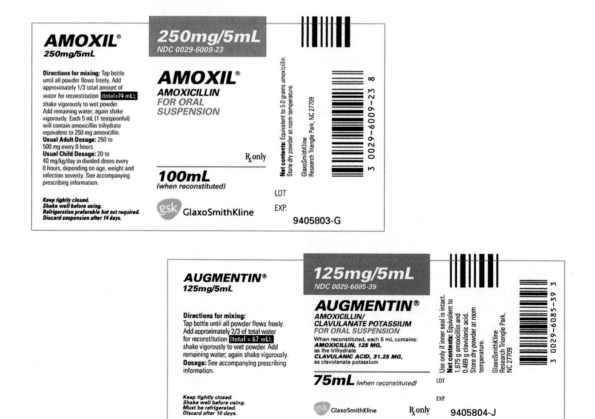

	mL	Suspension

3. Prepare a 0.1 mg dosage of digoxin. _____ _____

4. Prepare 100 mg of Vantin®. _____ _____

5. Prepare 5 mg of Lomotil®. _____ _____

6. Prepare 250 mg of tetracycline. _____ _____

7. Peri-Colace® 3 tsp is ordered. How many mL is this? _____ _____

8. Prepare 120 mg of acetaminophen. _____ _____

9. Prepare 187 mg of antibiotic "A." _____ _____

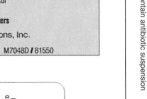

19

473 mL   NDC 0003-0815-50

125 mg per 5 mL
SUMYCIN SYRUP
Tetracycline
Oral Suspension USP

125 mg per 5 mL tetracycline hydrochloride equivalent

Caution: Federal law prohibits dispensing without prescription

6505-00-656-1344

Each 5 mL (teaspoonful) contains tetracycline equivalent to 125 mg tetracycline hydrochloride, buffered with potassium metaphosphate

Usual pediatric dosage: 10-20 mg per lb of body weight daily in 4 divided doses
See insert

Shake well before using

Keep tightly closed • Protect from light
Store below 30° C (86° F)

Contents should be used within 2 months after bottle is opened since some discoloration may occur

Dispense in tight, light-resistant containers

E. R. Squibb & Sons, Inc.
Princeton, NJ 08540
Made in USA   M7048D / 81550

Usual dose—Pediatric patients: 20 to 40 mg per kg a day (40 mg per kg in otitis media) in two divided doses. Adults: 375 mg two times a day. See literature for complete dosage information.
Contains antibiotic equivalent to 3.74 g in a pleasantly flavored mixture.
Prior to mixing: Store at controlled room temperature 59° to 86°F (15° to 30°C).
Directions for mixing: Add 62 mL of water in two portions to the dry mixture in the bottle. Shake well after each addition. Each 5 mL will then contain antibiotic suspension equivalent to 187 mg.

150 mL (when mixed)

Sample
ANTIBIOTIC
"A"
For Oral Suspension

187 mg per 5 mL

CAUTION—Federal (USA) law prohibits dispensing without prescription.

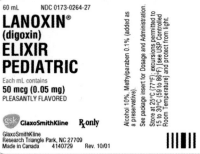

60 mL   NDC 0173-0264-27

LANOXIN®
(digoxin)
ELIXIR
PEDIATRIC

Each mL contains
50 mcg (0.05 mg)
PLEASANTLY FLAVORED

gsk GlaxoSmithKline   R x only

GlaxoSmithKline
Research Triangle Park, NC 27709
Made in Canada   4140729   Rev. 10/01

Alcohol 10%, Methylparaben 0.1% (added as a preservative).
See package insert for Dosage and Administration.
Store at 25°C (77°F); excursions permitted to 15 to 30°C (59 to 86°F) [see USP Controlled Room Temperature] and protect from light.

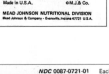

NDC 0087-0730-01
DROPS
TEMPRA®
ACETAMINOPHEN
10% SOLUTION
ANALGESIC
1/2 FL. OZ. (15 ML.)
Mead Johnson

TO RELIEVE DISCOMFORT DUE TO COLDS, SIMPLE HEADACHES, MINOR ACHES AND PAINS.
Each 0.6 ml. of TEMPRA® drops contains 60 mg. (1 grain) of acetaminophen and 10% alcohol.
Your physician is the best source of counsel and guidance in illness when pain or fever is present.
KEEP THIS AND ALL MEDICATIONS OUT OF THE REACH OF CHILDREN.
Made in U.S.A.   ©M.J.& Co.
MEAD JOHNSON NUTRITIONAL DIVISION
Mead Johnson & Company · Evansville, Indiana 47721 U.S.A.

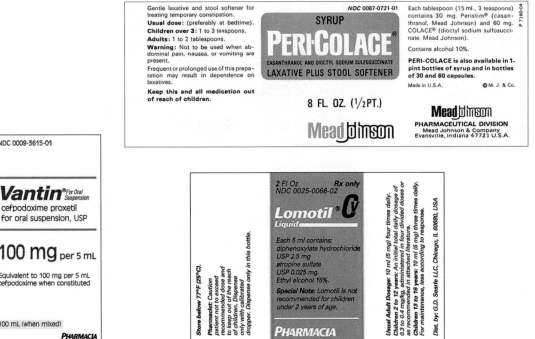

Gentle laxative and stool softener for treating temporary constipation.
Usual dose: (preferably at bedtime).
Children over 3: 1 to 3 teaspoons.
Adults: 1 to 2 tablespoons.
Warning: Not to be used when abdominal pain, nausea, or vomiting are present.
Frequent or prolonged use of this preparation may result in dependence on laxatives.

Keep this and all medication out of reach of children.

NDC 0087-0721-01
SYRUP
PERI-COLACE®
CASANTHRANOL AND DIOCTYL SODIUM SULFOSUCCINATE
LAXATIVE PLUS STOOL SOFTENER

8 FL. OZ. (1/2 PT.)

Mead Johnson

Each tablespoon (15 ml., 3 teaspoons) contains 30 mg. Peristim® (casanthranol, Mead Johnson) and 60 mg. COLACE® (dioctyl sodium sulfosuccinate. Mead Johnson).

Contains alcohol 10%.

PERI-COLACE is also available in 1-pint bottles of syrup and in bottles of 30 and 60 capsules.

Made in U.S.A.   © M. J. & Co.

Mead Johnson
PHARMACEUTICAL DIVISION
Mead Johnson & Company
Evansville, Indiana 47721 U.S.A.

R x only   NDC 0009-3615-01
See package insert for dosage and complete product information.
Warning: Not for injection
Store unconstituted product at controlled room temperature 20° to 25°C (68° to 77°F) [see USP]. Store constituted suspension in a refrigerator 2° to 8°C (36° to 46°F). Shake well before using. Keep container tightly closed. The mixture may be used for 14 days. Discard unused portion after 14 days.
Directions for mixing: Shake bottle to loosen granules. Add approximately 1/2 the total amount of distilled water required for constitution (total water = 57 mL). Shake vigorously to wet the granules. Add remaining water and shake vigorously.
Each 5 mL of suspension contains cefpodoxime proxetil equivalent to 100 mg cefpodoxime.
U.S. Patent No. 4,668,783
Licensed from Sankyo Company, Ltd., Japan
Made by
Pharmacia N.V./S.A., Puurs - Belgium
For
Pharmacia & Upjohn Company
A subsidiary of Pharmacia Corporation
Kalamazoo, MI 49001, USA
815 120 206
5Q7474

Vantin® For Oral Suspension
cefpodoxime proxetil
for oral suspension, USP

100 mg per 5 mL

Equivalent to 100 mg per 5 mL cefpodoxime when constituted

100 mL (when mixed)

PHARMACIA

Store below 77°F (25°C).

Pharmacist: Caution patient not to exceed recommended dose and to keep out of the reach of children. Dispense only with calibrated dropper. Dispense only in this bottle.

2 Fl Oz   Rx only
NDC 0025-0066-02

Lomotil®
Liquid   Cv

Each 5 ml contains:
diphenoxylate hydrochloride USP 2.5 mg
atropine sulfate USP 0.025 mg.
Ethyl alcohol 15%.

Special Note: Lomotil is not recommended for children under 2 years of age.

PHARMACIA

Usual Adult Dosage: 10 ml (5 mg) four times daily.
Children 2 to 12 years: An initial total daily dosage of 0.3 to 0.4 mg/kg, administered in four divided doses or as recommended in attached literature.
Children 13 to 16 years: 10 ml (5 mg) three times daily.
For maintenance, less according to response.

Dist. by: G.D. Searle LLC, Chicago, IL 60680, USA

Use the labels provided to calculate the dosages. Calculate to hundredths.

PART II

10. Prepare a 20 mg dosage of meperidine. _____

11. A dosage of morphine 10 mg has been ordered. _____

12. Draw up a 100 mg dosage of clindamycin. _____

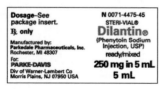

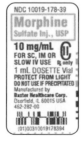

PART III

13. Prepare a 40 mg dosage of meperidine. _____

14. A dosage of Dilantin 50 mg has been ordered. _____

15. Prepare a 6 mg dosage of morphine. _____

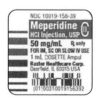

ANSWERS

1. 5 mL; suspension	**5.** 10 mL	**9.** 5 mL; suspension	**13.** 0.8 mL
2. 2.5 mL; suspension	**6.** 10 mL; suspension	**10.** 0.8 mL	**14.** 1 mL
3. 2 mL	**7.** 15 mL	**11.** 0.67 mL	**15.** 0.6 mL
4. 5 mL; suspension	**8.** 1.2 mL	**12.** 0.67 mL	

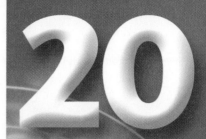

Pediatric Intravenous Medications

Pediatric IV medication administration involves a challenge and a responsibility that is multifaceted. Infants and children, particularly under the age of 4, are incompletely developed physiologically, and drug tolerance, absorption, and excretion are ongoing concerns. In addition, infants and acutely ill children can tolerate only a narrow range of hydration, making administration of IV drugs, which are diluted for administration, a critical and exact skill. Drug dilution protocols may specify a range for dilution, and on many occasions the smallest possible volume may have to be used in order not to overhydrate a child. Dosage and dilution decisions may have to be made on a day-to-day or even dose-to-dose basis and will involve the team effort of nurse, physician, and pharmacist. In addition, the suitability of any flow rate calculated for administration must be made on an individual basis. For example, a calculated flow rate of 100 mL/hr for a 2-year-old child is too high a rate to administer.

The fragility of infants' and children's veins, and the irritating nature of many medications, mandate careful site inspection for signs of inflammation and infiltration. This should be done immediately before, during, and after each infusion. Signs of inflammation include redness, heat, swelling, and tenderness. Signs of infiltration include swelling, coldness, pain, and lack of blood return in the IV tubing. Either complication necessitates discontinuing the IV and restarting it at a new site.

IV medication guidelines are always used to determine drug dosages, dilutions, and administration rates. In this chapter, all examples and problems are representative of actual rates.

Methods of IV Medication Administration

Intravenous medications may be administered over a period of several hours, or on an **intermittent** basis involving several dosages in a 24-hour period. When ordered to infuse over several hours, medications are usually added to an IV solution bag. Adding the drug to the IV bag may be a hospital pharmacy or staff nurse responsibility, but, in any event, it is not a complicated procedure. The steps for adding the drug to the solution are as follows:

STEP 1 Locate the type and volume of IV solution ordered.

STEP 2 Measure the dosage of drug to be added.

STEP 3 Use strict aseptic technique to add the drug to the solution bag through the medication port.

STEP 4 Mix the drug thoroughly in the solution.

STEP 5 Label the IV solution bag with the name and dosage of the drug added.

STEP 6 Add your initials with the time and date you added the drug.

STEP 7 Hang the IV and set the flow rate for the infusion. Chart the administration when it is hung.

For intermittent administrations the medication may also be prepared in small-volume solution bags or using a calibrated burette, such as the one illustrated in Figure 20-1. Because the total capacity of burettes is between 100 and 150 mL, calibrated in 1 mL increments, exact measurement of small volumes is possible.

Regardless of the method of intermittent administration, medication infusion is **routinely followed by a flush**, to make sure the medication has cleared the tubing, and that the total dosage has been administered. The volume of the flush will vary depending on the length of IV tubing from the medication source, that is, the burette or syringe, to the infusion site. If a primary line exists, the medication may be administered IVPB (IV piggyback) via a secondary line. If no IV is infusing, a saline or heparin lock (heplock) is frequently in place and used for intermittent administration.

When IV medications are diluted for administration, it is necessary to determine hospital policy on **inclusion of the medication volume as part of the volume specified for dilution**. For example, if 20 mg has a volume of 2 mL, and it is to be diluted in 30 mL, does this mean you must add 28 mL of diluent to the burette, or 30 mL?

Hospital policies may vary, but in all examples and problems in this chapter **the drug volume will be treated as part of the total diluent volume**.

Medication Administration via Burette

When a burette is used for medication administration, the entire preparation is usually done by staff nurses. Volumetric pumps are used to administer intermittent IV medications to infants and children. When these are used, the alarm will sound each time the burette empties to signal when each successive step is necessary. For example, it will sound when the medication has infused and the flush must be started, and again when the flush is completed.

Let's look at some sample orders and go step by step through one procedure that may be used.

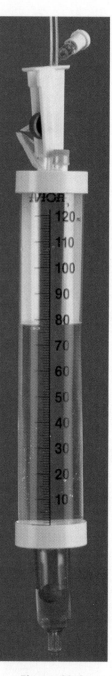

Figure 20-1

EXAMPLE **1**

A dosage of **250 mg in 15 mL** of D5 1/2NS is to be infused over **30 minutes**. It is to be followed with a **5 mL flush of D5 1/2NS**. A volumetric pump will be used, and the tubing is a **microdrip** burette.

STEP 1   Read the drug label and determine what volume the 250 mg dosage is contained in. Let's assume this is 1 mL.

STEP 2   The dilution is to be 15 mL. Run a total of 14 mL of D5 1/2NS into the burette, then add the 1 mL containing the dosage of 250 mg. This gives the ordered volume of 15 mL. Roll the burette between your hands to mix the drug thoroughly with the solution.

STEP 3   Calculate the flow rate for this microdrip.

Total volume = **15 mL**   Infusion time = **30 min**

Use DA to calculate mL/hr rate.

$$\frac{mL}{hr} = \frac{15\ mL}{30\ min} \times \frac{60\ min}{1\ hr} = \textbf{30 mL/hr}$$

STEP 4   Set the pump to infuse 30 mL/hr.

STEP 5   Label the burette to identify the drug and dosage added. Attach a label that states "medication infusing." This makes it possible for others to know the status of the administration if you are not present when the infusion is complete and the pump alarms.

STEP 6   When the medication has infused, add the 5 mL D5 1/2NS flush. Remove the "medication infusing" label and attach a "flush infusing" label. Continue to infuse at the 30 mL/hr rate until the burette empties for the second time.

STEP 7   When the flush has been completed, restart the primary IV, or disconnect from the saline/heparin lock. Remove the "flush infusing" label. Chart the dosage and time.

EXAMPLE **2**

An antibiotic dosage of **125 mg in 1 mL** is to be **diluted in 20 mL** of D5 1/4NS and infused over **30 min**. A **flush of 15 mL** D5 1/4NS is to follow. A volumetric pump will be used.

STEP 1   125 mg has a volume of 1 mL. Add 19 mL of D5 1/4NS to the burette, add the 1 mL of medication, and mix thoroughly.

STEP 2   Calculate the mL/hr flow rate.

Total volume = **20 mL**   Infusion time = **30 min**

$$\frac{mL}{hr} = \frac{20\ mL}{30\ min} \times \frac{60\ min}{1\ hr} = \textbf{40 mL/hr}$$

STEP 3 Set the pump to infuse 40 mL/hr.

STEP 4 Label the burette with the drug and dosage, and attach a "medication infusing" label.

STEP 5 When the medication has infused, start the 15 mL flush. Remove the "medication infusing" label and add the "flush infusing" label.

STEP 6 When the flush has completed, restart the primary IV or disconnect from the saline lock. Remove the "flush infusing" label. Chart the dosage and time.

EXAMPLE 3

An antibiotic dosage of **50 mg** has been ordered diluted in **20 mL** of D5W to infuse over **20 min**. A **15 mL flush** of D5W is to follow. A pump will be used.

STEP 1 Read the medication label to determine what volume contains 50 mg. You determine that 50 mg is contained in 2 mL.

STEP 2 Run 18 mL of D5W into the burette and add the 2 mL containing 50 mg of drug. Roll between your hands to mix thoroughly.

STEP 3 Calculate the flow rate in mL/hr necessary to deliver the medication.

Total volume = **20 mL**   Infusion time = **20 min**

$$\frac{mL}{hr} = \frac{20\ mL}{20\ min} \times \frac{60\ min}{1\ hr} = \textbf{60 mL/hr}$$

STEP 4 Set the rate at 60 mL/hr.

STEP 5 Label the burette with the drug name and dosage, and attach a "medication infusing" label.

STEP 6 When the medication has cleared the burette, add the 15 mL D5W flush. Continue to run at 60 mL/hr. Remove the "medication infusing" label and replace with a "flush infusing" label.

STEP 7 When the burette empties for the second time, restart the primary IV, or disconnect from the saline lock. Remove the "flush infusing" label. Chart the dosage and time administered.

EXAMPLE 4

An IV medication dosage of **100 mcg** has been ordered **diluted in 35 mL** of NS and infused in **50 min**. A **10 mL flush** is to follow. A pump will be used.

STEP 1 Read the medication label to determine what volume contains 100 mcg: 100 mcg = 1.5 mL.

STEP 2 Run 33.5 mL of NS into the burette, and add the 1.5 mL of medication. Roll the burette between your hands to mix thoroughly.

STEP 3 Calculate the mL/hr flow rate.

Total volume = **35 mL**   Infusion time = **50 min**

$$\frac{mL}{hr} = \frac{35 \text{ mL}}{50 \text{ min}} \times \frac{60 \text{ min}}{1 \text{ hr}} = \textbf{42 mL/hr}$$

STEP 4 Set the flow rate at 42 mL/hr.

STEP 5 Label the burette with the drug name and dosage and a "medication infusing" label.

STEP 6 When the medication has cleared the burette, add the 10 mL flush. Continue to run at 42 mL/hr. Replace the "medication infusing" label with the "flush infusing" label.

STEP 7 When the burette empties of the flush solution, restart the primary IV, or disconnect from the saline lock. Remove the "flush infusing" label, and chart the dosage and time administered.

PROBLEM

Determine the volume of solution that must be added to the burette to mix the IV drugs. Then calculate the flow rate in mL/hr for each administration.

1. An IV medication of 75 mg in 3 mL is ordered diluted to 55 mL to infuse over 45 min.

   Dilution volume _____ mL/hr _____

2. A dosage of 100 mg in 2 mL is diluted to 30 mL of D5W to infuse in 20 min.

   Dilution volume _____ mL/hr _____

3. The volume of a 10 mg dosage of medication is 1 mL. Dilute to 40 mL and administer over 50 min.

   Dilution volume _____ mL/hr _____

4. A dosage of 15 mg with a volume of 3 mL is to be diluted to 70 mL and administered in 50 min.

   Dilution volume _____ mL/hr _____

5. A medication of 1 g in 4 mL is to be diluted to 60 mL and infused over 90 min.

   Dilution volume _____ mL/hr _____

ANSWERS **1.** 52 mL; 73 mL/hr **2.** 28 mL; 90 mL/hr **3.** 39 mL; 48 mL/hr **4.** 67 mL; 84 mL/hr
5. 56 mL; 40 mL/hr

Comparing IV Dosages Ordered with Average Dosages

Knowing how to compare dosages ordered with average dosages for a particular medication is a nursing responsibility.

 Dosages of IV medications are calculated on the basis of body weight, or BSA.

Average dosages may be listed in terms of mg, mcg, or units per day, or per hour. BSA in m^2 is most often used to calculate chemotherapeutic drugs, which are administered only by certified nursing staff. The following examples will demonstrate how to use average dosage to check dosages ordered.

EXAMPLE 1

A child weighing **22.6 kg** has an order for **500 mg** of medication in 100 mL of D5W **q.12.h.** The normal dosage range is **40–50 mg/kg/day**. Determine if the dosage ordered is within the normal range.

STEP 1 Calculate the normal daily dosage range for this child.

$$40 \text{ mg/day} \times 22.6 \text{ kg} = \textbf{904 mg}$$
$$50 \text{ mg/day} \times 22.6 \text{ kg} = \textbf{1130 mg}$$

STEP 2 Calculate the dosage infusing in 24 hr.

$$500 \text{ mg in } 12 \text{ hr} = \textbf{1000 mg in 24 hr}$$

STEP 3 Assess the accuracy of the dosage ordered.

The 500 mg in 12 hr is within the 904–1130 mg/day dosage range.

EXAMPLE 2

A child with a body weight of **18.4 kg** is to receive a medication with a dosage range of **100–150 mg/kg/day**. The order is for **600 mg** in 75 mL of D5W **q.6.h.** Determine if the dosage is within normal range.

STEP 1 Calculate the normal daily dosage range.

$$100 \text{ mg/day} \times 18.4 \text{ kg} = \textbf{1840 mg/day}$$
$$150 \text{ mg/day} \times 18.4 \text{ kg} = \textbf{2760 mg/day}$$

STEP 2 Calculate the daily dosage ordered.

The dosage ordered is 600 mg q.6.h. (4 doses).

$$600 \text{ mg} \times 4 = \textbf{2400 mg/day}$$

STEP 3   Assess the accuracy of the dosage ordered.

The dosage ordered, 2400 mg/day, is within the normal range of 1840–2760 mg/day.

20

EXAMPLE 3

A child weighing **17.7 kg** is receiving an IV of **250 mL** of D5W containing **2000 units** of heparin, which is to infuse at **50 mL/hr**. The dosage range of heparin is **10–25 units/kg/hr**. Assess the accuracy of this dosage.

STEP 1   Calculate the dosage range per hour.

$$10 \text{ units/kg/hr} \times 17.7 \text{ kg} = \textbf{177 units/hr}$$
$$25 \text{ units/kg/hr} \times 17.7 \text{ kg} = \textbf{442.5 units/hr}$$

STEP 2   Calculate the dosage in units infusing per hour.

$$\frac{\text{units}}{\text{hr}} = \frac{2000 \text{ units}}{250 \text{ mL}} \times \frac{50 \text{ mL}}{1 \text{ hr}} = \textbf{400 units/hr}$$

STEP 3   Assess the accuracy of the dosage ordered.

The IV is infusing at a rate of 50 mL per hour, which is 400 units/hr. The normal dosage range is 177–442.5 units/hr. The dosage is within normal range.

EXAMPLE 4

A child weighing **32.7 kg** has an IV of **250 mL** of D5 1/4S containing **400 mcg** of medication to infuse over **5 hours**. The normal range for this drug is **1–3 mcg/kg/hr**. Determine if this dosage is within the normal dosage range.

STEP 1   Calculate the hourly dosage range.

$$1 \text{ mcg/kg/hr} \times 32.7 \text{ kg} = \textbf{32.7 mcg/hr}$$
$$3 \text{ mcg/kg/hr} \times 32.7 \text{ kg} = \textbf{98.1 mcg/hr}$$

STEP 2   Calculate the dosage infusing per hour.

$$400 \text{ mcg} \div 5 \text{ hr} = \textbf{80 mcg/hr}$$

STEP 3   Assess the accuracy of the dosage ordered.

The dosage of 80 mcg/hr infusing is within the normal range of 32.7–98.1 mcg/hr.

Calculate the normal dosage range to the nearest tenth and the dosage being administered for the following medications. Assess the dosages ordered.

1. A child weighing 24.4 kg has an IV of 250 mL of D5W containing 2500 units of a drug. The dosage range for this drug is 15–25 units/kg/hr. The pump is set to deliver 50 mL/hr.

   Dosage range per hr _____   Dosage infusing per hr _____

   Assessment _____

2. A solution of D5W containing 25 mg of a drug is to infuse in 30 min q.6.h. The dosage range is 4–8 mg/kg/day. The child weighs 18.7 kg.

   Dosage range per day _____   Daily dosage ordered _____

   Assessment _____

3. An IV solution containing 125 mg of medication is infusing. The dosage range is 5–10 mg/kg/dose, and the child weighs 14.2 kg.

   Dosage range per dose _____   Assessment _____

4. A child weighing 14.3 kg is to receive an IV drug with a dosage range of 50–100 mcg/kg/day in two divided doses. An infusion of 50 mL of D5W containing 400 mcg to run 30 min has been ordered.

   Daily dosage range _____   Daily dosage ordered _____

   Assessment _____

5. A dosage of 4 mg (4000 mcg) of drug in 500 mL of D5 1/2S is to infuse over 4 hours. The dosage range of the drug is 24–120 mcg/kg/hr, and the child weighs 16.1 kg.

   Dosage range per hr _____   Dosage infusing per hr _____

   Assessment _____

6. A child weighing 20.9 kg is to receive a medication with a normal dosage range of 80–160 mg/kg/day, in divided doses q.6.h. The IV ordered contains 500 mg.

   Dosage range per day _____   Daily dosage ordered _____

   Assessment _____

7. A child weighing 22.3 kg is to receive 750 mL of D5 1/45 containing 6 g of a drug, which is to run over 24 hours. The dosage range of the drug is 200–300 mg/kg/day.

   Dosage range per day _____   Assessment _____

8. An IV of 50 mL of D5W containing 55 mcg of a drug is infusing over a 30-min period. The child weighs 14.9 kg and the dosage range is 6–8 mcg/kg/day, q.12.h.

   Dosage range per day _____   Daily dosage ordered _____

   Assessment _____

9. A child weighing 27.1 kg is to receive a medication with a normal range of 0.5–1 mg/kg/dose. An IV containing 20 mg of medication has been ordered.

   Dosage range per dose _____   Assessment _____

10. An IV medication of 60 mcg in 200 mL is ordered to infuse over 2 hr. The normal dosage range is 1.5–3 mcg/kg/hr. The child weighs 16.7 kg.

    Dosage range per hr _____   Dosage infusing per hr _____

    Assessment _____

Summary

This concludes the chapter on administration of IV drugs to infants and children. The important points to remember from this chapter are:

IV medications may be ordered to infuse over a period of several hours, or minutes.

IV medications are diluted for administration, and it is important to determine hospital policy on inclusion of the medication volume as part of the total dilution volume.

A flush is used following medication administration to make sure the medication has cleared the tubing and the total dosage has been administered.

The volume of flush solution on intermittent infusions will vary depending on the amount needed to clear the infusion line.

Average dosage ranges are used to assess dosages ordered.

Pediatric IV medication administration requires constant assessment of the child's ability to tolerate dosage, dilution, and rate of administration.

Children's veins are very fragile, and intravenous sites must be checked for inflammation and infiltration immediately before, during, and following each medication administration.

20

Summary Self-Test

Determine the volume of solution that must be added to a calibrated burette to mix the IV drugs. The medication volume is included in the total dilution volume. Calculate the flow rate in mL/hr for each infusion.

	Volume of diluent	mL/hr rate
1. An IV antibiotic of 750 mg in 3 mL has been ordered diluted to a total of 25 mL of D5W to infuse over 40 minutes.	_____	_____
2. A dosage of 500,000 units of a penicillin preparation with a volume of 4 mL has been ordered diluted to 50 mL D5 1/2NS to infuse in 60 min.	_____	_____
3. A dosage of 1.5 g/2 mL of an antibiotic is to be diluted to a total of 40 mL of D5W and administered over 40 min.	_____	_____
4. An antibiotic dosage of 200 mg in 4 mL is to be diluted to 50 mL and administered over 70 min.	_____	_____
5. A dosage of 20 mg in 2 mL has been ordered diluted to 30 mL, to be infused over 35 min.	_____	_____
6. A dosage of 25 mg in 5 mL has been ordered diluted to 40 mL and administered in 50 min.	_____	_____

7. A 10 mg in 2 mL dosage has been ordered diluted to 20 mL to infuse over 30 min.
      _____   _____

8. A medication dosage of 800 mg in 4 mL is to be diluted to 60 mL and infused over 80 min.
      _____   _____

9. A dosage of 0.5 g in 2 mL is to be diluted to 40 mL and run in 30 min.
      _____   _____

10. A medication of 1000 mg in 1 mL is to be diluted to 15 mL and administered over 20 min.
      _____   _____

11. A dosage of 40 mg in 4 mL is to be diluted to 50 mL and administered in 90 min.
      _____   _____

12. A 2 g in 5 mL dosage has been ordered diluted to a total of 90 mL and administered in 45 min.
      _____   _____

13. An 80 mg dosage with a volume of 2 mL is to be diluted to 80 mL and administered in 60 min.
      _____   _____

14. A 60 mg dosage with a volume of 4 mL is ordered diluted to 30 mL and run over 20 min.
      _____   _____

15. A 5 mg per 2 mL dosage is to be diluted to 80 mL and administered in 50 min.
      _____   _____

16. The dosage ordered is 0.75 g in 3 mL to be diluted to 30 mL. Run in over 40 min.
      _____   _____

17. A medication of 100 mg in 2 mL is ordered diluted to 30 mL and run in 25 min.
      _____   _____

18. The dosage ordered is 100 mg in 1 mL to be diluted to 50 mL. Run in over 45 min.
      _____   _____

19. A 30 mg dosage in 1 mL has been ordered diluted to 10 mL to infuse in 10 min.
      _____   _____

20. A dosage of 250 mg in 5 mL has been ordered diluted to 40 mL and infused in 60 min.
      _____   _____

Calculate the normal dosage range to the nearest tenth and the dosage being administered for the medications. Assess the dosages ordered.

21. A child weighing 15.4 kg is to receive a dosage with a range of 5–7.5 mg/kg/dose. The solution bag is labeled 100 mg.

      Dosage range _____   Assessment _____

22. The order is for 200 units in 75 mL. The child weighs 13.1 kg and the dosage range is 15–20 units/kg per dose.

      Dosage range _____   Assessment _____

23. A dosage of 1.5 mg in 20 mL has been ordered b.i.d. The normal dosage range is 0.1–0.3 mg/kg/day in two divided doses. The child's weight is 12.4 kg.

      Dosage range per day _____

      Daily dosage ordered _____   Assessment _____

24. A dosage of 400 mg in 75 mL of medication is to be infused q.8.h. The normal range is 15–45 mg/kg/day, and the child weighs 27.9 kg.

      Dosage range per day _____

      Daily dosage ordered _____   Assessment _____

25. A child weighing 15.7 kg is to receive a medication with a normal hourly range of 3–7 mcg/kg. A 250 mL solution bag containing 350 mcg is infusing at a rate of 50 mL/hr.

                Dosage range per hr _____   Dosage infusing per hr _____

                                                Assessment _____

26. A child weighing 19.6 kg is to receive a medication with a normal dosage range of 60–80 mg/kg/day. A 90 mL infusion containing 375 mg has been ordered q.6.h.   Dosage range per day _____

                Daily dosage ordered _____   Assessment _____

27. Two infusions of 250 mL each containing 300 mg of medication are to infuse continuously over a 24-hr period (250 mL q.12.h.). The child receiving the infusion weighs 11.7 kg, and the normal dosage range of the drug is 50–100 mg/kg/day.

                Dosage range per day _____   Daily dosage ordered _____

                                                Assessment _____

28. The order is for 100 mL of D5W containing 150 mg of medication to infuse q.8.h. The normal dosage range is 3–12 mg/kg/day, and the child weighs 40.1 kg.   Dosage range per day _____

                Daily dosage ordered _____   Assessment _____

29. A child has an infusion of 250 mL containing 500 units of medication to run at 50 mL/hr. The normal dosage range is 10–25 units/hr. The child weighs 10.3 kg.   Dosage range per hr _____

                Dosage infusing per hr _____   Assessment _____

30. The normal dosage range of a drug is 0.5–1.5 units/hr. A child weighing 10.7 kg has a 150 mL volume of solution containing 45 units infusing at a rate of 20 mL/hr.   Normal dosage range per hr _____

                Dosage infusing per hr _____   Assessment _____

31. A child weighing 12.5 kg is receiving an IV of 2500 units of heparin in 250 mL of D5W at 40 mL/hr. The normal dosage range for heparin is 10–25 units/kg/hr.   Normal dosage range per hr _____

                Dosage infusing per hr _____   Assessment _____

32. A child with a weight of 10 kg is to receive a medication with a normal dosage range of 60–80 mg/kg/day. The order is for 200 mg q.6.h.

                              Normal dosage range per day _____

                Daily dosage ordered _____   Assessment _____

33. A 0.5 g medication in 100 mL of D5W q.6.h. Normal dosage range is 100–200 mg/kg/day. The child weighs 15 kg.

                              Normal dosage range per day _____

                Daily dosage ordered _____   Assessment _____

34. A continuous IV of 500 mL with 20 mEq KCl is infusing at 30 mL/hr. The dosage for potassium chloride is not to exceed 40 mEq/day.

                                    Dosage infusing per hr _____

            Dosage infusing per day _____   Assessment _____

35. A 24-kg child is receiving 116 mg per hr of medication IV for 3 hours. Dosage range for this drug is 10–20 mg/kg/day.

                              Normal dosage range per day _____

        Dosage received after 3 hours _____   Assessment _____

36. A 25% solution of medication is infusing at 15 mL/hr for a total of 6 hours. Normal dosage for children is 5–25 g/day.

Grams infused after 6 hr _____ Assessment _____

37. The usual dosage of a medication for children is 50 mg/kg/24 hr in equally divided doses. Order: infuse 50 mL with 290 mg q.6.h. The child weighs 51 lb.

Normal dosage per day _____ Daily dosage ordered _____

Assessment _____

38. Order: 500 mL D5RL with 30 mEq KCl to infuse at 40 mL/hr. A maximum of 10 mEq/hr of KCl should not be exceeded and the total 24-hr dosage should not exceed 40 mEq/day.

Dosage infusing per hr _____ Dosage infusing per day _____

Assessment _____

39. A child weighing 30 kg has an IV of 100 mL of D5W containing 600 mcg of medication to infuse over 2 hours. The normal range for this drug is 2–4 mcg/kg/hr. Normal dosage range per hr _____

Dosage infusing per hr _____ Assessment _____

40. 150 mL with 18 mg of medication is ordered to infuse over 10 hours. The normal range for this drug is 0.2 mg–0.6 mg/kg/hr. The child weighs 9 kg. Normal dosage range per hr _____

Dosage infusing per hr _____ Assessment _____

ANSWERS

1. 22 mL; 38 mL/hr	16. 27 mL; 45 mL/hr	26. 1176–1568 mg/day; 1500 mg; normal	33. 1500–3000 mg/day; 2000 mg; normal
2. 46 mL; 50 mL/hr	17. 28 mL; 72 mL/hr	27. 585–1170 mg/day; 600 mg; normal	34. 1.2 mEq/hr; 28.8 mEq/day; normal
3. 38 mL; 60 mL/hr	18. 49 mL; 67 mL/hr	28. 120.3–481.2 mg/day; 450 mg; normal	35. 240–480 mg/day; 348 mg; normal
4. 46 mL; 43 mL/hr	19. 9 mL; 60 mL/hr	29. 103–257.5 units/hr; 100 units/hr; normal	36. 22.5 g/6 hr; normal
5. 28 mL; 51 mL/hr	20. 35 mL; 40 mL/hr	30. 5.4–16.1 units/hr; 6 units/hr; normal	37. 1160 mg/day; 1160 mg; normal
6. 35 mL; 48 mL/hr	21. 77–115.5 mg/dose; normal	31. 125–312.5 units/hr; 400 units/hr; too high	38. 2.4 mEq/hr; 58 mEq/day; too high
7. 18 mL; 40 mL/hr	22. 196.5–262 units/dose; normal	32. 600–800 mg/day; 800 mg; normal	39. 60–120 mcg/hr; 300 mcg; too high
8. 56 mL; 45 mL/hr	23. 1.2–3.7 mg/day; 3 mg; normal		40. 1.8–5.4 mg/hr; 1.8 mg; normal
9. 38 mL; 80 mL/hr	24. 418.5–1255.5 mg/day; 1200 mg; normal		
10. 14 mL; 45 mL/hr	25. 47.1–109.9 mcg/hr; 70 mcg; normal		
11. 46 mL; 33 mL/hr			
12. 85 mL; 120 mL/hr			
13. 78 mL; 80 mL/hr			
14. 26 mL; 90 mL/hr			
15. 78 mL; 96 mL/hr			

Illustration Credits

The publisher would like to thank the following companies for providing drug labels, package inserts, and syringe images for use in this text.

Chapter 6
Courtesy of Abbott Laboratories:
Synthroid
Courtesy of American Pharmaceutical Partners:
Potassium Chloride
Courtesy of AstraZeneca:
Toprol-XL
Courtesy of Aventis:
Carafate, Diabeta, Lasix, Trental
Courtesy of Bayer Pharmaceuticals:
Cipro
Courtesy of Bristol–Myers Squibb:
Sinemet
Courtesy of Eli Lilly and Company:
Ceclor, Prozac liquid, V-Cillin
Courtesy of Endo Pharmaceuticals:
Percocet
Reproduced with permission of GlaxoSmithKline Group of Companies, All Rights Reserved:
Amoxil, Augmentin, Eskalith, Lanoxin, Stelazine, Tagamet, Thorazine
Courtesy of King Pharmaceuticals, Inc.:
Procanbid
Courtesy of McNeil Consumer and Specialty Pharmaceuticals:
Synthroid, Tylenol
Used with permission of Merck and Company Inc.:
Aldomet, Blocadren, HydroDiuril, Prinivil
Courtesy of Novartis:
Brethine, Lopressor
Courtesy of Parke–Davis:
Lopid, Nitrostat
Registered trademark of Pharmacia and G.D. Searle, wholly owned subsidiaries of Pfizer Inc. All Rights Reserved. Courtesy of Pfizer Inc.:
Antivert, Aricept, Feldene, Glucotrol, Minipress, Neurontin, Procardia
Courtesy of Pharmacia Corporation, Peapack, NJ:
Aldactone, Azulfidine, Calan SR, Flagyl, Halcion, Lomotil, Micronase, Vantin, Xanax
Courtesy of Roxane:
Dexamethasone
Courtesy of Schwarz Pharma:
Dilatrate-SR, Verelan
Courtesy of UCB Pharma, Inc.:
Lortab

Courtesy of Valeant Pharmaceuticals:
Librium

Chapter 7
Courtesy of Becton, Dickinson and Company:
3 mL, 0.5 mL, 5 mL, 10 mL syringes
Courtesy of Tyco Healthcare:
6 mL, 12 mL, 20 mL syringes

Chapter 8
Courtesy of American Pharmaceutical Partners:
Calcium Gluconate, Cyanocobalamin, Dexamethasone Sodium Phosphate, Furosemide, Gentamicin, Heparin, Lidocaine, Potassium Chloride, Sodium Bicarbonate, Sodium Chloride
Courtesy of American Regent Laboratories, Inc.:
Epinephrine
Courtesy of Baxter Healthcare Corporation:
Diazepam, Fentanyl, Meperidine, Methotrexate, Morphine, Robinul
Reproduced with permission of GlaxoSmithKline Group of Companies, All Rights Reserved:
Thorazine
Courtesy of International Medication Systems, Ltd.:
Amphastar-IMS, Atropine Sulfate
Courtesy of King Pharmaceuticals:
Bicillin C-R, Pitocin, Tigan
Courtesy of Merck and Company:
Cogentin
Courtesy of Ortho-McNeil Pharmaceuticals:
Haldol
Courtesy of Pfizer Inc. Used with permission:
Pfizerpen, Terramycin, Vistaril
Courtesy of Pharmacia Corporation, Peapack, NJ:
Cleocin Phosphate, Depo-Provera

Chapter 9
Courtesy of Apothecon:
Nafcillin Sodium
Courtesy of Bedford Laboratories, Bedford, Ohio, 800-562-4797:
Cytarabine
Courtesy of Bristol-Myers Squibb:
Velosef
Courtesy of Eli Lilly and Company:
Kefzol, Vancocin HCl

Courtesy of Pfizer Inc. Used with permission:
    Pfizerpen, Zithromax
Courtesy of Pharmacia Corporation, Peapack, NJ:
    Solu-Medrol, Vantin

Chapter 10
Courtesy of Eli Lilly and Company:
    Humulin L, Humulin U, Humulin 70/30, Humulin
    50/50, NPH Iletin, Regular Iletin
Courtesy of Novo Nordisk Pharmaceuticals:
    Novolin N, Novolin R, Regular Purified Pork

Chapter 11
Courtesy of Abbott Laboratories:
    Aminophylline
Courtesy of American Pharmaceutical Partners:
    Calcium Gluconate, Cyanocobalamin,
    Dexamethasone, Furosemide, Gentamicin, Heparin
    Sodium, Lidocaine, Methotrexate, Potassium
    Chloride, Robinul, Sodium Chloride
Courtesy of American Regent Laboratories, Inc.:
    Epinephrine
Courtesy of Baxter Healthcare Corporation:
    Duramorph, Fentanyl, Meperidine, Methotrexate,
    Morphine, Naloxone, Robinul
Courtesy of Bristol–Myers Squibb:
    Pronestyl
Courtesy of Cetus Oncology:
    Doxorubicin Hydrochloride
Courtesy of Eli Lilly and Company:
    Nebcin
Courtesy of Endo Pharmaceuticals, Inc.:
    Narcan, Nubain
Courtesy of GlaxoSmithKline Group of Companies,
All Rights Reserved:
    Thorazine
Courtesy of International Medication Systems, Ltd.:
    Amphastar-IMS, Atropine Sulfate
Courtesy of King Pharmaceuticals, Inc.
    Bicillin C-R, Pitocin, Tigan
Courtesy of Merck and Company, Inc.:
    Cogentin
Courtesy of Ortho-McNeil Pharmaceuticals:
    Haldol
Courtesy of Parke–Davis:
    Dilantin
Courtesy of Pfizer, Inc. Used with permission:
    Vistaril
Courtesy of Pharmacia Corporation, Peapack, NJ:
    Cleocin Phosphate, Depo-Provera
Reproduced with permission of the copyright owner
Schering Corporation. All Rights Reserved:
    Celestone, Trilafon

Chapter 12
Courtesy of Bayer Pharmaceuticals:
    Mithracin dosage instructions

Courtesy of Bristol–Myers Squibb:
    Principen, Veetids, Fungizone dosage and
    administration instructions, Velosef dosage and
    administration instructions
Courtesy of Eli Lilly and Company:
    Ceclor, Kefzol, Vancocin HCl dosage and
    administration instructions
Used with permission of GlaxoSmithKline Group of
Companies, All Rights Reserved:
    Amoxil, Ancef dosage and administration
    instructions, Ticar dosage and administration
    instructions, Zinacef dosage and administration
    instructions
Courtesy of Novartis Pharmaceutical Corporation:
    Mezlin dosage and administration instructions
Courtesy of Pharmacia Corporation:
    Solu-Medrol dosage and administration instructions
Courtesy of Wyeth:
    Omnipen-N dosage and administration instructions

Chapter 13
Courtesy of Bedford Laboratories, Bedford, Ohio,
800-562-4797:
    Vinblastine sulfate dosage and administration
    instructions
Courtesy of Bristol–Myers Squibb:
    BiCNU dosage and administration instructions,
    Blenoxane dosage and administration instructions,
    Mutamycin dosage and administration instructions,
    Paraplatin dosage and administration instructions,
    Platinol dosage and administration instructions

Chapter 16
Abbott Laboratories Inc.:
    Venoset IV sets

Chapter 18
Courtesy of American Pharmaceutical Partners:
    Heparin Sodium
Courtesy of Eli Lilly and Company:
    Heparin sodium
Courtesy of Pharmacia Corporation, Peapack, NJ:
    Heparin sodium

Chapter 19
Courtesy of Baxter Healthcare Corporation:
    Meperidine, Morphine
Courtesy of Bristol–Myers Squibb:
    Peri-Colace, Sumycin, Tempra
Courtesy of Eli Lilly and Company:
    Ceclor
Courtesy of GlaxoSmithKline Group of Companies,
All Rights Reserved:
    Amoxil, Augmentin, Lanoxin
Courtesy of Parke-Davis. Used with permission:
    Dilantin
Courtesy of Pharmacia Corporation, Peapack, NJ:
    Cleocin Phosphate, Lomotil, Vantin

Index

E

Electronic infusion devices
 heparin, 262, 265, 268
 IV therapy, 200, 201–3, 206
 IV medications, 244, 258
 patient-controlled analgesia
  devices, 204–5, 207
 pediatric IV medications, 280–83
 programming, 202
 syringe pumps, 203, 207
 titration of IV medication, 244,
  254, 258
 Volumetric pumps, 200, 201–3, 206
Enteric coated medications
 medication labels, reading, 55
 pediatric medications, 275
Equations. *See* dimensional analysis
 (DA); fraction equations
Errors, common. *See also* legal
 responsibility
 incorrect dosages, 59
 metric system dosages, 43–44
 programming volumetric pumps,
  202
 syringes, minim scale on, 74, 79, 87
Expiration dates and times
 medication labels, reading, 57
 reconstitution of powdered drugs,
  110, 113, 115
Eye medications, 47

F

Flushing IV tubing, 280, 287
Fraction equations
 decimal fractions, 25–28, 31–34
  multiple numbers, 28–30, 31, 32–34
  whole number, 22–25
Fractions, decimal. *See* decimal
 fractions

G

Gelatin capsules, 55
Generic (official) names of
 medications, 56, 57, 66
Grams, metric system, 37, 38, 44

H

Height
 body surface area, 182–84
 IV solution placement, 197, 198,
  206, 207, 208
Heparin
 heplocks (heparin locks), 200, 206,
  207, 208, 280

international units, 47, 262–69
 intravenous administration
  calculations, 262–69
 tuberculin (TB) syringes, 80
Household measures, 50, 51
Human (recombinant DNA) insulin,
 122–24
Hyperalimentation, 206

I

Indwelling, intermittent infusion ports
 adult, 200, 201, 206, 207, 208
 pediatric, 280
Infiltration of IV sites, 279, 287
Injection ports on IV tubing, 196, 206
Insulin
 combined, premixed, 123
 combining types, 129–30, 131
 international units, 47, 122–35
 measuring dosages, 122–35
 regular, 122, 123, 125, 129–30
 syringes, 74, 122, 125–29, 131
 types of, 122–24, 129–30, 131
Intermittent administration of
  medications
 indwelling infusion ports, 200, 201,
  206, 207, 208
 pediatric, 279, 280, 287
International (Système International
  d'Unités) (SI) system of
  measurement. *See* metric,
  international (SI) system
International units
 drug measurement, 47–48, 50, 51,
  95
 heparin, 47, 262–69
 insulin, 47, 122–35
Intramuscular injections, 273, 275,
 276, 278
Intravenous (IV) flow rates
 calculation of, 209–21
 heparin, 265–68
 hourly, 222–24, 236–38
 IV therapy, introduction to, 195,
  196, 197
 medication infusion, 244–54, 258,
  259–61
 regulating, 218–19
 titration of medication, 244,
  254–58, 259–61
Intravenous (IV) fluids
 heparin, pre-mixed, 262, 263, 268
 introduction to, 205–6, 207
 percentage measures, 47
Intravenous (IV) infusion times
 calculating, 222–30, 232–38
 completion, 222, 230–38

labeling, 232–35, 236, 239–43
Intravenous (IV) medications
 bolus (push) administration, 200
 infusion of, 244–61
 parenteral medication labels, 91, 97
 piggyback administration, 197–99,
  206
Intravenous (IV) pumps. *See*
 electronic infusion devices
Intravenous (IV) therapy. *See also*
 electronic infusion devices
 burettes, 200, 206, 213, 280–83
 intermittent locks, 200, 201, 206,
  207, 208
 IV fluids, introduction to, 205–6, 207
 pediatric intermittent locks, 280
 primary lines, 195–97, 206, 207, 208
 secondary lines, 197–99, 206, 207
Intravenous (IV) tubing
 flow rates, calculation of, 209–21
 flushing, 280, 287
 infusion time, calculating, 224–30,
  236–38
 microdrip tubing, 209, 214, 219,
  228, 244
 primary lines, 195–97, 206
 secondary lines, 197–99, 206
IV topics. *See* specific intravenous
 (IV) topics

L

Labels, drug
 body weight dosage calculation,
  169–72, 176
 heparin IV, 262–64
 insulin dosages, 122–24, 131
 IV infusion and completion times,
  232–35, 236, 239–43
 oral medications, 55–73
 parenteral medications, 91–108
 powdered drugs, reconstitution of,
  110, 113, 115
Legal responsibility. *See also* errors,
 common; questions to ask
 giving correct dosages, 167, 170,
  171, 176
 medication labels, reading, 59
 reconstitution of powdered drugs,
  110, 115
Length, metric system, 37, 38
Liters, 37, 38, 39, 44
Lo-dose insulin syringes, 125–26

M

Measurement
 dosage strength, 56

Dimensional Analysis for Meds Learning Program, Third Edition
Anna M. Curren

WINDOWS PLATFORM
System Requirements
Microsoft Windows 98, Windows ME, Windows 2000, Windows NT, or Windows XP

Pentium III 450 MHz or faster processor

64 MB RAM (128 MB recommended)

8× speed CD-ROM drive (12× speed or faster recommended)

Sound Blaster or equivalent sound card

Video card capable of displaying 800×600 images in millions of colors

Set-Up Instructions
1. Insert CD into your CD-ROM drive.
2. If the presentation doesn't start automatically:
   a. Double-click on the My Computer icon.
   b. Double-click on the CD-ROM drive (labeled DA_MEDS).
   c. Double-click the CLICK_ME.EXE icon to run.

Windows AutoPlay Enabled: The CD-ROM is AutoPlay enabled. If you wish to bypass the AutoPlay feature, hold down the shift key while the CD-ROM is loading. To access additional shortcut commands, right-click on the CD-ROM icon.

MACINTOSH PLATFORM
System Requirements
Mac OS 9.1 and higher, or OS X 10.1 and higher

350 MHz G3 or faster processor

64 MB RAM (128 MB recommended)

8× speed CD-ROM drive (12× speed or faster recommended)

Video card capable of displaying 800x600 images in millions of colors

Set-Up Instructions
1. Insert the CD-ROM into your CD-ROM drive.
2. If the presentation doesn't start automatically:
   a. Double-click the DA_Meds icon.
   b. Double-click the CLICK ME icon to run.

Macintosh CarbonLib: CarbonLib is a Macintosh Extension that allows software to be run on both OS X and the 9.x operating system. Macromedia Flash MX requires CarbonLib 1.5 or later to run on Mac OS 9.x. To use Macromedia Flash MX in Classic mode either download CarbonLib 1.5 from Apple's download center or CarbonLib can also be upgraded with Apple's Software Update service. With OS X use System Preferences > System > Software Update and for OS 9.x use the Control Panel > Software Update.

ENHANCING PERFORMANCE
1. The Dimensional Analysis for Meds Learning Program is optimized for 32-bit (millions/true color) displays with a resolution of 800×600. Refer to the user's manual that came with your computer to adjust these settings.
2. To increase performance of the program, exit all other applications.
3. Some screen savers may reduce performance. If you are experiencing poor performance, disable your screen saver.
4. Some network connections may reduce performance. If you are experiencing poor performance, disconnect your computer from your network.
5. Performance can be enhanced by copying the contents of the CD-ROM to your hard drive. This requires approximately 215 MB of free hard drive space.

international treaties, including the Berne Convention and the Universal Copyright Convention. Nothing contained in this Agreement shall be construed as granting the End User any ownership rights in or to the Licensed Content.

3.2 Thomson Delmar Learning reserves the right at any time to withdraw from the Licensed Content any item or part of an item for which it no longer retains the right to publish, or which it has reasonable grounds to believe infringes copyright or is defamatory, unlawful, or otherwise objectionable.

4.0 PROTECTION AND SECURITY

4.1 The End User shall use its best efforts and take all reasonable steps to safeguard its copy of the Licensed Content to ensure that no unauthorized reproduction, publication, disclosure, modification, or distribution of the Licensed Content, in whole or in part, is made. To the extent that the End User becomes aware of any such unauthorized use of the Licensed Content, the End User shall immediately notify Thomson Delmar Learning. Notification of such violations may be made by sending an e-mail to delmarhelp@thomson.com.

5.0 MISUSE OF THE LICENSED PRODUCT

5.1 In the event that the End User uses the Licensed Content in violation of this Agreement, Thomson Delmar Learning shall have the option of electing liquidated damages, which shall include all profits generated by the End User's use of the Licensed Content plus interest computed at the maximum rate permitted by law and all legal fees and other expenses incurred by Thomson Delmar Learning in enforcing its rights, plus penalties.

6.0 FEDERAL GOVERNMENT CLIENTS

6.1 Except as expressly authorized by Thomson Delmar Learning, Federal Government clients obtain only the rights specified in this Agreement and no other rights. The Government acknowledges that (i) all software and related documentation incorporated in the Licensed Content is existing commercial computer software within the meaning of FAR 27.405(b)(2); and (2) all other data delivered in whatever form, is limited rights data within the meaning of FAR 27.401. The restrictions in this section are acceptable as consistent with the Government's need for software and other data under this Agreement.

7.0 DISCLAIMER OF WARRANTIES AND LIABILITIES

7.1 Although Thomson Delmar Learning believes the Licensed Content to be reliable, Thomson Delmar Learning does not guarantee or warrant (i) any information or materials contained in or produced by the Licensed Content, (ii) the accuracy, completeness or reliability of the Licensed Content, or (iii) that the Licensed Content is free from errors or other material defects. THE LICENSED PRODUCT IS PROVIDED "AS IS," WITHOUT ANY WARRANTY OF ANY KIND AND THOMSON DELMAR LEARNING DISCLAIMS ANY AND ALL WARRANTIES, EXPRESSED OR IMPLIED, INCLUDING, WITHOUT LIMITATION, WARRANTIES OF MERCHANTABILITY OR FITNESS OR A PARTICULAR PURPOSE. IN NO EVENT SHALL THOMSON DELMAR LEARNING BE LIABLE FOR: INDIRECT, SPECIAL, PUNITIVE OR CONSEQUENTIAL DAMAGES INCLUDING FOR LOST PROFITS, LOST DATA, OR OTHERWISE. IN NO EVENT SHALL THOMSON DELMAR LEARNING'S AGGREGATE LIABILITY HEREUNDER, WHETHER ARISING IN CONTRACT, TORT, STRICT LIABILITY OR OTHERWISE, EXCEED THE AMOUNT OF FEES PAID BY THE END USER HEREUNDER FOR THE LICENSE OF THE LICENSED CONTENT.

8.0 GENERAL

8.1 Entire Agreement. This Agreement shall constitute the entire Agreement between the Parties and supercedes all prior Agreements and understandings oral or written relating to the subject matter hereof.

8.2 Enhancements/Modifications of Licensed Content. From time to time, and in Thomson Delmar Learning's sole discretion, Thomson Delmar Learning may advise the End User of updates, upgrades, enhancements and/or improvements to the Licensed Content, and may permit the End User to access and use, subject to the terms and conditions of this Agreement, such modifications, upon payment of prices as may be established by Thomson Delmar Learning.

8.3 No Export. The End User shall use the Licensed Content solely in the United States and shall not transfer or export, directly or indirectly, the Licensed Content outside the United States.

8.4 Severability. If any provision of this Agreement is invalid, illegal, or unenforceable under any applicable statute or rule of law, the provision shall be deemed omitted to the extent that it is invalid, illegal, or unenforceable. In such a case, the remainder of the Agreement shall be construed in a manner as to give greatest effect to the original intention of the parties hereto.

8.5 Waiver. The waiver of any right or failure of either party to exercise in any respect any right provided in this Agreement in any instance shall not be deemed to be a waiver of such right in the future or a waiver of any other right under this Agreement.

8.6 Choice of Law/Venue. This Agreement shall be interpreted, construed, and governed by and in accordance with the laws of the State of New York, applicable to contracts executed and to be wholly preformed therein, without regard to its principles governing conflicts of law. Each party agrees that any proceeding arising out of or relating to this Agreement or the breach or threatened breach of this Agreement may be commenced and prosecuted in a court in the State and County of New York. Each party consents and submits to the nonexclusive personal jurisdiction of any court in the State and County of New York in respect of any such proceeding.

8.7 Acknowledgment. By opening this package and/or by accessing the Licensed Content on this Web site, THE END USER ACKNOWLEDGES THAT IT HAS READ THIS AGREEMENT, UNDERSTANDS IT, AND AGREES TO BE BOUND BY ITS TERMS AND CONDITIONS. IF YOU DO NOT ACCEPT THESE TERMS AND CONDITIONS, YOU MUST NOT ACCESS THE LICENSED CONTENT AND RETURN THE LICENSED PRODUCT TO DELMAR LEARNING (WITHIN 30 CALENDAR DAYS OF THE END USER'S PURCHASE) WITH PROOF OF PAYMENT ACCEPTABLE TO THOMSON DELMAR LEARNING, FOR A CREDIT OR A REFUND. Should the End User have any questions or comments regarding this Agreement, please contact Thomson Delmar Learning at delmarhelp@thomson.com.